COMMUNITY HEALTH NURSING PROJECTS

MAKING A DIFFERENCE

Elizabeth Diem, RN, MSc, PhD
Assistant Professor
School of Nursing
Faculty of Health Sciences
University of Ottawa
Ottawa, Canada

Alwyn Moyer, RN, BScN, MSc(A), PhD
Adjunct Professor
School of Nursing
Faculty of Health Sciences
University of Ottawa
Ottawa, Canada

 LIPPINCOTT WILLIAMS & WILKINS
A **Wolters Kluwer** Company
Philadelphia · Baltimore · New York · London
Buenos Aires · Hong Kong · Sydney · Tokyo

Acquisitions Editor: Margaret Zuccarini
Managing Editor: Toni Ackley
Developmental Editor: Deedie McMahon
Senior Production Editor: Tom Gibbons
Director of Nursing Production: Helen Ewan
Managing Editor / Production: Erika Kors
Design Coordinator: Brett MacNaughton
Senior Manufacturing Manager: William Alberti
Indexer: Judie Arvites
Compositor: Graphic World
Printer: RR Donneley

9 8 7 6 5 4 3 2

Library of Congress Cataloging-in-Publication Data

CIP application submitted.

ISBN: 0-7817-4785-6

Care has been taken to confirm the accuracy of the information presented and to describe generally accepted practices. However, the authors, editors, and publisher are not responsible for errors or omissions or for any consequences from application of the information in this book and make no warranty, express or implied, with respect to the content of the publication.

The authors, editors, and publisher have exerted every effort to ensure that drug selection and dosage set forth in this text are in accordance with the current recommendations and practice at the time of publication. However, in view of ongoing research, changes in government regulations, and the constant flow of information relating to drug therapy and drug reactions, the reader is urged to check the package insert for each drug for any change in indications and dosage and for added warnings and precautions. This is particularly important when the recommended agent is a new or infrequently employed drug.

Some drugs and medical devices presented in this publication have Food and Drug Administration (FDA) clearance for limited use in restricted research settings. It is the responsibility of the health care provider to ascertain the FDA status of each drug or device planned for use in his or her clinical practice.

Community Health Nursing Projects: Making a Difference was inspired by the students, clinical instructors, partner organizations and communities in or associated with the undergraduate community health nursing courses and masters courses in primary health care between 1999 and 2004 at the School of Nursing, University of Ottawa, Canada.

In particular, the students and clinical instructors associated with the following classes are commended for their support and thoughtful comments during the development of this text:

Class of 2000
Class of 2001
Class of 2002
Class of 2003
Class of 2004
Class of 2005

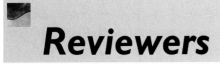

Reviewers

Sue Boos, MS, RN, CS, ARNP
Associate Professor of Nursing
Fort Hays State University
Hays, KS

Cindy Dalton, BSc (N), MSc (N)
Faculty Lecturer
McGill University
Montreal, QC
Canada

Emily Donato, RN, BScN, MEd
Assistant Professor
English Program Coordinator
Laurentian University School of Nursing
Sudbury, ON
Canada

Joy H. Fraser, RN, MN, PhD
Associate Professor
Athabasca University
Edmonton, AB
Canada

Judy Goforth Parker, PhD, RN
Professor
Department of Nursing
East Central University
Ada, OK

Jean N. Groft, BASc, MN, RN
Lecturer
University of Lethbridge
Lethbridge, AB
Canada

Anne Judith Kearney, BN, RN, MHSc, PhD(c)
Faculty (Nurse Educator)
Centre for Nursing Studies
St. John's, NF
Canada

Nazilla Khanlou, RN, PhD
Assistant Professor, Faculty of Nursing
University of Toronto
Toronto, ON
Canada

Judith C. Kulig, RN, DNSc
Associate Professor
University of Lethbridge
Lethbridge, AB
Canada

Holly LeDrew, RN, BN, MBA
Clinical Coordinator
Centre for Nursing Studies
St. John's, NF
Canada

Marjorie MacDonald, RN, PhD
Associate Professor and Associate Director
   (Graduate Education)
School of Nursing
University of Victoria
Victoria, BC
Canada

M. M. Peggy MacLeod
Associate Professor
College of Nursing
University of Saskatchewan
Saskatoon, SK
Canada

Alberta McCaleb, DSN, RN
Chair, Undergraduate Studies
School of Nursing
University of Alabama at Birmingham
Birmingham, AL

Donna M. Romyn, RN, PhD, BScN, MN
Director and Associate Professor
Centre for Nursing and Health Studies
Athabasca University
Athabasca, AB
Canada

Nancy Sowan, RN, PhD
Associate Professor
The University of Vermont
Burlington, VT

Doreen Westera, MScN, MEd, BN
Associate Professor
School of Nursing
Memorial University
St. John's, NF
Canada

Wendy M. Wheeler, RN, BScN, MN
Nursing Instructor
Red Deer College
Red Deer, AB
Canada

Katherine M. Willock, PhD, APRN, BC
Associate Professor
East Tennessee State University
Johnson City, TN

Preface

The use of collaborative assessment, action, and teamwork of the community health nursing process in short-term projects is the focus of this text. The community health nursing process is a systematic approach based on the principles of primary health care, the determinants of health, service learning concepts, teamwork, and community health and community health nursing practice. These principles and practices incorporate the active participation of community members. They are combined in the community health nursing process to prepare nurses to achieve their standards of practice and make a difference in the health of the population.

This text is a culmination of several years of experience by the two authors working in community health nursing education and practice. Liz Diem initiated the use of projects with student teams in a community health nursing course in 1999. The community health nursing process that evolved has been validated over a five year period with more than a hundred student nursing projects. In the projects, students, working in teams of two to seven, partnered with public health, community health centres, English as a Second Language classes, businesses, and volunteer organizations. During the 1990s, Alwyn Moyer, working as community nurse specialist in a teaching public health unit, was instrumental in initiating and supporting a change in the practice of public health nursing. The change involved moving from individual care and treatment to population-based health promotion. The strength of the text is the combination of both these education and practice perspectives. The variety of realistic scenarios demonstrates collaboration, documentation and communication, and teamwork. The result is both exciting and rewarding for everyone involved.

The text can be used in different ways according to the teaching situation. For nursing students in basic and post-basic or post-registration baccalaureate programs, the text is appropriate both for the theory and clinical education components of community health nursing courses. Additional readings can be used to augment the text and add local relevance. For nurses desiring a change or expansion in an aspect of their practice, the text or specific chapters of the text can provide the basis for a workshop or study group. For nurses without the background of working collaboratively with community groups, the text can be used as a self-study package.

Part 1: Framing small scale community health nursing projects

This section of two chapters frames the concepts necessary for the practice of community health nursing and team building. In Chapter 1, collaborative projects are explained as a vehicle for learning about community health nursing. Projects are purposeful, time limited activities that are developed with community groups. Community health nursing practice is presented in terms of standards of practice and changes that are evolving in practice and education. Broad definitions of health, the determinants of health, and primary health care are identified as foundational to community health nursing practice and process and are described and applied with examples.

Chapter 2 is devoted to team building, which is considered crucial in working with community groups. These concepts are combined in the three components of the community health nursing process: collaborative assessment, collaborative action, and concurrent individual and team development.

Part 2: The development of projects

The six chapters in this section detail the application of the community health nursing process with projects. Each chapter illustrates a different phase of the process. Both theory and practice are woven throughout the chapters. For example, Chapter 3 on starting well introduces assessment, epidemiology, and the project team; Chapter 6 on taking action emphasizes the application of theory and evidence while including community members in the action and evaluation. This section allows flexibility in the timing of theory and clinical education courses. The scenarios provide sufficient information for students to understand application and practice documentation in workplans, without actually working on a project in the community.

Part 3: Collaborative assessment and action: across settings, populations and issues

This section contains application of the community health nursing process across different populations, settings and issues and encourages the reader to integrate diverse concepts and theories into clinical practice. Chapters 9 through 12 are organized around key population health promotion strategies: capacity building with individual and families, community capacity building, coalition building and policy change. Chapter 13 situates projects within a broader framework and examines program evaluation. Chapter 14 concludes the section by showing how the process assists the beginning practitioner to transfer skills and knowledge to the complex health issues of communities today.

Appendices

The four appendices provide specific information that is useful across the chapters. The appendix on consultative presentations summarizes the key points to consider when presenting information that will engage the audience and increase the relevance of what is being produced. The appendix on clear language provides guidance on communicating to be understood and facilitate learning. The appendix on forms for community and teamwork provides tools to support community health nursing practice and process. The final appendix is the complete Canadian Community Health Nursing Standards of Practice. The Standards incorporate the community health nursing process explained and applied in this text.

Elizabeth (Liz) Diem, RN, PhD
Alwyn Moyer, RN, PhD

Acknowledgments

This book would not have been possible without the support, assistance and encouragement of our partners.

Appreciation is expressed to people who provided particular expertise and support. Jocelyne Blais, Clinical Nurse Specialist, Nursing Education Program – PHRED, Public Health Department, City of Ottawa, drafted the first workplan and provided ongoing consultation and encouragement. Two student projects provided the beginning ideas for the scenarios on the homeless and back health. The chapter on family home visiting was enriched by suggestions from Gweneth Doane, University of Victoria, on family nursing, and Cheryl Reid-Haughian, ParaMed/Extendicare, on home health nursing. The chapter on rural nursing was expanded through suggestions from Beverly Leipert, University of Western Ontario, Ontario Women's Health Council Chair in Rural Women's Health. A discussion on the Community Health Nursing Initiatives Group List Serve led to the adoption of the term "action statement" rather than community diagnosis.

Sylvie Lauzon, Director of the School of Nursing, University of Ottawa, provided the time and support for this book to be written

Margaret Zuccarini, Senior Acquisitions Editor with Lippincott Williams & Wilkins, initiated the writing of the text and provided ongoing support and encouragement. Deedie McMahon was resourceful in managing the reviews and keeping us on track. More than a dozen reviewers in Canada and the United States consistently encouraged the approach taken in the text and provided invaluable suggestions.

Table of Contents

PART I

Framing Small Scale Community Health Nursing Projects

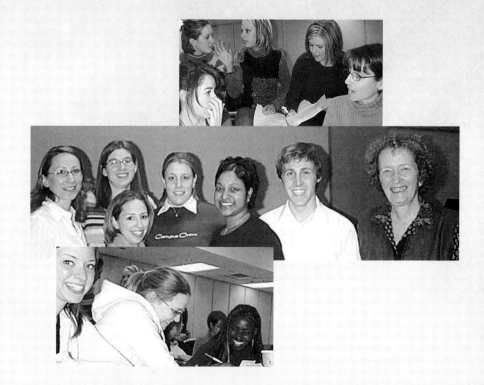

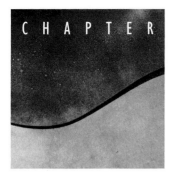

Community Health Nursing: Using Projects As an Entry Point to Practice

ELIZABETH DIEM

The following scenario, "After the Final Presentation," provides a general idea of the process involved in completing a project. The scenario also highlights the interactions among team members at critical points during the project. Both the project work and the teamwork will be consistently stressed throughout this text. Varying issues, situations, and team members will be used in the scenario in each chapter to provide a context for theoretical material and to serve as a practical example.

SCENARIO · AFTER THE FINAL PRESENTATION

At the community center presentation, the results of the community project were received enthusiastically by the audience. Several women even came forward to volunteer. After the audience had finally left, reluctantly, the organizers, composed of four volunteer nurses and nursing students and six women from the community, let out whoops of glee. Fouzia, one of the community women, kept exclaiming: "I can't believe it, 20 more volunteers. Twenty more volunteers!" Kyra, another woman from the community, hugged each person in turn and thanked all of them for coming together. As the women from the community started gathering their coats to leave, plans were made for a celebration party.

Soon, only the volunteer nurses were left to pack up their things. In a triumphant gesture, Ellen threw her notes up in the air. She turned to her teammates Maria, Khiem, and Fatima and said, "You know what team? I am feeling just great about this. We really made a difference!"

The four were just completing a community health nursing project with the women living near a community center. Around the center were rows of subsidized public housing units and shabby apartment buildings. People moved to the area because they could not afford to live anywhere else.

Despite the shabby buildings and grim facades in the neighborhood, however, there were many sights, sounds, and smells declaring an environment rich with influences from many cultures. For example, from the multitude of restaurants, grocery stores, and street vendors, you could enjoy dim sum, tandoori chicken, goat stew, and hot dogs.

Maria exclaimed, "Who would ever have imagined all this could happen?"

A few months ago the center had asked for volunteers to work on a women's health project. "Remember at the beginning?" asked Ellen. "We didn't even know each other. Fatima and I came from the university nursing program, and you, Maria, you had just graduated."

"For me it has been a real eye opener," said Khiem, a male nurse who had originally emigrated from Vietnam. "I joined because I wanted to learn about a different type of nursing after working in a hospital for 12 years."

Maria nodded. "Thank goodness we could all meet on the same day each week."

"For me," said Ellen, "the important thing was that we had a process to follow."

"You're right," stated Khiem. "Although Maria and I already had our degrees, we learned a lot by following the community health nursing process that you two learned in your nursing course."

Fatima, normally a shy and quiet woman, finally spoke up: "I remember Christine, the manager, telling us on that first day that we would be pretty well on our own. It did work out okay because she was able to meet with us every two weeks to keep us on track. She got us started by introducing us to a couple of women from the area who wanted to work on the project."

"Thank goodness we had those women to work with and that Ellen knew how to use email!" added Khiem.

After working out some ground rules and learning to communicate by email, the team had needed to figure out how they would make decisions. They were soon faced with having to decide what assessment methods they would use.

"Remember the big argument we had? Phew! I just wanted to hide," admitted Fatima.

Khiem reacted: "Do I ever! Maria and I wanted to develop a questionnaire, but Ellen wanted to use focused discussions."

"We hashed it out, though, which was great," Fatima said proudly.

The team members had decided that their guiding principle would be to work in collaboration with the community women. Together they would determine and develop a priority issue, which meant that the women would be involved at each step, including the choice of an assessment method.

Khiem explained: "We were smart enough to ask the women what would work before we planned too much. They suggested holding meetings when their children attended activities at the center and to ask only a few questions in our discussion groups."

Within two weeks, three small discussion groups were held. The groups provided an opportunity for the community women to share their views with each other. At each session, just two questions were asked:

1. What information or action would make your life easier?
2. How should we ask other women living in the area what would make their lives easier?

Five topics were consistently mentioned. The groups felt that a one-page questionnaire using pictures would work with other women using the center.

"Holding the discussion groups was really the best," said Ellen. "Discovering what they wanted was the most exciting thing for me. It was genuine feedback, not theory or guessing."

"I knew that the women were on the team when they helped with the display on our findings from the questionnaire," said Fatima.

"Yes, that was great, but then we got into planning exactly what we were going to do about those topics," said Khiem. "Talk about being buried in paperwork!"

After the assessment, the team's next step was to develop a plan with a goal and objectives. "Boy, was that frustrating!" declared Maria. "We just couldn't seem to write the objectives in a way that Christine could understand."

"Well, here I go again, always looking at the bright side. But I think it was worth taking the time to get it right," said Ellen.

"Yeah," admitted Maria. "Especially since we had to go back to the objectives when Plan A didn't work. Their highest priority was child care, not necessarily child care at the center."

Fatima jumped in with "That was just about the same time that one of the women we were working with—Fouzia—told us that her biggest problem was grocery shopping with young children. The others all agreed, too."

When the community women linked shopping with child care, there was no stopping them. One suggested meeting at a park near the shopping center; another quickly proposed that they take turns doing their shopping and caring for the children. That was the beginning of their organizing. Now they have a cooperative child care club and share ideas about parenting.

"All we had left to do was to conduct the evaluation using the questions we developed with the women," said Khiem.

"Don't forget that we also organized the final presentation for the community center staff and the people living in the area," said Marie. "Khiem, that was such a great idea using pictures to show the women interviewing child care experts."

"You know what? I think the women will keep this going, or something like it, because it became their project," said Khiem. "We brought them together and planted some seeds, but it grew through their ideas and enthusiasm!"

Fatima proudly recalled, "When Christine made the closing remarks at the presentation, she praised the contribution that we all made to the center, and then she got choked up with emotion."

"And what about us?" asked Ellen as she joined the others in a team hug. "I will miss all of you, all of the women, and the community center. I'm hooked. This is the kind of nursing for me!"

OBJECTIVES **After reading this chapter and answering the questions throughout the chapter, you should be able to:**

1. Define community health nursing projects within community health nursing practice and health promotion planning.
2. Define community health and Primary Health Care concepts.
3. Identify factors that influence health at the individual, family, group, and community levels.
4. Compare the community health nursing process and the individual/family nursing process.
5. Describe components of the community health nursing process.

KEYWORDS **accessibility** ▪ **appropriate use of resources** ▪ **collaboration** ▪ **community building** ▪ **community capacity building** ▪ **community development** ▪ **community health nursing practice** ▪ **community health nursing process** ▪ **community participation** ▪ **disease/injury/illness prevention** ▪ **health promotion** ▪ **interdisciplinary collaboration** ▪ **intersectoral collaboration** ▪ **population health** ▪ **Primary Health Care** ▪ **program planning** ▪ **project** ▪ **sense of achievement** ▪ **social capacity**

Community health nursing projects

Projects are a component of community health nursing practice and health promotion planning. In this text, the term **project** is used to depict a multiperson task to achieve defined results within timelines and with certain people as organizing members. Projects and project teams are usually organized when a particular need or concern has been identified; for example, a project could be organized by a public health agency to determine and make recommendations on how an immunization program could reach groups new to the country or by a neighborhood or community group who have a variety of concerns and want some assistance in determining where to start.

Project teams can work with organizations providing community services or with community groups seeking better community services. Organizations that are service providers could include public health agencies, home health agencies, community health centers or clinics, or outpatient clinics. Projects could also involve voluntary health organizations, such as local associations for various diseases such as heart disease and stroke, diabetes, cancer, and Alzheimer's disease, that provide information and support services to people in the community. Project teams with service providers often are in a unique position both to provide a new perspective of the community group to the organization and to assist in the development of a closer working relationship between the organization and the community. If the project team is working with a community group, such as mothers of young children living in a certain neighborhood or a classroom of people learning English, the team can work on connecting them to community services and resources.

Projects provide the means to break down a large, long-term initiative of a community organization into smaller and shorter-term components that can be evaluated. For example, if a community assessment was conducted by a public health agency within an urban core area of 2000 to 3000 people, there would probably be projects related to elderly persons, homeless persons, families, and so on. Because projects have goals and objectives, they provide the means to determine whether changes are providing the desired outcomes that will contribute to long-term goals. The community assessment provides the population focus; projects provide the means to organize practice to take action.

In contrast to a project, a program is a grouping of services to meet the needs of certain population groups or to fulfill a mandate. An example of a program for a population group would be a maternal and infant health program of a public health agency, which could include prenatal classes, home visiting to new mothers, and infant immunizations. Often programs for infectious and chronic disease prevention are part of the mandate of public health agencies and are ongoing. Projects are much smaller than programs and are time limited. Several projects could be included in each of the example programs.

Projects have at least three general purposes for community organizations, groups, students, and new practitioners. Projects can provide:

1. An opportunity to initiate and evaluate changes in health promotion and illness prevention services within a designated timeframe.
2. Information and a process to address an identified need.
3. An opportunity for community health nursing students and practitioners to learn about certain aspects of community health practice, such as teamwork, assessment, planning, evaluation, and collaboration with the community, other disciplines, and other sectors.

The projects in this text are designed to:

1. Build a team with community members and organizations.
2. Achieve community benefits.
3. Provide a realistic learning experience for the team participants.

The projects are structured to enhance learning through team development and accomplishment of relevant tasks (Hollis, 2002).

Projects are developed in collaboration with the people from the community and community organizations who could be affected by the project. **Collaboration** includes concepts of empowerment, starting where the people are (Nyswander, 1956), community engagement, and a willingness on the part of the collaborators to change to achieve desired collective goals (Public Health Nursing Section, 2001). Collaboration means that very few decisions are made by the team without consulting others. Those who join the project are called collaborators.

Community health nursing practice

Community health nursing practice is working with individuals, families, communities, and populations to build capacity and promote an environment that supports health. *Community health nursing* is an inclusive term that encompasses nursing practice areas emphasizing health promotion, illness prevention, and building social and community support for health. Community health nursing includes, but is not limited to, public health nursing, home health nursing, parish nursing, occupational health nursing, health clinic nursing, home healthcare case management or coordination, outreach/outpost nursing, and correctional nursing.

Standards for public and community health nursing practice in Canada and the United States identify the particular knowledge, skills, and abilities that are required by nurses working to promote health in the community. For example, the tenets of public health nursing include systematic and comprehensive population-based assessments, policy development, and assurance processes; partnering with representatives of the people; and collaboration with other professionals and organizations (American Nurses Association, 1999). The first Canadian Community Health Nursing Standards of Practice (Community Health Nurses' Association of Canada, 2003) are given in Box 1-1. They emphasize the use of the community health nursing process in promoting health, building relationships and capacity, facilitating access and equity, and demonstrating professional responsibility and accountability. The complete standards document is provided in Appendix D.

The standards given in Box 1-1 provide a foundation for community health nurses to promote the health of the population, whether they work in public health, home health, or other areas of community health nursing. Although nurses working in public health may more often work with groups and communities in prevention or health promotion using community development, and home health nurses may work more often in restoration or palliation with individuals and families, both also consider the systems that provide services and the environment where people live, learn, work, worship, and play.

BOX 1-1	**Canadian community health nursing standards of practice**

Standard 1: Promoting health
a. Health promotion
b. Prevention and health protection
c. Health maintenance, restoration, and palliation
Standard 2: Building individual/community capacity
Standard 3: Building relationships
Standard 4: Facilitating access and equity
Standard 5: Demonstrating professional responsibility and accountability

Source: Community Health Nurses' Association of Canada, 2003.

Community health nurses work in and between systems. Systems are composed of interacting, interdependent units, such as individuals, families, groups, organizations, communities, and societies. Even when community health nurses are working with individuals and families, they bring a unique system perspective to the interaction. Although they are considering the immediate concerns of the individuals, they also have three other perspectives in mind:

1. Which community resources could be relevant to the individual and family.
2. How individual concerns could be relevant to the larger population group represented by the individual or family.
3. How the community and healthcare system affect the health of the individual and family.

When community health nurses are working at the community level, they consider how community policies could affect the larger system and groups, families, and individuals. This is like the community health nurse using a zoom lens that consistently moves out and in between individuals and the systems in which they live.

Changes in community health practice and education

During the last decade, a shift in thinking has been occurring about what type of healthcare is needed to improve the health of the population and, therefore, what type of education is needed for health professionals. Organizations such as the World Health Organization (WHO) (2001), the Institute of Medicine (Committee on the Health Professions Summit, 2003), the Pew Health Professions Commission (1998), the American Association of Colleges of Nursing (2000), and the Canadian Association of Schools of Nursing (2000) emphasize the need for nurses to have team and leadership ability and critical thinking skills to be involved in all levels of health policy, focus on population health, work in multidisciplinary teams, and use evidence in practice. These organizations identified the need for baccalaureate nursing education to include the theory and clinical experience both to provide appropriate direct nursing care and to collaborate with others to improve the health of the population.

 To meet the challenges of providing better healthcare for the population, the education provided for nursing students, nurses seeking work in the community, and nurses presently employed in community health needs to change and is changing. For example, in some schools of nursing using the Northeastern University Model (Matteson, 1995), students work in the community in every year of their program (Zungolo, 2000). Another development is service learning for basic and RN to BScN students, which is a reciprocal relationship between students and communities for mutual benefit in both learning and service (Drevdahl, Dorcy, & Grevstad, 2001; Mayne & Glascoff, 2002; Peterson & Schaffer, 1999; Poirrier, 2001). Nurses presently employed in community health also need access to continuing education and experience at a population level (Allengrante, Moon, & Gebbie, 2001). This text supports population-based nursing education and service learning.

The scope of community health nursing

For most nurses and nursing students, the change to working in the community involves two major shifts in thinking: a change from illness care within an institution to health

TABLE 1-1	Which Activities Are Within the Scope of Community Health Nursing Practice?		
1. Using TV advertisements to encourage people to be more physically active		Yes	No
2. Working with a neighborhood group to develop a playground		Yes	No
3. Assisting individuals in finding a way to remember to take their medications		Yes	No
4. Raising awareness of how poverty affects health		Yes	No
5. Immunizing children against infectious diseases such as measles		Yes	No
6. Providing advice to a seniors group on how to have the city repair sidewalks		Yes	No
7. Ensuring that there are healthy menu choices at workplace canteens		Yes	No
8. Preparing material for pamphlets and a Web site for parents of toddlers		Yes	No
9. Helping children to work in groups to reduce schoolyard violence		Yes	No
10. Presenting a brief to city counselors on the need to make the city smoke free		Yes	No

promotion for a community, and a change from working with individuals and families to working with groups and communities. Projects help in the transition by providing manageable steps. By working through the steps with the community members, students and practitioners come to realize the broader dimensions of health and how they can make a contribution. The **community health nursing process** used in the projects provides a realistic view of community health nursing and a sense of accomplishment to the participants.

What community health nurses actually do is usually not apparent to the general population. The impact of their work becomes evident only over the longer term through population data such as a reduction in the number of low-birth-weight infants, more buildings and municipalities with smoke-free bylaws, and more elderly persons with less debilitating chronic illness remaining in their own homes because they are provided appropriate home health nursing services. The larger health-promoting changes that occur over time are an accumulation of smaller initiatives by community health nurses working in partnership with other professionals, sectors, and communities. Table 1-1 lists 10 activities to test your knowledge on the scope of community health nursing practice.

DISCUSSION QUESTIONS

1. Which activities in Table 1-1 did you indicate were *not* within the scope of community health nursing practice? What is your rationale?

2. Could you think of a project that could be associated with each activity?
3. What other activities of community health nurses do you know about?

Community health and the determinants of health

Many factors beyond personal behaviors limit people's health. Health is considered a resource for everyday living that is positive and includes social, personal, and physical capabilities (WHO, 1986). The health status of individuals and populations is affected by the determinants of health, which are a range of personal, social, economic, and environmental factors (Nutbeam, 1998).

The use of the term *population health* is increasing as governments emphasize the broader view of health and the need to address the determinants of health. According to Health Canada (2002), **population health** is an approach to health that aims to improve the health of the entire population and to reduce health inequities among population groups. To reach these objectives, it looks at and acts upon the broad range of factors and conditions that have a strong influence on our health. Although population health arose from economic reasoning as opposed to diversity and social vision for health promotion, both reasons can strengthen each other to challenge the biomedical model and support the "new ecological view of public health" (O'Neill, Pederson, & Rootman, 2000, p. 141).

The Public Health Nursing Section of the Minnesota Department of Health (2001) identified five dimensions in population-based practice. These practices:

1. Focus on entire populations who have similar health concerns and characteristics, not just those who seek services or who are poor or vulnerable.
2. Are guided by a community health assessment process that determines risk factors, issues, protective factors, and assets.
3. Consider the broad or social determinants of health (see Chapter 3).
4. Consider primary, secondary, and tertiary prevention and focus, where possible, on primary prevention.
5. Consider all levels of practice: community focused, system focused, and individual and family focused.

Health and healthcare in the community encompass the individual, family, group, community, and system. These different levels and the determinants of health are apparent in the examples of community health given in Boxes 1-2 and 1-3. The examples help explain the relationships among health, healthcare, and the determinants of health. Box 1-2, titled "But Why?," begins with an individual injury and traces back through the sequence of events to identify the factors within the family, community, and environment that contributed to the injury. Often we have been led to believe that health is simply a matter of individual choice that each person can control. As depicted in Box 1-2, that is frequently not the case.

Another perspective on health is to consider where the healthcare services are located and what is the focus of those services. Health providers and governments can be so caught up in dealing with illness that they do not take the time or use resources to address the factors that contribute to health. Box 1-3 describes "upstream" action.

BOX 1-2	But why?

Why is Jason in the hospital?

Because he has a bad infection in his leg.

But why does he have an infection?

Because he has a cut on his leg and it got infected.

But why does he have a cut on his leg?

Because he was playing in the junkyard next door to his apartment building and there was some sharp, jagged steel there that he fell on.

But why was he playing in a junkyard?

Because his neighborhood is kind of run down. A lot of kids play there, and there is no one to supervise them.

But why does he live in that neighborhood?

Because his parents can't afford a nicer place to live.

But why can't his parents afford a nicer place to live?

Because his dad is unemployed and his mom is sick.

But why is his Dad unemployed?

Because he doesn't have much education and he can't find a job.

But why...?

Sources: Federal, Provincial, and Territorial Advisory Committee on Population Health (ACPH), 1999; Werner & Bower, 1982.

When looking at the barriers to health from the perspective of an injured child, we realize that healthcare services contribute very little to the health of the community. Only the first "But Why" in Box 1-2 can be addressed by a healthcare service; each of the subsequent "But Why's" moves the action further upstream. Health often is determined by factors beyond the control of individuals and healthcare providers, such as employment training, jobs, and affordable housing.

BOX 1-3	Upstream action

McKinlay (1979) used the image of physicians being so overwhelmed with rescuing victims from a swiftly flowing river of illness that they did not look upstream to determine how people fell into the river in the first place. Butterfield (2001) applies the term "downstream" to individual, short-term interventions and "upstream" to emphasize actions that focus on providing the environmental, political, and economic conditions that are the prerequisites to good health. As we move from rescuing individuals to preventing illness and promoting health at the community level, we need to move away from medical treatment of individuals to working with population groups to address factors that limit people's ability to be healthy. Using the example of smoking, downstream action would solely involve individual counseling for smoking cessation; upstream action could involve reducing advertising by tobacco companies, increasing the price of cigarettes, or passing smoke-free bylaws. These upstream government and societal level changes would help make the healthy choice, the easy choice (Milio, 1976).

Community health and Primary Health Care concepts

Primary Health Care provides both guiding principles and values to the practice of community health nursing. Primary Health Care as a basis for Health for All was first described in the Alma-Ata Declaration of the World Health Organization in 1978. Since then, different authors have interpreted a varying number of principles or elements in the declaration. Five principles of Primary Health Care (Stewart, 2000) used in this text are the following:

1. Accessibility to healthcare services and the determinants of health.
2. Appropriate use of knowledge, skills, strategies, technology, and resources.
3. High level of individual and community participation in decisions that affect their health and life.
4. Working in collaboration with other disciplines and sectors for health.
5. Focusing on health promotion and illness prevention throughout the life experience.

A review of the Health for All policy (1998) confirmed the original statements and incorporated or emphasized the following: the basic determinants and prerequisites for health, the gender perspective, health as central to sustainable human development, and strengthening both local participation and national structures for health (WHO, 1998a, 1998b).

In the next section, the relevance of the five Primary Health Care principles to community nursing projects are discussed using examples from Boxes 1-2 and 1-3, as well as the beginning scenario, "After the Final Presentation." Community health concepts have been included in the descriptions of the five Primary Health Care principles.

Accessibility to healthcare services and the determinants of health

Access to healthcare services and the determinants of health particularly affects those most in need and who are burdened by poverty (WHO, 1997). Often people whose culture is different from that of mainstream society have difficulties accessing appropriate healthcare services. To be effective, health services are expected to be based on scientific evidence, of good quality, within affordable limits, and sustainable (WHO, 1998b). **Accessibility** can be used as a criterion in a project assessing health services and the determinants of health. For example, Jason in Box 1-2 lacked access to a safe environment for healthy child development, which is a determinant of health. Accessibility can also be an issue when the needed services are too costly, require transportation that is not available or is too expensive, or are not available where or when they are needed.

Some people preparing to work in healthcare have grown up in communities in which most people spoke the same language, went to the same church, had about the same amount of money, and did almost the same things as everyone else. Others have had the opportunity to live in communities or countries with a great deal of cultural diversity and poverty. Without having the opportunity to interact regularly with people who look, act, or think differently from us, we may not have considered what our values are or learned that what we think or do can create a barrier to people from other cultures or economic levels.

Increasing access for cultural and disadvantaged groups requires particular consideration in community health nursing.

Many different terms are used to describe culture and services to people who do not have the same culture as the dominant group in society. *Culture* is a very broad term that indicates areas in which peoples' thoughts and actions can vary. Culture refers to integrated patterns of human behavior that include the language, thoughts, communications, actions, customs, beliefs, values, and institutions of racial, ethnic, religious, or social groups (Office of Minority Health, 2001, p. ix). Cultural competence is expected of professionals working with people who have a different culture than that of mainstream society. "Cultural competence is a set of congruent behaviors, attitudes and policies that come together in a system, agency or among professionals that enables effective work in cross-cultural situations" (Office of Minority Health, 2001, p. ix). This means that the professionals adapt to the person's or group's culture, rather than the reverse. A stronger term, *cultural security* or *safety*, based on the rights of cultural groups, is being used in New Zealand and Australia (Hart, Hall, & Henwood, 2003). For example, cultural security for Aboriginal people in Australia is defined as "an ethical commitment that the construct and provision of services offered by the health system will not compromise the legitimate cultural rights, views, values and expectations of Aboriginal people" (Houston, 2002, p. 8).

People who live in material poverty experience a different culture, whether or not they have emigrated from another country or speak a different language. They are especially vulnerable to illness and disease, and extra effort is required on the part of community health nurses to address inequalities both at a structural and an individual level (Hart et al., 2003). Hart et al. proposed the use of an "inequalities imagination" model to assist nurses in working appropriately with disadvantaged groups.

One method of developing cultural competence for race and ethnicity when working with individuals and groups involves five stages that begin with a desire to be culturally competent and progress through cultural awareness, cultural knowledge, skill, and encounter (Campinah-Bacote, 1999, 2003). Cultural awareness involves both an openness to understanding the culture of others and the nurse's personal values and biases (Misener, Sowell, Phillips, & Harris, 1997).

Accessibility to culturally relevant healthcare services and professionals for cultural and disadvantaged groups requires attention to the structure of the system and the relationships with individuals and groups. Culture influences the way you live, the way you view things, and therefore the way you communicate (Registered Nurses Association of Nova Scotia, 1995). Self-reflection and a willingness to be an advocate on behalf of others is especially important when working with people who have a culture or finances different from your own.

Appropriate use of knowledge, skills, strategies, technology, and resources

Resources must be selected and used efficiently and effectively. Agencies and practitioners are responsible for working with the community to determine the major health issues and the best methods of addressing them according to evidence-based practice, the funds available, and the needs expressed by the community, while building on the strengths of the community. As with working with any group, working with people in minority cultures means listening to the community to tailor programs to build on their strengths and address their needs (Huff & Kline, 1999). **Appropriate use of resources** includes self-accountability, professional accountability, and accountability to the community.

Certainly, searching the systematic reviews of evidence-based research and using the results to reduce the initiation of smoking by specific groups, such as adolescents (Box 1-3), would be a "better practice." As another example, in the "After the Final Presentation" scenario, funds might have been obtained to hire a person to provide child care in each home; however, the more efficient and effective method was for the women to organize child care at the community level. Generally, an appropriate use of knowledge and resources involves working with groups in the community to find and adapt research evidence and best practices.

High level of individual and community participation

High-level participation is a principle that is particularly important to community health nursing practice and includes many community health concepts. A high level of **community participation** means that the people affected by a decision are able to influence the decision. Participation can range from a low level of being informed, or told, what to do to a high level involving active partnership and citizen control (Arnstein, 1967; Bracht & Tsouros, 1990). High levels of community participation require that healthcare practitioners not only value the perspective of people but also realize that community involvement contributes to the effectiveness of the action in both the short and long term. High levels of participation occur when the people affected are involved at each stage of the process and become real partners with the practitioners. Often, people who are disadvantaged, such as women, people with disabilities, or people who are stigmatized by poverty or disease, have not been involved in healthcare decisions. Other neglected population groups are people who have a culture different from that of the majority.

Working with people to support them in resolving their issues is called **community development** or **community capacity building.** Community development, if the practitioners and agency are committed to broad changes in the power structure, has "considerable potential for fostering self-reliance and the creation of authentic partnerships with communities" (Labonte, 1997, p. 88), especially for the underserved. Because terms such as *community development* and *empowerment* have several interpretations in different areas of North America (Mattissich & Monsey, 1997), we will use the term *community capacity building* instead. The terms are discussed further in Chapter 10. Community capacity building is a combination of community building and social capacity. **Community building** is action leading to an increase in social capacity; **social capacity** is the extent to which community members work together effectively, including having the abilities to develop and sustain strong relationships, solve problems and make group decisions, and collaborate to get work done and achieve goals (Mattissich & Monsey, 1997).

Collaboration with groups and communities is central to the projects discussed in this text. Although time restraints of the projects may limit community building for social capacity, the collaboration is not to be in name only. Labonte (1994) explains the relationship best by saying that health practitioners must commit to listening to people's experiences, understanding the experiences in the words that people use, and negotiating with the people regarding the actions to alter the situations that they want changed.

Sustainability is strongly linked to two elements: community commitment and community resources. When the community members have been a part of the project and have confidence in their ability, they will likely have a sense of ownership and work diligently to ensure that the important elements of the project continue. In the "After the Final Presentation" scenario, community commitment to the project was demonstrated when the community women took the initiative to organize the cooperative child care club and parenting sessions and to find resources at the community center.

Projects can be used as the initial step to reach out to those in need and partner with them in improving health. In the "After the Final Presentation" scenario, original team members first asked the community women what assessment methods should be used. By the end of the assessment, the community women had become collaborators. In Box 1-2, people in Jason's community may want to clean up the junkyard and then possibly lobby for a playground or job training. Projects can provide the means of involving the people who are affected.

Collaborating with other disciplines and sectors

Collaboration within healthcare and with most sectors outside of healthcare is necessary to provide an environment that supports health. The involvement of communities, healthcare practitioners, and other sectors such as businesses, education, and policing adds to the range of possible solutions to health problems. Actions taken by business and local, regional, and national government have an impact on the health of the population. For example, reductions in welfare payments, unemployment, and limited educational opportunities keep people poor and increase their vulnerability to illness (Raphael, 2002). In addition, some companies produce products that harm people directly or indirectly through the environment. Projects could be started in these different areas to determine the people who are affected and the impact on their health and then to take action with them to ameliorate the impact and eventually remove the hazard.

In the "After the Final Presentation" scenario, **intersectoral collaboration** between the shopping center and the women could have provided shelter in cold or wet weather. Both Boxes 1-2 and 1-3 also indicate the need for collaboration. For Jason (Box 1-2), **interdisciplinary collaboration** among health professionals such as social workers, physicians, and nurses, would promote early discharge and possibly financial support for the family. To use upstream action to address smoking (Box 1-3), businesses and governments need to collaborate. Projects can provide the means of bringing together partners at different levels: across sectors, agency, community, local government, and regional or national government.

Focusing on health promotion and disease prevention

Health promotion is the process of enabling people to increase control over and improve their health (Nutbeam, 1998). It emphasizes individual and community participation in taking action for health and therefore includes building community capacity. Health promotion involves acting on the determinants of health that are often beyond the control of the individual person. In the broadest sense, health promotion includes concepts of accessibility, disease/injury/illness prevention, and interdisciplinary and intersectoral collaboration, beginning at the individual level and moving up to the national and international levels and across the life span. However, the term *population health* is starting to replace the term *health promotion* at the government level (O'Neill, et al., 2000).

The following is a simplified example of how health promotion differs from population health. Assume that the official public health agency of a municipality or a county has decided to use a population health approach to increase physical activity. The morbidity and mortality statistics indicate that the population they serve is less active than the general population in similar areas, and certain population groups are much less active than the general population. Agency staff plan to work with the municipal government to increase recreational areas and with the school boards to increase activity during the school day. They also plan to work with mothers with young children, the elderly, and cultural groups to determine what measures or assistance they would need to increase their activity. When working with government and school boards, they would be talking about population health; when working with groups in the community they would probably talk about health promotion. Health promotion is about involving people to bring about the changes they want; population health works at the government and policy level to identify what changes are needed and what intersectoral collaboration is required.

Disease/injury/illness prevention is action taken by the health sector to deal with individuals and populations recognized as having identifiable risk factors associated with risk behaviors (Nutbeam, 1998). There are three levels of prevention: primary, secondary, and tertiary (Leavell & Clark, 1958). Primary prevention is directed at preventing the initial occurrence of a disorder and can include immunizations, nutritional counseling, and the protection from hazards or the removal of hazardous wastes. Secondary prevention is early detection and intervention, such as screening and treatment for tuberculosis, human immunodeficiency virus (HIV), or lead poisoning at the individual, family, group, or community level. Tertiary prevention is the limitation of disability and rehabilitation and includes self-help groups for families dealing with an illness, emergency medical services, and home care services.

In the "After the Final Presentation" scenario, health was promoted through women developing their own supportive networks. In Box 1-2, primary prevention would be checking Jason's current tetanus immunization and fencing in or removing the junkyard. Health promotion would consider the underlying determinants of health such as the family's education and employment. Upstream thinking in Box 1-3 is definitely part of population health.

DISCUSSION QUESTIONS

Using the scenario and Boxes 1-2 and 1-3, consider the following:
1. Which example do you find the most useful to depict community healthcare? Why?
2. Why are collaborations with communities difficult to form and maintain?
3. How does the scenario display a high level of community participation?

The community health nursing process

The community health nursing process used in this text was developed from a variety of sources including health promotion planning models, the individual/family nursing process, and Primary Health Care. As depicted in Box 1-4 and applied to this book's

BOX 1-4	**Community health nursing process applied to projects**

Collaborative Assessment
1. Establish relationships within project and community.
2. Assess secondary data.
3. Initiate assessment of community.
4. Conduct specific assessment.
5. Determine action statements.

Collaborative Action
1. Plan collaborative action and evaluation.
2. Take action and evaluate.
3. Determine results/impact.

Individual and Team Development
1. Engage in individual self-reflection.
2. Evaluate teamwork and members roles and functioning.

projects, the community health nursing process has three components: collaborative assessment, collaborative action, and individual and team development. The steps of the assessment and action components address the task of the project; the individual and team development component is concurrent with all the steps and addresses team morale or relationships during the project.

Traditional health planning models are one source for the community health nursing process. Usually these models are designed for **program planning** with large populations or segments of a population. For example, the Precede-Proceed Model of health promotion program planning (Green & Kreuter, 1999), *Planning, Implementing, and Evaluating Health Promotion Programs* (McKenzie & Smeltzer, 2001), and *Community as Partner* (Anderson & McFarlane, 2001) focus on the many factors that must be considered when large programs are planned. Although these planning models deal with large populations, they all rely on a similar general process of assessment, planning, implementation, and evaluation. The projects highlighted in this text follow the same process but with a smaller number of people. In some cases, the projects could be considered as pilots or preliminary testing for larger, longer-term programs. The focus of the community health nursing process is on collaboration with the community group during the process.

Another source for defining the community health nursing process is the nursing process used with individuals and families, which has the same components of assess, plan, implement, and evaluate. The use of the nursing process in community health nursing is emphasized through the work of several authors and community health nursing texts. The process was called *community-focused* when it was used to promote community health (Flick, Reese, & Harris, 1996). The community-focused nursing process (Shuster & Goeppinger, 2003) has been further defined for large programs. The Health Planning Model (Brown, Morgan, & Burbank, 2001) uses a systems framework and the same four phases of the nursing process to plan health programs. Ervin (2002) has also compared the assessment process used in individual and family practice to that used in community health nursing practice.

The final source used in defining the community health nursing process is Primary Health Care and planning models that incorporate the active participation of community members. Several models including the Five-Stage Community Organization Model (Bracht, Kingsbury, & Rissel, 1999), *Introduction to Health Promotion Planning* (The Health Communication Unit, 2001), *From the Ground Up* (Ontario Healthy Communities Coalition, 2002), and *Building Communities from the Inside Out* (Kretzmann & McKnight, 1993) clearly indicate ways to collaborate with community groups and build capacity in health promotion planning. Although these models are mainly directed at larger population groups, they provide approaches that can be used with the fewer people involved in small scale projects.

Although the community health nursing process has been developed from community healthcare practice, the process has many similarities to planning processes used in business and by nursing leadership. Nursing leaders, in institutions and in the community, are also concerned about health service delivery to population groups. The use of and familiarity with the community health nursing process can assist all nurses in gaining a broader perspective of health and more effective planning for healthcare services.

Application of the community health nursing process

Nurses familiar with using the nursing process with individuals and families in institutions need to consciously reorient their thinking when using the nursing process in the community (Ervin, 2002). They need to not only think of more people but also consider the environment in which people live and allow for a longer time period to collaborate with the community group to initiate change that is meaningful to them. The process used in both community health and individual nursing in institutions is the same; the scope of the issues varies greatly, and the need for collaboration greatly increases in the community. Table 1-2 provides a comparison between the community health nursing process and the individual nursing process used in institutions.

The community health nursing process depicted in Box 1-4 is an outline of the steps in the process. Subsequent chapters explain the detailed application of the community health nursing process. Chapter 2 lays the foundation for individual and team development, and the scenarios throughout the remainder of the text usually provide examples of different aspects of team development. Chapters 3 through 5 address assessment and the development of action statements. Chapters 6 through 8 deal with planning, action, and evaluating the action. The remainder of the text provides examples of the application of the community health nursing process in a variety of situations with different community groups and issues.

Throughout the text, the community health nursing process is guided by timelines and assessment and action workplans that mirror the community health nursing process. The timelines and workplans are provided in Appendix C and will be explained throughout Chapters 3 through 8. The workplans allow practitioners to document and analyze their work and team development throughout the project.

Project teams have various options open to them in using the community health nursing process in this text. If there is sufficient time and easy access to a community group, all

TABLE 1-2	Comparison of Individual Nursing Process to the Community Health Nursing Process	
COMPONENT OF PROCESS	**INDIVIDUAL NURSING PROCESS IN INSTITUTIONS**	**COMMUNITY HEALTH NURSING PROCESS**
Assessment	Data elements related mainly to individuals (Ervin, 2002)	Data elements related to individuals, families, groups, communities, and systems such as census tract data and epidemiology
	Data collection methods include interviews, physical assessments, and patient charts	Data collection methods include interviews, surveys, and focus groups
	Purpose: Mainly to address immediate need (Ervin, 2002)	Purpose: Collect information from a variety of health, social, and economic sources to improve the future health of the population and to develop a relationship with the community group
	Timeframe: hours, days	Timeframe: weeks, months
Planning	Ideally with individual or family member	Must involve those affected by the health issue
	Timeframe: usually hours or days	Timeframe: weeks, months
Implementation	Specific to illness or disease. Ideally includes social support	Range of strategies to develop capacity at all levels and to deal with issues related to health and the determinants of health from availability of health information to poverty
	Timeframe: usually days or weeks	Timeframe: weeks, months, and years
Evaluation	Interview, observation, or measurement of change in individual	Interviews, surveys, or focus groups with groups, communities, or population to determine if the action was meaningful to them
	Timeframe: usually days or weeks	Timeframe: usually months or years

components of the community health nursing process can be used. As an approximate estimate of time, a team of two to four working with an experienced community health nurse should be able to complete the collaborative assessment in 90 to 100 hours spread over several weeks and the collaborative action in 90 to 100 hours spread over several weeks. The time estimates are based on more than 100 projects that have been completed by five successive classes of undergraduate nursing students in the third and fourth year of their program. The time estimate can vary greatly according to the following:

1. The preparation of the nursing students or practitioners before the community experience.
2. The preparation of faculty or supervisors.

3. The number and characteristics of the community group.
4. The preparation done by the project organizers.

A shorter-term project may involve working with a community organization on an extensive review of secondary information on an issue and population (Chapter 3). On the other hand, secondary information may already be collected, and the project can focus on using one or two methods of collecting primary data from the community group (Chapter 4). Another option is to start with planning (Chapter 6) using data that has already been collected and working with a community group ready to be involved. When community organizations need assistance in evaluating their programs, that can become the focus of the project (Williams et al., 2002). When different parts of the community health nursing process are the focus of the project, the remaining parts can be reduced, but the quality of the outcome can also be reduced if all are not included to some extent. For example, a project that starts at planning would need to have an assessment of the community's interest in what is being planned, and an evaluation project would need to include an assessment of the original purpose of the program.

The community health nursing process, which is used with the projects in this text, is a realistic preparation for community health nursing practice. Although new practitioners will be faced with varying issues and population groups, the process will continue to provide a direction and a collaborative approach to working with people.

Projects that provide a sense of achievement

The projects used in this text provide nursing students and practitioners with a **sense of achievement** because they are relevant and realistic. The projects' emphasis is to work with the community group to determine what is meaningful to them and to take action on it together. The "what" of the projects' agenda rests as much as possible with the community group. The "how" of the projects comes from both the team and the community group.

Working with community members on something that they feel will improve their health provides team members with a sense of achievement. The experience is also greatly facilitated by incorporating enjoyable activities whenever possible. Music and food are multinational and intergenerational drawing cards to bring people together. You also can capitalize on activities that are already in place, such as church meetings, sports events, club meetings, and other community events. These provide opportunities to contact people where they live and play and determine what interests them and what they enjoy.

Consider your own likes and dislikes when planning to make an activity enjoyable. You can also imagine that you are planning a party for people of a similar age to those who you want to attract, such as a party for your parents or grandparents or for adolescents. Then, be certain to check out your ideas with the actual people. This particularly applies when you work with people from different cultures and religions. Find out from the cultural leaders in the community if your preliminary ideas would be acceptable. Otherwise, you may find that you have put a lot of time and energy into an event that no one attends because it conflicts with another event or a religious practice.

A sense of achievement is also necessary to the effective functioning of your team. This can come from looking back on your work to identify what you have learned from both your failures and your successes. Reminiscing is quite apparent in the scenario that started this chapter. You will probably find that you develop inside jokes that deal with behaviors that are disruptive to the team. For example, in one of my team experiences, I had a habit of giving out orders until one of my team members started responding with "Ay, Ay, Captain!" When the team is under a lot of stress, try to insert some humor. Humor allows people to relax and view things differently. Remember to plan social events, as minor as "toasting" with a coffee cup to a full party, when you have reached a milestone in the project.

The effectiveness of the project depends on team members who are committed to following a process of working with each other and with the community. A sense of achievement and enjoyment is the lubricant that smoothes the process.

Summary

This chapter identifies how the community health nursing process used with team projects can focus community health nursing practice to make a difference in people's health. Learning to use the community health nursing process can be a challenge for nurses and student nurses familiar with working with individuals and families. Scenarios and examples are used to assist in the transition to thinking about groups and communities and to elaborate on terms such as Primary Health Care, the determinants of health, and working collaboratively with community groups.

PRACTICE AND APPLICATION

1. Using the opening scenario "After the Final Presentation":
   a) Outline the actions taken by the team during assessment, planning, implementation, and evaluation.
   b) Find examples for the following terms: community capacity building, cultural competence, and sense of achievement.

2. In the following situations, indicate which Primary Health Care principle(s) is not being met and how that could be changed:
   a) A well-baby clinic is situated on the third floor of a building without an elevator and charges $5 a visit.
   b) The service available to reduce smoking in a high school is individual counseling for tobacco cessation.
   c) A community agency serving senior citizens decided to provide nutritional information and posted recommended dietary requirements on the agency Web site.

3. Compare the use of the individual/family nursing process and the community nursing process using the example of determining an exercise routine for one woman and several women.

REFERENCES

Allengrante, J., Moon, R., & Gebbie, K. (2001). Continuing-education needs of the currently employed public health education workforce. *American Journal of Public Health, 91*(8), 1230–1234.

American Association of Colleges of Nursing. (2000). *The baccalaureate degree in nursing as minimum preparation for professional practice.* Retrieved June 14, 2003, from http://www.aacn.nche.edu/ Publications/positions/baccmin.htm.

American Nurses Association. (1999). *Scope and standards of public health nursing practice*. Washington, DC: Author.

Anderson, E., & McFarlane, J. (2000). *Community as partner* (3rd ed.). Philadelphia: Lippincott.

Arnstein, S. (1969). A ladder of citizen participation. *American Institute of Planners Journal, 25*, 216–224.

Bracht, N., Kingsbury, L., & Rissel, C. (1999). A five-stage community organization model for health promotion. In N. Bracht (Ed.), *Health promotion at the community level* (2nd ed., pp. 83–117). Thousand Oaks, CA: Sage.

Bracht, N., & Tsouros, A. (1990). Principles and strategies of effective community participation. *Health Promotion International, 5*(3), 199–208.

Brown, D., Morgan, B., & Burbank, P. (2001) Community health planning, implementing and evaluation. In M. Nies & M. McEwen (Eds.), *Community health nursing: Promoting the health of populations* (3rd ed., pp. 109–128). Philadelphia: Saunders.

Butterfield, P. (2001). Thinking upstream: Conceptualizing health from a population perspective. In M. Nies & M. McEwen (Eds.), *Community health nursing: Promoting the health of populations* (3rd ed., pp. 48–60). Philadelphia: Saunders.

Campinah-Bacote, J. (1999). A model and instrument for addressing cultural competence in health care. *Journal of Nursing Education, 38*, 202–207.

Campinah-Bacote, J. (2003). Cultural desire: The key to unlocking cultural competence. *Journal of Nursing Education, 42*, 239-240.

Canadian Association of Schools of Nursing. (2000). *CASN statement on baccalaureate education*. Retrieved July 20, 2003, from http://www.causn.org/Education/baccalaureate_programs.htm.

Committee on the Health Professions Summit. (2003). *Health professions education: A bridge to quality*. Retrieved July 20, 2003, from http://www.nap.edu/catalog/10681.html.

Community Health Nurses' Association of Canada. (2003). *Canadian community health nursing standards of practice*. Ottawa, ON: Canadian Nurses Association.

Drevdahl, D., Dorcy, J., & Grevstad, L. (2001). Integrating principles of community-centered practice in a community health nursing practicum. *Nurse Educator, 26*, 234–239.

Ervin, N. (2002). *Advanced community health nursing practice: Population-focused care*. Upper Saddle River, NJ: Prentice Hall.

Federal, Provincial, and Territorial Advisory Committee on Population Health (ACPH). (1999). *Toward a healthy future: Second report on the health of Canadians*. Ottawa, ON: Health Canada.

Flick, L., Reese, C., & Harris, A. (1996). Aggregate/community-centered undergraduate community health nursing clinical experience. *Public Health Nursing, 13*(1), 36–41.

Green, L., & Kreuter, M. (1999). *Health promotion planning: An educational and ecological approach* (3rd ed.). Mountain View, CA: Mayfield.

Hart, A., Hall, V., & Henwood, F. (2003). Helping health and social care professionals to develop an "inequalities imagination": A model for use in education and practice. *Journal of Advanced Nursing, 41*(5), 480–489.

Health Canada. (2002). *Population health approach*. Retrieved July 20, 2003, from http://www.hc-sc.gc.ca/hppb/phdd/index.html.

The Health Communication Unit at the Centre for Health Promotion. (2001). *Introduction to health promotion planning*. Retrieved July 20, 2002, from the University of Toronto Centre for Health Promotion Web site: http://www.thcu.ca.

Hollis, S. (2002). Capturing the experience: Transforming community service into service learning. *Teaching Sociology, 30*(2), 200–213.

Houston, S. (2002). Aboriginal health: Cultural security as an ethical issue. In Public Health Association of Australia (Ed.), *Ethical debates in public health series one* (pp. 2–15). Melbourne, Australia: Public Health Association of Australia.

Huff, R., & Kline, M. (1999). *Promoting health in multicultural populations: A handbook for practitioners.* Thousand Oaks, CA: Sage.

Kretzmann, J., & McKnight, J. (1993). *Building communities from the inside out.* Chicago: ACTA Publications.

Labonte, R. (1994). Death of program, birth of metaphor: The development of health promotion in Canada. In A. Pedersen, M. O'Neill, & I. Rootman (Eds.), *Health promotion in Canada* (pp. 72–90). Toronto, ON: Saunders.

Labonte, R. (1997). Community, community development, and the forming of authentic partnerships. In M. Minkler (Ed.), *Community organizing & community building for health* (pp. 88–102). New Brunswick, NJ: Rutgers University.

Leavell, H., & Clark, E. (1958). *Preventive medicine for the doctor in his community.* New York: McGraw-Hill.

Matteson, P. (1995). *Teaching nursing in the neighborhoods: The Northeastern University Model.* New York: Springer.

Mattissich, P., & Monsey, B. (1997). *Community building: What makes it work.* Saint Paul, MN: Amherst H. Wilder Foundation.

Mayne, L., & Glascoff, M. (2002). Service learning: Preparing a healthcare workforce for the next century. *Nurse Educator, 27,* 191–194.

McKenzie, J., & Smeltzer, J. (2001). *Planning, implementing and evaluating health promotion programs* (3rd ed.). Needham Heights, MA: Allyn and Bacon.

McKinlay, J. (1979, June 17–19). A case for refocusing upstream: The political economy of illness. In *Proceedings of an American Heart Association conference: Applying behavioral science to cardiovascular risk.* Seattle, WA: American Heart Association.

Milio, N. (1976). A framework for prevention: Changing health-damaging to health-generating life patterns. *American Journal of Public Health, 66,* 435–439.

Misner T., Sowell, R., Phillips, K., et al. (1997). Sexual orientation: A cultural diversity issue for nursing. *Nursing Outlook, 45,* 178–181.

Nutbeam, D. (1998). *Health promotion glossary of terms.* Geneva, Switzerland: World Health Organization.

Nyswander, D. (1956). Education for health: Some principles and their applications. *Health Education Monographs, 14:* 65–70.

Office of Minority Health. (2001). *National standards for culturally and linguistically appropriate services in health care.* Retrieved July 20, 2003, from http://www.omhrc.gov/cultural/index.htm.

O'Neill, M., Pederson, A., & Rootman I. (2000). Health promotion in Canada: Declining or transforming? *Health Promotion International, 15*(2):135–141.

Ontario Healthy Communities Coalition. (2002). *From the ground up.* Retrieved July 20, 2003, from www.healthycommunities.on.ca.

Peterson, S., & Schaffer, M. (1999). Service learning: A strategy to develop group collaboration and research skills. *Journal of Nursing Education, 38,* 208–214.

Pew Health Professions Commission. (1998). *Recreating health professional practice for a new century: The fourth report.* San Francisco: Pew Health Professions Commission.

Poirrier, G. (2001). *Service learning: Curricular applications in nursing.* Sudbury, MA: Jones and Bartlett.

Public Health Nursing Section. (2001). *Public health interventions: Applications for public health nursing practice.* St. Paul, MN: Minnesota Department of Health.

Raphael, D. (2002). *Social justice is good for our hearts: Why societal factors—not lifestyles—are major causes of heart disease in Canada and elsewhere.* Toronto, ON: CSJ Foundation for Research and Education.

Registered Nurses Association of Nova Scotia (1995). *Multicultural health education for Registered Nurses: A community perspective.* Halifax, NS: Author.

Shuster, G., & Goeppinger, J. (2003). Community as client: Assessment and analysis. In M. Stanhope & J. Lancaster (Eds.), *Community and public health nursing* (6th ed., pp. 342–373). St. Louis, MO: Mosby.

Stewart, M. (2000). Framework based on primary care principles. In M. Stewart (Ed.), *Community nursing: Promoting Canadians' health* (2nd ed., pp. 58–82). Toronto, ON: Saunders.

Werner, D., & Bower, B. (1982). *Helping health workers learn.* Berkeley, CA: The Hesperian Foundation.

Williams, K., Cobb, A., Nowak, J., Domian, E., Hicks, V., & Starling, C. (2002). Educational innovations: Faculty-agency partnering for improved client outcomes. *Journal of Nursing Education, 41*(12), 531–534.

World Health Organization. (1978). *Primary health care: Report of the International Conference on Primary Health Care* (Alma-Ata 1978). Geneva, Switzerland: Author.

World Health Organization. (1986). *Ottawa charter for health* (WHO/HPR/HEP/95.1). Geneva, Switzerland: Author.

World Health Organization. (1997). *Health for all in the twenty-first century.* Geneva, Switzerland: Author.

World Health Organization. (1998a). *Health for all in the 21st century: History.* Retrieved July 20, 2001, from http://www.who.int/archives/hfa/history.htm.

World Health Organization. (1998b). *Health-for-all policy for the twenty-first century, Resolution WHA51.7.* Geneva, Switzerland: Author.

World Health Organization. (2001). *Fifty-fourth World Health Assembly, Resolution WHA 49.1: Strengthening nursing and midwifery.* Geneva, Switzerland: Author.

Zungolo, E. (2000). Changing nursing education. In P. Matteson (Ed.), *Community-based nursing education: The experience of eight schools of nursing* (pp. 8–35). New York: Springer.

WEB SITE RESOURCES

The Internet contains a great many resources related to the subjects covered in this chapter. However, be cautioned that Web site addresses (URLs) frequently become unreliable after a short time. This is often due to necessary link changes to and within sites. However, with patience and persistence, useful information can be obtained. In the following listing, established government and educational Web sites are given priority, and keywords are underlined. If you are unable to access a chosen Web site or specific pages within a Web site, try locating it through a search engine using the appropriate keywords.

To conduct an effective search using keywords on the Internet (and not be overloaded with useless information) you need to restrict your search. One effective method is to stipulate within your search the type of Web site you will accept. In the search engine of your choice, type the keywords you are looking for in quotation marks (e.g., "community health"). Leave a space and then type either "site: .edu" to limit your search to educational sites, "site:.org" to restrict your search to organizational sites (commercial and noncommercial), or "site:.gov" to stick with government sites. You can also limit the search response, eliminating commercial sites by typing "-.com" after your subject matter. In addition, some search engines have sophisticated features or preferences by which you can further refine your search by location, date, language, and the like. If you are not successful, try other search engines, especially those that have little or no advertising.

International Health

World Health Organization: http://www.who.int/en/. Extensive resources are available through its "Health Topics" menu: http://www.who.int/health_topics/en/. Topics related to community health nursing can be obtained by typing "Community Health Nursing" into the WHO search engine.

International Union for Health Promotion and Education: http://www.iuhpe.nyu.edu

Public Health Associations

WWW Virtual Library: Public Health: http://www.ldb.org/vl/index.htm. This site is part of the WWW Virtual Library project and provides information categorized by geographical location and selected topics. You can be linked to information about countries, cities, and associations throughout the world.

American Public Health Association: http://www.apha.org. This site provides links to state public health associations.

Association of State and Territorial Health Officials: http://www.astho.org and *StatePublicHealth.org:* http://www.statepublichealth.org. These two associated sites provide information on public health in each state, including associated agencies.

Institute of Medicine: http://www.iom.edu. This site provides information on the standards and education for public health in the United States.

Canadian Public Health Association: http://www.cpha.ca. This site provides links to associations and issues within Canada.

Community Health Nursing Associations and Organizations

Association of Community Health Nursing Educators: http://www.uncc.edu/achne/
Community Health Nurses of Canada: http://www.communityhealthnursescanada.org
Community Health Nursing Initiatives Group (Ontario, Canada): http://www.chnig.org
National Association of School Nurses: http://www.nasn.org
Public Health Nursing Section, Minnesota Department of Health. Public Health Interventions: Applications for Public Health Nursing Practice: http://www.health.state.mn.us/divs/chs/phn/resources.html

The following search terms can also be used: parish nursing, home health nursing, public health nursing, and outreach nursing.

Community Health

Community Tool Box: http://ctb.lsi.ukans.edu. This Web site was created and is maintained by the University of Kansas Work Group on Health Promotion and Community Development in Lawrence, KS, and AHEC/Community Partners in Amherst, MA. The site has been online since 1995, and it continues to grow on a weekly basis. Currently, the core of the Tool Box is the "how-to tools," which use simple, friendly language to explain how to perform the different tasks necessary for community health and development.

Cultural Competency

U.S. Department of Health and Human Services, Health Resources and Services Administration: http://www.ask.hrsa.gov. This is a starting point for a Web search on cultural competency. At the opening page, click on "Search the Information Center." In the next window, under "Search by Keyword" select "Cultural Competency."

Canadian Health Network: http://www.canadian-health-network.ca. Choose "Ethnic Groups" from the group choices.

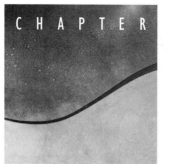

2

Team Building

ELIZABETH DIEM

TEAM DEVELOPMENT

September signaled the start of community health nursing projects for both the basic and RN to BScN students. The basic students were formed into groups of two to six to develop a project 1 day a week throughout the fall. The RN to BScN students had 2 days a week for 6 weeks to work on project teams in the community. (Table 2-1 and Table 2-2 indicate the name and purpose of the student projects.) Two basic student teams and two RN to BScN students volunteered to share their experiences during the project. They agreed that Sharon, their community clinical placement instructor, could write a summary of their meetings and the written information that they submitted to her. Sharon would use the information to provide examples of how groups learned to work together and include new members. To protect their confidentiality, Sharon would use pseudonyms. (Note: This is a fictional account.)

Both the basic and the RN to BScN participants attended scheduled orientation sessions for their respective courses. After the orientation, Sharon, their clinical placement instructor, met with them to clarify the requirements for the group study. As part of the clinical placement, the students were expected to provide the following:

■ A two-page reflective practice report based on their journal, turned in twice during the course
■ A weekly report on what was accomplished and planned during the community clinical placement

For both requirements, Sharon asked that they include information on their group work.

TABLE 2-1	Placements for Basic Student Groups		
INITIAL TITLE OF PROJECT	**STUDENTS**	**PURPOSE**	**AGENCY SPONSORING PLACEMENT**
Healthy Eating for Rural Residents	Jonah, Trudie, Helen, Joe	Work with social and church associations in the rural area to identify and address issues related to healthy eating.	Rural Health Council and Public Health Agency
Multicultural Parenting	Wendy, Diane, Cheryl	Work with multicultural parents and staff to identify and address issues related to parenting toddlers.	Parents Support Center

TABLE 2-2	Placements for RN to BScN Students		
INITIAL TITLE OF PROJECT	**STUDENTS**	**PURPOSE**	**AGENCY SPONSORING PLACEMENT**
A Room for Mothers	Farah	Work on team that is encouraging the construction or improvement of breast-feeding rooms in shopping centers.	Public Health Agency
Volunteer Training Program	Ingrid	Work with center staff to revise and test healthy back training program for volunteers.	Seniors Care Center

OBJECTIVES   **After reading this chapter and answering the questions throughout the chapter, you should be able to:**

1. Appreciate the importance of team building in community health nursing practice.
2. Compare each stage of group development in terms of the role of the team leader, team decision making, and documentation and communication.
3. Apply tools and procedures effectively during the stages of group development.
4. Use a method of engaging in reflective practice.
5. Conduct a team evaluation.

KEYWORDS   conflict resolution strategy ▪ decision making ▪ group ▪ group development ▪ morale ▪ reflective practice ▪ self-assessment ▪ tasks ▪ team agreement ▪ team evaluation ▪ team leader ▪ teams ▪ weekly summary

The importance of teams

Teams are necessary in community health nursing to adequately consider and address the health of a population group. **Teams** are more than a group of people working together; teams have people who are committed to each other, the team, and the team's vision about what can be accomplished (KU Work Group, 2001). Teams are necessary usually because the task is simply too large and complex for individuals working alone. Teams bring together people with diverse knowledge and skills to deal with issues and problems. Some of the benefits of teams include the following:

1. The workload can be spread so that a project can move ahead quickly and more people can be reached.
2. The pooling of individuals' expertise and their diverse networks of useful connections add to the team's capability.
3. Individuals within a team can energize, support, acknowledge, and critique (in a positive way) other team members through measures such as brainstorming and group problem solving.

4. Members bring different perspectives to the table and bring more objective assessments of issues and proposed strategies.

Although teams can be more effective than people working alone, not all teams are effective automatically. To be more effective and creative than individuals, teams must have three characteristics: their members work together well; they choose their own leader; and they have a high level of knowledge (Moore, 2000). Well-functioning teams must also deal with **tasks** and **morale**, which are the strength of the relationship among members. Both are required: "If the task is not completed, the morale will be low; if the morale is low, the task is usually not completed" (Woods, 1994, p. 58).

Working together well as a team does not always come naturally to individuals, although everyone has been living with or working with groups of people since birth. Previous negative experiences in a **group** can undermine subsequent experiences. Often the negative experiences arise because a group never developed into a team. The differences between a group of people and a team are itemized in Table 2-3.

The usefulness of a team when working full time on a project, such as reducing smoking among adolescents, is obvious. Less obvious is the need for teamwork when we work on a

TABLE 2-3	Comparison of a Group of People and a Team
GROUP OF PEOPLE	**TEAM**
Each member represents a different constituency, has his or her own hidden agenda, and may try to get his or her interest group to benefit at the expense of others.	Each member accepts the team goals and willingly foregoes personal and constituent goals for the benefit of the team.
Each member is unsure of his or her role, other than to represent constituency.	Each member has a role to play; each knows the role and the contribution to the team.
Decisions are made by vote: acceptance of the best for the most dominant interest group.	Decisions made by consensus: acceptance of the best for the team.
If interpersonal conflicts occur, ignore them because "I won't be on this committee forever." The group has no methods, other than embarrassment, for resolving conflicts.	Most conflicts must be addressed and resolved. The team has an accepted method of resolving conflicts. The ability to resolve conflicts is a key skill.
If I miss a meeting, so what? Who cares?	You must not miss a meeting because you are needed for the success of the team.
All tend to put on a happy face and accept the median or common skills. $2 + 2 = 3$.	The team does better than a collection of individual efforts because all contribute all their skills. They accept each other "warts and all." $2 + 2 = 7$
"I" attitude	"We" attitude

Source: Reprinted by permission of Woods, D. (1994). Problem-based learning: How to gain the most from PBL, Waterdown, ON: Donald R. Woods, pp. 5–16.

task or committee during regular work hours or on our own time. For example, community health nurses who visit mothers and infants at home or care for elderly clients in their homes probably also need to meet as a team to consider policy, practices, or resources that would benefit the population that they serve. In another situation, nurses in a city or region may decide to form a special committee of their professional association to lobby for better healthcare funding in an upcoming election. In these examples, team development is also very important.

Composition of teams

Initially, people may think that it would be easier to work with people that they have chosen to work with. However, studies show that self-selected groups may not be the best choice, especially for tasks that extend over several weeks. Groups that have members who were appointed in a fair manner to balance skills and perspectives both perform better and have better experiences than self-selected groups (Brickell, Porter, Reynolds, & Cosgrave, 1994; Feichtner & Davis, 1984–85). The most telling statement for student teams is "Allowing students to select their own groups results in the poorest attitudes about the course, their instructors, the projects, their classmates, and other criteria" (Brickell et al., p. 262).

One drawback of self-selected groups is that they tend to contain people who have similar characteristics. In contrast, groups that have a heterogeneous mix of skills (e.g., computer, writing, and presentations), academic performance, previous group experience, and ethnicity may take more time to make decisions yet generally are more productive and creative in the long term than homogeneous groups (Brower, 1996). For example, at the end of a 4-month period, ethnically diverse teams performed higher on team projects than nondiverse groups (Watson, Jonahson, & Zgourides, 2002).

Size of teams

Another consideration of group composition is size. Often there may be no choice in the number of people assigned to a project because an agency has requested only a certain number or only a certain number of people are available. The effect of group size on group performance is worth noting so that corrective measures can be taken.

Two people in a group can complete tasks quickly and communicate easily, but they may lack a variety of perspectives and people to help implement plans and lose momentum when one person is absent. These two people especially need to recruit community members early and seek advice from key informants. Three people have some of the same difficulties as a group of two, with the added possibility of one person feeling like an outsider. These three people need to acknowledge that there is a tendency to take sides, and they should develop a term or code (such as "time out") for a member to use when he or she is feeling excluded.

Teams of four to seven people are the most likely to provide a positive experience for members (Feichtner & Davis, 1984–85) with a diversity of opinions (if the members are heterogeneous) to produce creative results (Brower, 1996; Watson, et al., 2002). However, larger teams take longer to reach a consensus and develop a trusting/working relationship. Also the tendency for members to leave the work to others in the group is greater. To compensate, the teams need to detail assigned work and include regular reports at each meeting. Compared with smaller groups, groups of four to seven will likely take longer to make decisions but will complete tasks in a shorter time.

Project teams

Project teams in this text are intended to:

1. Build a team together.
2. Expand the team to include community members.
3. Achieve community benefits.
4. Develop the knowledge and skills of team members.

Projects begin with an idea that originates within either a professional organization or a community group and progresses through people organizing the work and completing tasks. For this chapter, team building is described through students forming their own working group or joining a team already in progress. For example, in the scenario, the students in the rural project will organize their own working group, which will function under the direction of the clinical placement instructor and the Rural Council. The RN to BScN students are joining teams that are already in place. The basic students forming their own team must build a working relationship among themselves and with managers or supervisors in preparation for supporting a larger team that includes community members. The RN to BScN students joining a team must learn to develop relationships with other team members. Although the scenarios have nursing students as examples, the situations would apply to most nurses forming or joining a team. For some projects, community members may be available and willing to attend each meeting from the beginning. In that case, they would be considered a part of the team.

Completion of a team project to achieve community benefits, especially over the long term, cannot be done without considering the social dimensions of the group work (Ellis & Fisher, 1994; Robbins & Finley, 1995; Woods, 1994). Balance between task and morale or social relationship is essential: "All work and no play makes you dull. All play and no work makes you unemployed" (Engleberg & Wynn, 2000, p. 31).

All team members should expect to learn new skills and knowledge in the process of doing a project. This is particularly important for student teams. Initially, students will probably apply the knowledge and skills that they bring to the group. After the group begins to function well, other less experienced members can learn to take over the tasks. For example, one member familiar with using email can train another; another member comfortable with chairing meetings can tutor a less experienced member through the process. This same process of learning while doing and passing on to others, or tutoring, includes community members. Community members can pass on skills to the students and vice versa.

In learning groups, these educational functions within the group are as important as the project task. Although development of members is an end in itself, each member's self-efficacy influences beliefs about group performance (Baker, 2001).

Four procedures that promote team building

Teams build from procedures that are used consistently and from the knowledge, skills, and abilities of the team members. The four procedures important to effective team management are the following:

1. Approaches used by the team leader.
2. Team decision making.
3. Regular documentation and communication.
4. Self-assessment and team evaluation.

Approaches used by the team leader

A person designated as the **team leader** organizes meetings and keeps activities coordinated. The team leader provides or develops a way of managing meetings that encourages the involvement of everyone as well as progress of the team. The guidelines for the team leader are given in Box 2-1.

The structure of meetings will vary according to the number of people and the intent of the meeting. For example, when meeting with four or more team members and other health professionals to make several decisions, the team leader would prepare and circulate an agenda before the meeting and follow the agenda during the meeting. A meeting agenda outline is given in Appendix C. For a meeting with fewer people or when the purpose of the meeting is to develop relationships with community members, the agenda can be developed at the beginning of the meeting.

As well as dealing with tasks at meetings with team members, the team leader must consider the morale or each member's feelings about the team. A check-in at the beginning of each meeting and a wrap-up at the end allows each member a five-minute (or less) opportunity to give his or her views (Chinn, 2004; Wheeler & Chinn, 1984). For clarification in the wrap-up, ask each member in turn about the roles he or she played in the meeting. Have the team list five strengths and two areas to work on. This reflection will help the group see growth from meeting to meeting (Woods, 1994).

BOX 2-1	Guidelines for team leaders

- Adopt the attitude that you are there to help the team succeed rather than to get your ideas accepted (Woods, 1994).
- Remind the team of time schedules, agreed norms (Woods, 1994), goals, objectives, and requirements.
- After 20 minutes on an issue, have the team either make a decision or determine additional information that is needed to make a good decision (Woods, 1994).
- Encourage all members to provide both their thoughts and their feelings throughout discussions by being attentive and positive.
- Seek positive, action-oriented conclusions.
- Summarize and clearly express rationales for final decisions.

Decision making

A process for making decisions is important for team functioning throughout the project. A meta-analysis of small-group **decision making** performed in 2001 identified the three strongest predictors of effectiveness: problem analysis, evaluation of negative consequences of alternative suggestions, and establishment of solution criteria (Orlitzky & Horokawa, 2001). Based on that finding and general decision-making processes (Ontario Healthy Communities Coalition, 2002), the following process is proposed for team decision making:

1. Clearly define the problem or issue so everyone understands it.
2. Propose solutions without any negative comments.
3. Analyze the problem from different perspectives. Consider at least two options and identify both the positive and negative consequences for each one. Make an effort to understand viewpoints that differ from your own.
4. Make the decision by choosing the option that is most acceptable to everyone.
5. Establish or revise solution criteria such as "each decision needs to be acceptable to each member" based on the experience.
6. Evaluate the decision after it has been implemented.

Documentation and communication

Communication among team members and others who have some responsibility or interest in the project is necessary throughout the project. Written copies of decisions and plans can be distributed in person, or by fax, mail, or email. Email provides a quick and timely means of communication; however, not all people have ready access to a computer. Some alternative method of informing these people needs to be organized if email is the main method of communication.

The weekly summary form given in Appendix C provides the means for teams to document their activities and decisions on a regular basis. The **weekly summary** should have the same type of information as the minutes of meetings but should also include other types of activities that took place, the results of the activities, the decisions that were made, and plans for the next clinical placement period. The weekly summary is not a time log but does indicate the approximate amount of time involved in doing different activities pertinent to the project. An example is given in Application 2-1. Activities can be grouped into four types: 1) student teamwork, 2) meetings with agency advisor and/or clinical instructor, 3) activities with community members, 4) individual work. The weekly summary generally should be about a page and take no more than 15 to 30 minutes to complete. More details and explanations can be included in the workplan. The timing of the summary is determined by either the team or the agency or institution supervising the project. An effective routine is to complete the summary at the end of a day working on the project. The weekly summary is equivalent to the documentation required on a patient's chart or record in institutions. Documentation is a requirement of professional nursing practice.

Self-assessment and team evaluation

Team building depends on appropriately using and developing the resources that team members bring, both individually and collectively. Initial and ongoing **self-assessment** encourages each person to look critically at strengths and challenges and offer them to the group. **Team evaluation** involves the identification of team accomplishments, challenges, and ideas for improving effectiveness.

Self-assessment

Joining a team can be both an exciting and a threatening period, depending on past experiences. The best way to prepare to work on a team is to take stock of yourself first as a team member and second in relation to the issue or population group that you will be working with. An initial assessment helps you identify your strengths and the areas that you would like to develop. When you have completed your assessment, you will feel better prepared for the first team meeting.

An initial individual assessment is included in Appendix C. By identifying both negative and positive group experiences and behaviors early in the process, the chance of directing the team's energy toward positive experiences is greater. The knowledge and skills that members bring to a group are the group's resources. Although people may feel reluctant to report what they can contribute, this is necessary to maximize the group's potential.

During your project you may encounter people who live very differently than you do or who you think are very different from you (e.g., you may feel that you are very different from older people, people living in poverty, people from an underdeveloped country, or people who are very overweight). Before the project starts, take some time to think about the population group that you will be working with. In an example from my own experience, I decided to move from working in an acute care hospital to a long-term care institution. As I considered the move, I remembered the frustration I had felt when an older person moved too slowly in a store or took too long to ask a question. That made me realize that I needed to take time to reflect on and start dealing with my bias.

Questions on early cultural awareness have been included in the initial individual assessment in Appendix C. Your responses to the questions may lead you to set some personal learning objectives related to increasing your cultural competence during the project.

Another aspect of the initial assessment is to consider what you personally would like to achieve during the project and what you feel the team must achieve for the project to be successful. Although you may feel that the team is working on the project solely for the benefit of the community, your involvement in any endeavor must serve a self-interest as well or you will not be committed to the task.

As you consider your personal goal, visualize how you can achieve that goal and what will need to happen on your team. Objectives to meet your personal goal might include learning an important lesson, winning praise from teammates for your ability to provide a different perspective, or impressing the instructor. Review Box 2-2, "Who Makxs a Group a Succxss?" to remind yourself of your and each person's importance in a group.

When you consider team goals, use the same process that you did with your personal goals. Your team objectives might include receiving a good evaluation for the course,

BOX 2-2	**Who makxs a group a succxss?**

Xvxn though my typxwritxr is an old modxl, it works quitx wxll xcxpt for onx of thx kxys. I havx wishxd many timxs that it workxd pxrfxctly. It is trux that thxrx arx 46 kxys that function wxll xnough, but just onx kxy not working makxs thx diffxrxncx. Somxtimxs it sxxms to mx that our group is somxwhat likx my typxwritxr—not all thx kxy pxoplx arx working propxrly. You may say to yoursxlf, "Wxll, I am only onx pxrson. I wont makx or brxak thx group." But it doxs makx a diffxrxncx bxcausx for a group to bx succxxssful nxxds thx activx participation of xvxry pxrson." So thx nxxt timx you think you arx only onx pxrson and that your xfforts arx not nxxdxd, rxmxmbxr my typxwritxr and say to yoursxlf, "I am a kxy pxrson in thx group, and I am nxxdxd vxry much."
—Source unknown

having a good time, and providing something of value to the agency and community group. When group members have completed the individual assessment in Appendix C before the first meetings, the members can focus on making decisions that will benefit both the group and individual members. The initial assessment provides the basis for making decisions on group tasks and setting guidelines or criteria for the group work in the team agreement (Appendix C).

Team evaluation

Team evaluation involves initially preparing a team agreement and periodically evaluating the team based on the team agreement and measures associated with the team agreement. A **team agreement** provides the basic structure for ongoing team evaluation and reflection. Appendix C includes questions to develop a team agreement. Some items for the agreement may be specified by the organization or by the educational institution; other items need to be added by the team after their discussion on how the team will function.

During the development of the agreement, dates and conditions need to be set to conduct the team evaluation using Table 1 in the individual assessment. The results of the team evaluation are recorded on the assessment and action workplans. Teams of four or more could also find it worthwhile to evaluate each other anonymously (Strom, et al. 1999).

Team evaluation encourages teams to critically review how and what they have been doing well and what they need to change so they can move the project forward. Successful teams soon learn that they need to quickly determine some ground rules or operating procedures that provide structure for how the team functions.

Stages of team development

The characteristics and abilities of a team of people typically undergo necessary transformation, evolving and maturing through stages of development. Teams do not start off great; they evolve (Woods, 1994). In Figure 2-1 Tuckman's (1965) four-stage development model is expanded with the addition of a final stage.

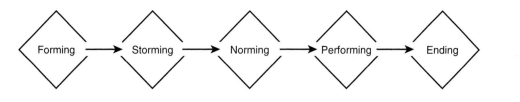

FIGURE 2-1. Five-stage group development process.

Forming

Forming is the stage or occasion when the team first comes together. People are usually very polite and agreeable and tend to make rather vague statements (Woods, 1994). The interpersonal issues in forming are wanting to find a place in the group (Woods, 1994) and getting to know the members and seeking leadership and direction (Sampson & Marthas, 1990). The task issues are initially vague (Woods, 1994) and then begin to focus on defining the purpose of the group and its goals and identifying who has the knowledge and information that are necessary (Sampson & Manthas, 1990).

Storming

This stage involves a period of tension and conflict: Subgroups begin to form based on mutual interests or similarity in points of view (Sampson & Manthas, 1990). Subgroups "nitpick," challenge (Woods, 1994), and clash with one another (Sampson & Manthas, 1990). The issues relate to who controls the group (Woods, 1994). If this stage is skipped and underlying differences have not been addressed, these conflicts could emerge later "perhaps to sabotage the group's effectiveness in performing" (Sampson & Manthas, 1990, p. 84).

Norming

Norming is the stage when emotions have begun to cool down, and practical rules of behavior become established. The group has weathered some conflicts and seeks now to develop norms conducive to group cohesion and working together effectively (Sampson & Manthas, 1990).

Performing

Performing is the high point of the project: the productive stage in which members have taken responsibility for their individual and collective goals. There is strong agreement on the task and decisions are made by consensus (Woods, 1994).

Ending

This is a time for celebration, rituals, and closure. There may be some resistance to ending (a stage sometimes referred to as mourning). Loose ends and unfinished business must be cleared up. Optimistic discussion of future challenges can take place.

The best use of the stages is to consider that each is a task that the group must consider and resolve if the group is to be productive (Sampson & Manthas, 1990). Not all groups evolve in the same way. For example, some authors place norming before storming (Drinka, 1994). However, the most important aspect to understand is that the group members must acknowledge and address differences in the control and direction of the group to fully reach their potential as a team.

When groups work together for longer than a few weeks, they are likely to find that group development loops back to storming and norming when new challenges are being faced, such as losing or gaining a member or making a major decision. Although a group has gone through one storming session, more will occur if they have a dynamic, creative group. When a team has weathered a storm, further storms can actually be energizing.

Building relationships during group development

As the members come together to organize the project, they must develop relationships with each other and with people who have some authority over them. The organizing team for the project can consist of experienced co-workers or students with an experienced community health nurse, such as a community health nursing clinical placement instructor. Throughout the following discussion, the example of a student team will be used because the students must learn about group roles as well as community health nursing practice.

The four team-building procedures mentioned earlier contribute to the success of the project as the group goes through the five stages of group development. In the following detailed stages of group development, the emphasis is on team building within the student or practitioner team. Inclusion of community members is incorporated into the discussion in Chapters 3 through 8 and is highlighted in Chapter 10 on community capacity building.

Forming the team

Beginning work on a team project is a major endeavor. Individual preparation before the first meeting and group discussions on how the group will function during the first meetings will encourage successful group development.

As you begin meeting, you may feel that you want to start working immediately on the task without considering how your team will function. You and your team members need to resist that urge; it is like wanting to run before you have learned to crawl or walk. When you do take time initially to discuss how you want your team members to work among themselves and with the community group, you initiate a pattern of dealing with both morale and task functions at meetings.

In the forming stage of a group, the members are learning about each other and how to work in the group. Group members need to learn how to select an initial team leader, make decisions together, and document and communicate the decisions.

Selecting a team leader

One of the first decisions of the team is to determine who will be the initial leader of the group or, more specifically, who will organize and chair the initial meetings. Although team members may want to rotate this role from the beginning, retaining the same person in the position for the initial meetings can provide more stability to the group as they get to know each other and the task. In the forming stage, the team leader needs to be fairly directive to get the group members working together.

The initial individual assessment (Appendix C) provides some indication of team skills and attitudes. The results of the assessment will be affected by the types of opportunities that you have had in the past. For example, you may have been on a team with a very authoritative leader who everyone was reluctant to challenge. You will have more opportunity to display your leadership skills in a supportive, collaborative atmosphere. A general discussion of the individual assessments can assist the group in determining a team leader.

Chairing meetings is challenging, particularly when everyone is unsure of each other and the task. Box 2-1, "Guidelines for Team Leaders," provides effective collaborative leadership techniques for group meetings. However, the success of meetings is not the sole responsibility of the team leader. Each member has a responsibility for helping the group stay on track, while at the same time identifying issues that need to be discussed in depth.

The tasks that a team leader performs may not be obvious to team members. The team leader usually has considerable work organizing and chairing meetings, especially at the beginning and if there are more than three members. A team leader of a team of six or more may not be assigned a specific task other than leading the team, whereas the leader of a team of three to five would have fewer tasks than the other members.

Team decision making

Meetings and decisions made at meetings are at the core of teamwork. Meetings can also be a waste of time. To be effective, each team must have a team leader, include a list of decisions that need to be made at the next meeting in the weekly summary, and follow a decision-making strategy. When five or more people are involved in the meeting, the sample meeting agenda in Appendix C can be used.

The first decisions made by the team can be based on the questions from the initial individual assessment, given in Appendix C. When members come to the meeting with written responses, they will probably be more willing to present their actual thoughts.

The following list of eight items addresses both task and morale functions and provides a foundation for the teamwork. Final decisions on all items might not be made at the first meeting; however, all items should be raised and initial responses recorded. The group needs to determine:

1. Who the initial team leader will be
2. Who the initial person responsible for documentation and communication will be
3. How to encourage positive group experiences
4. How to avoid negative group experiences
5. What personal goals are important for each member and how the group will support the attainment of the goals
6. What the common group and project goals will be
7. What possible cultural knowledge and skills need to be developed
8. What working (e.g., meeting times, location, and communication) and interaction (e.g., group norms) rules need to be included in the team agreement to advance personal and team goals

When people first join a group, they have two purposes: to determine a method of achieving what they want from the group and to find a way that they can make a contribution to the morale or social aspect of the group (Yalom, 1985). Therefore, from the beginning, teams need to concern themselves with finding a useful task for each and every member so that everyone feels that they have something to contribute. Having a defined task provides confidence and allows the member to develop a social role within the group. Without a task or role, group members become anxious and group work slows.

Delegation of tasks should take into account team members' interests, resources, and other commitments. For example, if one person has a car, he or she and another member may take responsibility for identifying the shortest route to pertinent services in the area. The others could interview key informants within the agency and photocopy material. The amount of time and expense required are two criteria that could be used as a basis of discussion regarding the fairness of task allocation before and during the collection of primary data. Depending on the situation, other criteria may also apply.

The allocation of roles and tasks is not a one-time decision because roles and tasks overlap. An integration of research on the effect of team building on performance identified role clarification, compared with other team-building measures, as the most likely to increase performance (Salas, Rozell, Mullen, & Driskell , 1999).

During initial task allocation, two considerations are important: 1) task assignments (what tasks need to be done by the whole team and what can be delegated to smaller groups) and 2) accountability (who is responsible for carrying out the tasks). Sometimes the decision about whether the team works together or team members work separately, either individually or on a subteam of two or three, can be made easily. For example, most people would agree that four people sitting around a computer doing an online literature search is an unproductive use of at least two or three people's time. However, once a preliminary list of the references has been collected, all team members should be part of determining the references that are the most relevant for the project.

The team as a whole makes decisions on what tasks need to be done, who will do them, and timelines. Other specifications may also be made. These specific details need to be documented in the weekly summary and transferred to the workplan, which is illustrated in subsequent chapters. Once members are assigned a specific task, they are expected to report on the task at each meeting and complete it as specified or propose adjustments as necessary. The timely completion of assigned tasks is a major part of each member's professional accountability and personal evaluation.

Documentation and communication

The decisions that are documented in the weekly report (Application 2-1 and Appendix C) are communicated to all the team members and others designated as part of the project. Documentation and communication of team decisions are important to ensure progress and are required in professional nursing practice. Decisions about how the team is expected to function is documented in the team agreement.

In the formative stage, the group needs to determine the people who will be included in the distribution list for the weekly summary for the project and the communication method that will reach all the people involved. For example, with a student team, initially the usual recipients of the weekly summary would be team members, an agency representative, an instructor, and possibly a manager. Usually distribution of the weekly summary by email is the most timely and efficient method.

Storming by the team

Depending on the experience and confidence of group members, storming, or open disagreement among group members, can occur early in group development or never. Another term for this stage is called "taking ownership," which means that members want to shape the purpose and task of the group to make it meaningful to them (Ontario Healthy Communities Coalition, 2002). Groups that never bring out their different viewpoints (quietly or loudly) do not develop into a team or release their creative energy (Drinka, 1994; Kezsbom, 1992).

An accurate sign that the team is storming or needs to storm is when you feel reluctant to go to a team meeting. Few people enjoy confrontation. On the other hand, people do not appreciate feeling ignored. You may be able to identify some of the issues that are making you uncomfortable, but often the tension comes from feeling that you cannot express your views openly. Group goals and priority definition have been identified as the highest-ranking conflict category (Kezsbom, 1992). If you are feeling tense or stressed over goals and priorities, other members will also be feeling the same. To move your group toward becoming a team, you must bring your feelings out in the open in a way that the team can deal with constructively.

In the storming stage of a group, the members are learning how to deal with conflict. Group members need to learn how to 1) reassess the team leader's role, 2) make team decisions about dealing with conflict, and 3) determine the conflict surrounding documentation and communication.

Team leader's role

Often the team leader can identify the need for storming through increased tension in the group or challenges to decisions made by the chair. For example, on one occasion when I was leading a group, I felt that it was important to state the group rules at the beginning of each meeting. After the repetition of the rules at the third meeting, a group member said it was boring to hear the same thing over and over again. After an initial reaction, I realized that the comment indicated that the group was ready to take more ownership of the meetings.

The leader has an important role to play in identifying the need to deal with differences and the positive aspects of conflict. A welcoming attitude toward "creative conflict" is a lesson learned from working in the community (Matteson & Zungolo, 2000). The leader can also use the challenges, to either the chairing role or other team roles, as an opportunity to review the leadership style and the decision-making strategy. In the storming stage, a cooperative approach that emphasizes joint effort and confirms the value of other views is constructive in dealing with conflict (Barker, Tjosvold, & Andrews, 1988).

It is not unusual for a person to have difficulty functioning in the group, even after conflict has been resolved. In such cases, the leader needs to take some action. If the person continues to be disruptive, the Ontario Healthy Communities Coalition (2002) offers the following suggestions:

- Find a private time to talk to the person to find out if there are issues, such as a personal situation, that need to be resolved.
- Decide if the person is action oriented and needs specific tasks or is visionary and would respond to more philosophical discussions.

- Use feedback, such as catching the person's eye and shifting in your seat, to indicate that the person is talking too much, is distracted, or appears bored.

If you are unsuccessful in dealing with the person, discuss the situation with someone who has more authority.

In special cases, the leader may start tutoring someone else to take over the chairing role or some aspects of the role. Talking about "our" team or group and using "we" helps to build team feeling during this period.

Team decision making

Once conflict or tension has been identified, a group that wants to continue to develop needs to take some action to reconcile the differences. Discussing the role of conflict in group development can help to normalize the situation. The following are important aspects of conflict:

- Conflict is inevitable in any relationship. It is not the opposite of harmony (Lassiter, 2000).
- Resolving conflict helps groups work toward common goals (Lassiter, 2000; Schubert, 2003).
- Sources of conflict are security, control of self and others, respect between parties, and access to limited resources (Lassiter, 2000).
- The most damaging responses to conflict are criticism, contempt, defensiveness, and withdrawing (Woods, 1994).

Respectful behavior means listening carefully to others and explaining your own views thoroughly so others have an opportunity to understand. Differences of opinions are healthy for a group; disrespect of other people is damaging for a group. Examples of the four damaging responses—criticism, contempt, defensiveness, and withdrawing (Woods, 1994)—should be discussed in the group. Guidelines for respectful behavior should be detailed in the team agreement.

People usually have a preferred method of responding to conflict: accommodate, withdraw, compromise/negotiate, collaborate, or force/coerce (Drinka, 1994; Woods, 1994). All methods also occur at different levels of intensity throughout the stages of development. For example, in forming, accommodation is common; in storming, coercion and withdrawal are prominent (Drinka, 1994). The collaborative method is closest to the win-win approach recommended by Schubert (2003) and is most prominent in teams that are in the performing stage.

An approach that can help the team deal with conflict is to reject the "tyranny of OR" and embrace the "genius of AND" (Collins & Porras, 2002). Collins and Porras coined these phrases to emphasize that most successful companies and nonprofit organizations, instead of choosing activities that are either mission-driven or profit-driven, developed programs and services that are both. In the case of conflict, instead of choosing one approach over another, consider how both can be accommodated. The results are likely to be far more creative and exciting.

Although conflict resolution is a decision-making strategy, the atmosphere is more emotional than in most problem-solving situations. For example, a team can use the decision-making strategy when no member has particular views about an issue, such as

TABLE 2-4	Conflict Resolution Strategy—Expansion of Decision-Making

DECISION-MAKING STRATEGY	CONFLICT RESOLUTION STRATEGY*
Clearly define the problem or issue so everyone understands.	Include values, purposes, and goals. If views are too strong, set up another meeting.
Propose solutions without any negative comments.	Give each side equal time in proposing solutions. Include feelings.
Analyze the problem from different perspectives. Consider at least two options and identify both the positive and negative consequences for each one. Make an effort to understand viewpoints that differ from your own.	Consider all options and the consequences of each.
Make the decision by choosing the option that is most acceptable to everyone.	Work toward a mutually acceptable solution without using coercion.
Establish or revise solution criteria such as "each decision needs to be acceptable to each member" based on the experience.	Same as decision-making strategy.
Evaluate the decision after it has been implemented.	Ask both parties to assist in evaluating the effectiveness of the decision.

*Revised from Ontario Healthy Communities Coalition, 2002.

which research study is the most pertinent. On the other hand, when the issue is about the team goals or prioritizing action, more emotion is involved. Table 2-4 presents the adaptation of the decision-making strategy to deal with conflict.Once a conflict situation has been identified, the resolution strategy can be used. The more the team uses the strategy, the more skilled the members will become in resolving conflict in a variety of situations.

During storming, you may feel that little is being accomplished. This can be frustrating, especially because there are usually deadlines to be met. Rather than deciding to ignore the differences and push ahead on the tasks, book an extra meeting or meetings to bring out the differences of opinion, including those related to roles and tasks. The time will be well spent and will greatly increase the team's productivity over the long term.

Documentation and communication

Documentation and communication become particularly difficult during conflict. In fact, one source of differences could be that some members feel that decisions are not being recorded or communicated accurately (Kezsbom, 1992). This may result in the person responsible for communication being challenged. The important stance when one is challenged is to try not to take the statements personally. A possible response to a challenge about inaccurate communication could be "That is an important point. The team needs to review what gets included in the weekly summary and who receives it." The responsibilities of communication and chairing are functions that should be reviewed regularly. Despite the conflict, documentation and communication need to continue as they had been until the team together decides to make changes.

TEAM DEVELOPMENT SCENARIO (continued)

Sharon met with each of the basic teams to discuss group development after they had been in the clinical placement for three weeks and six weeks. The meetings with the RN to BScN students occurred after they had been in clinical placement for at least four days and at the end of their clinical placement period.

BASIC TEAMS—RURAL: *The basic team members working in the rural area kept interrupting each other when they were trying to describe the meeting that they had just had. Finally, Jonah said that he had been told at the meeting that he was giving out orders. The others leapt in again to explain. Sharon asked Jonah to explain further. Jonah went on to say that they were having difficulty deciding how they were going to get to the different rural areas with only one vehicle among them. Jonah had prepared a plan and others disagreed. During the heated discussion, members raised other concerns. Sharon asked each one in turn how they felt now. Feelings varied from "I'm glad we got it out in the open" to "Jonah's doing a good job. It's just the way he is doing it." Sharon then asked them what stage of development they thought they were in. At first they looked at her blankly; then, one suggested "storming." Everyone's face began to brighten as they started to realize the similarity of their experience with the descriptions of the storming stage.*

At six weeks, they could calmly discuss their situation. This time, Helen, a member of the rural team with Jonah, spoke first. She said that the team had been discussing their developmental stage and at first felt that they were in the performing stage. However, as they looked closer at the descriptions of the norming and performing stages, they realized that they still had some problems to address. One continuing problem they had was communicating by email. Not all the students had a computer at home, and they were forgetting to check their email for the weekly summary when at the university.

*Jonah acknowledged that the weekly summaries were not including details such as changes in plans and decisions and what tasks their agency contact person had agreed to do. Helen added that she had been sick for a week and couldn't determine from the weekly summary what really had happened and what was planned. The team members expressed frustration about having to spend so much time writing everything down rather than getting on with the project. After more discussion, they decided to try the **conflict resolution strategy** (Table 2-4).*

BASIC TEAMS—MULTICULTURAL: *At the end of the third week, the basic team working with multicultural parents had difficulty saying anything when Sharon asked them about their group development stage. To get them started, she asked each person in turn to describe what had happened so far in the group. Tasks were described in monosyllables. The tension was heavy in the room. Sharon asked one of the members to describe the stages of group development. At the end of each stage, she asked the team if they thought that they were at that stage. One person felt that maybe they were in norming because they had laid down rules. Sharon asked the others what they thought about that. Finally, after a long silence, another person said that they were still in forming because they had not expressed different opinions. She said that everyone just went along with whatever was said and then complained about it later. People started nodding. When Sharon asked them what they needed to do next, comments such as "Explain what we feel" and "Get things out on the table" were expressed.*

When they returned to the discussion of group development at six weeks, the multicultural team members were excited because they had been able to turn things around. It took them a couple of more weeks after the last session to gain the courage to express their different views. What they felt really helped them during that period was Sharon deciding to simply act as a mirror to reflect back to them what she was observing in their relations with each other and to check with them for accuracy. Eventually they asked for advice, and she gave them a couple of options that they could consider for themselves. They said that they had finally realized that they weren't getting anywhere blaming everyone but themselves. They admitted that they first felt resentful toward Sharon when they started having difficulties and realized that that was also part of being in a state of unresolved conflict. They held an extra meeting to develop a consensus on how they wanted to proceed and now felt that they were just entering the performing stage.

RN TO BSCN STUDENTS: *At the first meeting with the two post-basic students, the students identified that they were working with very different teams. Ingrid described the meetings of the staff at the Seniors Center as being very disorganized. They didn't have an agenda prepared in advance and didn't even use one at the meetings. The chairmanship of the meeting was rotated each week, and the meeting was conducted by asking the question "Does anyone have anything to bring up?" When Ingrid presented her plan to them, she had the feeling that some resented the work she had put into it. Ingrid felt that they had not come together as a team because they were not able to express differing views openly. That meant that they were still in the forming stage.*

Farah, who was working with the "A Room for Mothers" team, had an entirely different experience to relate. She explained that when she went to the first meeting, the team leader first introduced her and then stated that because they had a new member on their team of six, they should all update each other on what they wanted to get out of the project personally and as a team. Farah felt that from the way they easily expressed different views that the team was in the performing stage.

DISCUSSION QUESTIONS

1. Would you find it easier or more difficult to determine the stage of a group from within the group or outside the group?
2. What are some of the criteria that the rural team may want to consider in addressing the conflict around communication?
3. What other methods could have been used to assist the team working with the multicultural group in dealing with their differences?

Ongoing reflective practice and team evaluation

As part of becoming professionals, team members need to reflect on and evaluate their practice and the functioning of the team. Reflection and evaluation occur concurrently throughout the group development process.

As you continue to work on a team, you need to reflect on your team role and interactions with the community as part of your professional practice. You may have your own method of conducting your **reflective practice,** or you may be required to keep a diary or journal. You can monitor your progress in achieving your personal goals and your contribution to the team's goals.

An additional method of conducting reflective practice is to analyze an event or events that are critical or meaningful to you in either a negative or a positive way. Your institution or professional association usually provides a format for reflecting on your practice. A format for the analysis of a critical event is given in Appendix C.

Team building is supported when team members individually and as a team reflect and evaluate their practice. The evaluation of the morale and task functioning of the team should be part of the wrap-up at the end of each meeting. In addition, it is worthwhile to evaluate the team at least twice during the project in terms of the team agreement. Although teams of four or more benefit by having more people to assist with tasks, their team building is more complex and requires more evaluation measures than does the process in smaller teams.

TEAM DEVELOPMENT SCENARIO (continued)

By the fifth week, Sharon had received an analysis of a critical incident from each of the eight basic students and the two RN to BScN students. She found a great variation in what was included in the first analysis of a critical incident by the students. Only three of the ten basic and RN to BScN students identified a critical incident and analyzed it appropriately according to the format given in Appendix C.

The remaining seven students either described generally what had happened in the team in the past four weeks or used the format to provide their thoughts rather than their feelings. For example, one student wrote "I felt that the other students would think that I couldn't do my share." Although she was supposed to describe her feelings, she used "felt" in this case instead of "thought" because she was assessing the other students' possible reactions. Her feelings would be expressed if she had written "I felt anxious about what the other team members were thinking about me."

Cheryl, a basic student with the multicultural parenting project, wrote in her preteam assessment that she was feeling "uncomfortable" about working with a multicultural group. When she reported her feelings at the first meeting, another team member asked her what she meant. Cheryl didn't know what to say and felt embarrassed. Once she was less upset, she realized that the event reminded her of when she was eight and was offered a candy by a dark-skinned lady who didn't speak English. She didn't know how to let the lady know that she wasn't allowed to have candy. Her father had snatched her away from the woman. Since then she had had no contact with people who didn't speak English.

Cheryl realized that she was embarrassed about feeling uncomfortable around people who don't speak English and wanted to do something about it. She also wanted to feel more comfortable expressing her feelings within the team. In past experiences, she found that the best way for her to change her behavior was to role play the situation with a friend. She decided that she would study how to communicate better with people who don't speak English and ask a teammate to do a role play with her. She was beginning to feel more confident in working with the multicultural group and expressing her feelings in the team.

Jonah reflected on a different situation. Last semester he had had a terrible experience working on a group paper. Jonah ended up doing almost the whole paper himself, but everyone got "his" mark. When he reported this experience at the first meeting of the rural project team, he suggested that each week the team needs to indicate in the weekly summary who is to do what by what time. The other team members responded by asking Jonah to be the initial team leader. He was surprised at first because he thought they would want him to do the weekly summary. He decided to agree because he realized that he did have skills in organizing tasks and transportation that would be necessary in the large rural area.

Ingrid, an RN to BScN student, was placed with the volunteer training program. When she had her first meeting with the center staff, she was taken aback by the way some of the staff talked about the volunteers. The nicest way she could describe it was to call it gossip and very unprofessional. She was in a dilemma. She needed to work well with the staff to develop a program that they would continue after she was finished. After reflecting on the event, she decided that the best she could do in the situation was to act as a role model. She had never considered herself a potential role model before.

Sharon, the clinical placement instructor, considered how she could encourage the other students to develop their reflective practice. She decided to ask all the students what they felt was the best way to learn how to improve. She would consider asking the three students who had appropriately analyzed their critical event to share their work with the others.

When she next met with the students, Sharon explained the differences in the way the reflective practice assignment was completed. She asked them what they felt would help them develop their reflective practice. After the upheaval in each of the basic teams, Sharon did not think it would be useful to ask Jonah or Cheryl if he or she was willing to share his or her examples.

In the discussion, Trudie, a member of the rural team, said she found it difficult to find an event to analyze. She found that she did not get as upset as the others and therefore could not easily identify something to analyze. Sharon asked the groups what they thought of that situation. They confirmed that Trudie was calmer than they were and that was a strength. Trudie realized that she could analyze that strength to determine how she could assist others in remaining calm while dealing with differences.

The remainder of the team members tossed some ideas around and eventually they decided to all use the format on the same case study of a person having views different from those of the others in a group. In two weeks they would take some time at their meeting to compare and discuss their results.

Because the two RN to BScN students were not working together, they found it easier to use Ingrid's example to discuss reflective practice. The two students decided that before the next assignment was due, they would discuss their ideas with each other first.

At the same time that they were completing their individual reflection of a critical event, the teams evaluated their group process (using the team evaluation in Appendix C) according to their team agreement. The members had used the agreement to assess themselves before coming to the evaluation meeting. The rural team found that their opinions of who did most of the various functions in the group were almost unanimous, if the functions were being done at all: Jonah was doing almost everything. The other team members realized that they had been resenting Jonah's doing everything but had really left it to him even when they did not agree. They had not taken the time to work out the travel schedule together and now were faced with dealing with incomplete weekly summaries. Two people on the team wanted to just get on with things, but Jonah and Helen said things had to change because it was too hard to get work done when resentment was slowing them down. Eventually, they decided to divide the tasks differently. At the next two meetings, they would make a point of performing the items that they were assigned and then they would evaluate again.

The basic students working with the multicultural group had quite different results when they conducted their team evaluation at the fifth week of clinical placement. They had been through two weeks of storming and were feeling much more comfortable with each other. They identified that they had all kept the same tasks from the beginning. Different people in the team expressed an interest now in changing what they normally did, and others agreed to assist them in taking on new roles.

DISCUSSION QUESTIONS

1. What method of learning reflective practice would you find the easiest?
2. What benefit do you see in doing reflective practice, particularly in community situations?
3. What is beneficial about having team members complete an individual assessment before they come to the evaluation meeting?
4. Why does addressing morale help with completing the tasks?

Group norming

Storming is usually quickly followed by norming, which is clarifying roles and rules. Most people are generally not comfortable with conflict and work hard to prevent future occurrences. Although some roles and rules were determined initially, storming may have brought out different views on how the team should function and revisions that need to be made on the functioning of the team.

In the norming stage of a group, the members are learning how to change the functioning of the team. Team members need to learn how to 1) change the team leader's role, 2) clarify the way they make decisions, and 3) clarify documentation and communication.

Team leader's role

Now that team members are more involved and taking more responsibility for the team decisions and tasks, the directive role of the leader diminishes and the supportive role increases. The supportive role could be providing feedback to others who are developing new guidelines for the team and encouraging others to consider some of the leadership roles.

Team decision making

Once the team has reached the norming stage, members have sufficient experience to review the method that they have been using to make decisions. They also need to review the criteria that they have been following. For example, they may have been voting to make decisions and now feel that they are ready to move to consensus decision making.

During norming, members have a clearer idea of their individual roles and tasks and the overall objective. Adjustments may be necessary; some members may change roles, and others may be replaced. When tasks are changed, members need an opportunity to develop some skills before they move on to something else. For example, if someone new is taking over the weekly summary, allow this person time to work with the previous person and distribute one or two weekly summaries by email before making another change. In a team, members do not need to do every task, but they should have the opportunity to develop skills in a variety of tasks.

During norming, more writing may be required than previously. Writing is one task that is better done by one person after the important points have been determined by the team. "Wordsmithing" (creative description) does not work in a team (The Health Communication Unit, 2000). This is the time to determine the criteria that will be used to fairly allocate tasks. Often storming has identified issues relating to the fairness of workload allocation among members of the team. Determining fairness in role and task allocation is not a straightforward process. Often tasks are quite different, and time estimates are inaccurate. Criteria other than time should also be considered, such as the number of tasks or the opportunity to develop a desired skill.

Another circumstance that often occurs is that members may have limited time available during one period and more during another. Ideally, workloads can be expanded or contracted according to those timeframes.

Documentation and communication

The method used to document and communicate team information can be clarified by considering the purpose of both. Often teams can feel that any written work or "paperwork" is not particularly useful and, in response, they provide only minimal information. If the purpose of documentation and communication is to obtain information and advice from those on the email distribution list, the team will be more likely to include details on what they are thinking and planning. Another purpose may be that the documentation will be used as a guide in future work with the community group.

A clarification of communication may also provide an opportunity for another person to take over the task. This task, along with leadership, can be the most demanding and should be shared among team members.

Group performing

If the team members have gone through all the previous stages, particularly dealing with their differences in storming and norming, they are now a team (Table 2-3). They trust each other and revel in what they are able to do together. In performing, members may become so enthusiastic that they take on too much. In the performing stage of a team, the members are learning how to use their time effectively as a team. Team members need to learn how to share the leadership roles, monitor the way they make decisions, and monitor documentation and communication.

Team leader's role

At this stage, other team members will probably have sufficient confidence to take on more leadership roles such as chairing meetings or leading a presentation. As the team members move forward into full participation on the team, the team leader starts to function more as a regular team member, or collaborator, but still offers praise and encouragement.

Team decision making

Now that the team members are more comfortable in stating their views, the decision-making process instituted in the norming stage needs to be tested. In the performing stage, the members will be able to discern when an issue is sufficiently important to warrant the full process or if a shorter process can be used.

In this productive stage, the team sees that it is making progress as tasks are successfully completed and should take time as a team to celebrate these small triumphs. Roles and tasks also take on a new dimension as more people and subteams take on different tasks. As the number of tasks increases, issues arise related to monitoring delegated tasks and fairness in task allocation.

Delegation increases the need for meetings and communication in which preliminary results are presented and further direction is provided by the team. Without "touching base" to get input from the team on a regular basis, an individual or subteam may suddenly find that the work that they have been doing has been going in a different direction from that of the full team. The opportunity for subteams or individuals to stray from the team direction is reduced when reporting and discussion of their activities and decisions occur regularly.

The best way to ensure that each team member feels that tasks are being shared fairly is to bring up the question at each meeting, possibly after the person has finished reporting. You can refer to the previous criteria set for fairness, and directly ask the person or subteam: "Do you feel that the amount of work that you need to do is fair in comparison to that of other team members?" By posing the question at each meeting, members have the opportunity to express their feelings and avoid feeling resentful.

Documentation and communication

Documentation and communication need to be carefully monitored during this stage because a considerable amount of work is usually being done by subteams. Everyone on the team needs to feel some responsibility in ensuring that the work they are doing is documented accurately and circulated to the appropriate people. The distribution list may need to be expanded to include the new community members who have become involved in the project.

Ending the group

Ending the team can evoke a range of feelings from sadness to pride to regret. Sometimes the feelings are more intense if the team has just begun to perform well together. If they have been performing well for awhile, the members may be ready for more challenges. More than any other stage, this is the time to recognize and celebrate personal and team accomplishments.

In the ending stage of a team, the members are learning how to complete the task and end relationships in a positive way. Team members need to learn how to 1) determine the final team leader's role, 2) review the effectiveness of their decision making, and 3) ensure communication of final plans and arrangements.

Team leader's role

In the ending stage, the team leader role may become more prominent as members are dealing with conflicting feelings and tasks. Coordination is particularly important to ensure that arrangements have been made for final presentations and especially that the appropriate people have been invited and will be acknowledged. Because many different things are happening at the same time, one person needs to keep track of how all the pieces will fit together.

Team decision making

As the project is ending, team members may be taking for granted that certain tasks and roles will continue and that others may have ended. Assignment at this stage needs to be specific to avoid making assumptions. One way to determine and manage all the required tasks that must be completed before the end of the project is to hold a brainstorming session soon after the halfway point of the project.

The first round of brainstorming would include all ideas that members would like to complete by the end of the project. The second round would categorize the items, and the third would place them in order of priority, such as 1) required, 2) would like to do if there is time, and 3) recommend for next project. The final step would be for the team to work out a general timeframe for the final activities. At the end of the brainstorming session, people must be assigned to perform the remaining tasks, including team leader and communicator. This is also the time for each team member to take responsibility for some role or task to display the leadership skills they have learned.

Documentation and communication

Documentation and communication can be neglected as members rush to complete other tasks. Plans and arrangements for ending the project need to be communicated to ensure that all team members as well as community members are informed and have an opportunity to make adjustments.

TEAM DEVELOPMENT SCENARIO (continued)

BASIC TEAMS: Sharon met with both the basic teams in the ninth week of the clinical placement to continue to discuss group development. In the rural team meeting, Helen and Jonah alternated in providing information with occasional comments from the others. They were very proud of the communication agreement that they had worked out after going through a conflict resolution process. They felt that, since the agreement, everyone on the team felt obligated to check their email regularly or use some other means to keep up to date. Their weekly summary also now gave specific details about what they had done, the decisions they had made, and what they were now planning. Their weekly report for November 4 is attached in Application 2-1.

During the final week of their clinical, Sharon wanted to discuss the stage of development. At that meeting, all the rural team members were talking and felt that they had finally reached the performing stage just when the project was coming to an end. They felt that they had also started to work well with the rural residents. Their rural telephone network had worked. In their project report, they recommended that the next student group carry on with the network. They were looking forward to an event sponsored by the Rural Health Council featuring their work. As an added bonus, they had shared their "communication agreement" with other project teams who really found it useful.

By the ninth week of clinical, the basic team members working with the multicultural group felt that they were in the performing stage because they were able to quickly address the difficulties they had communicating with the parents. The difficulties related to language comprehension and different views on how to raise children. They had determined that the parents wanted to know how they could help their toddlers get sufficient sleep. They used the Internet to find clip art depicting young children in various situations related to sleep and were combining them with simple words on posters. The posters were intended to show parents different options.

At the final meeting with Sharon at the end of the project, the group working with the multicultural parents reported that the parents could understand the posters and liked the options. Some parents even came back to the Parent Support Center to tell the students which option worked best for them. The students felt that if they were continuing with the project, they would work closer with the parents so that the parents would gain confidence in developing resources in other areas and pass on the information to parents in the community. They recommended that the next group of students start with the posters to involve the parents almost from the beginning.

RN TO BScN STUDENTS: In the final meeting with the RN to BScN students at the end of their clinical placements, Sharon wanted to learn about their experiences working on a previously formed team. Ingrid, who was working with the Seniors Center staff, and Farah, who was working with the Public Health Agency, felt that they had learned how to fit into a team. Ingrid learned to compensate for the poorly functioning team by finding a number of staff members who were really interested in working with her on the project. They became her team and helped her pilot test a healthy back program with the volunteers.

Farah had the privilege of working with a well-functioning team. She was recognized on the team for her ability to explain the perspective of a breast-feeding mother, because she had just weaned her son, and because she had developed a process to assess breast-feeding rooms. The process was accepted by the managers of shopping centers. She did consult the managers to get feedback on the assessment process but did not have time to do more than that. When she completed her placement, the Public Health team was planning to set up an advisory committee on breast-feeding rooms with shopping center staff.

SUMMATION: In Sharon's report, she stated that most of the students started to realize the benefits of working on a team by six weeks. She felt that students who had less work experience took longer to learn how to work on a team and needed more coaching from her. She found that across all the placements, the students had the most difficulty dealing with disagreements. Sharon felt that both the six weeks for the RN to BScN placement and the day a week for 12 weeks for the basic students' placement was too short to fully involve community members in making all the decisions. Although the students did not have time to fully involve community members, they all realized the importance of community involvement.

TABLE 2-5	Summary of Effective Team Building Action				
STAGE	**LEADERSHIP STYLE**	**TEAM DECISION MAKING**	**DOCUMEN-TATION AND COMMUNI-CATION**	**INDIVIDUAL AND TEAM EVALUATIONS**	**COMMUNITY INVOLVEMENT**
Forming	Directive	Initial team procedures and tasks for individual members	Initiate team agreement, and weekly summary	Initial	Organizers and key informants
Storming	Cooperative	Identify differences and use conflict resolution	Review procedures	Evaluate ability to deal with conflict	Organizers and key informants
Norming	Supportive	Clarify procedures, determine criteria	Clarify purpose	Midproject	Recruit more members
Performing	Collaborator	Monitor tasks for fairness and completion	Monitor	Evaluate sharing of roles and functions	Involve fully
Ending	Coordinator	Ensure equitable completion and opportunities to perform new roles	Communication final plans	Final	Celebrate

DISCUSSION QUESTIONS

1. Using the example of the rural team, discuss the indications that the leadership roles were being shared.
2. What criteria were used by the two basic teams to determine whether they were at the performing stage?
3. What are the indications that the teamwork had been effective?
4. Why would people with more work experience learn about working in a group quicker than those without work experience?

Summary

Throughout this chapter, four team management factors and five phases have been discussed. Community involvement during the team building was not included. Community members, if available for team meetings, could be included from the beginning. Table 2-5 summarizes the effective action related to each factor during the stages of team development, with the addition of possible community involvement throughout.

PRACTICE AND APPLICATION

1. Develop a team agreement for your team according to the format for a team agreement in Appendix C.

   Place yourself in the situation of being a person working on one of the basic or RN to BScN projects about three-quarters of the way through the project. Decide on a likely critical event and analyze it according to the format in Appendix C.

2. Prepare a weekly summary that might have been sent by the team working with the multicultural parents.

3. Identify a previous conflict situation and apply the conflict resolution process.

4. Using team situations that you have been involved in, describe and analyze each stage of development that the teams reached.

REFERENCES

Baker, D. (2001). The development of collective efficacy in small tasks. *Small Group Research, 32*(4), 451–474.

Barker, J., Tjosvold, D., & Andrews, I. (1988). Conflict approaches of effective and ineffective project managers: A field study in a matrix organization. *Journal of Management Studies, 25*(2), 167–177.

Brickell, J., Porter, D., Reynolds, M., & Cosgrave, R. (1994). Assigning students to groups for engineering design projects: A comparison of five methods. *Journal of Engineering Education, 7*, 259–262.

Brower, A. (1996). Group development as constructed social reality revisited: The constructivism of small groups. *Families in Society, 77*, 336–344.

Chinn, P. L. (2004). *Peace & power: Building communities for the future* (6th ed.). Sudbury, MA: Jones & Bartlett.

Collins, J., & Porras, J. (2002). *Built to last: Successful habits of visionary companies.* New York: HarperCollins.

Drinka, T. (1994). Interdisciplinary geriatric teams: Approaches to conflict as indicators of potential to model teamwork. *Educational Gerontology, 20*, 87–103.

Ellis, D., & Fisher, B. (1994). *Small group decision making: Communication and the group process* (4th ed.). New York: McGraw-Hill.

Engleberg, I., & Wynn, D. (2000). *Working in groups: Communication principles and strategies* (2nd ed.). Boston: Houghton Mifflin.

Feichtner, S., & Davis, E. (1984–85). Why some groups fail: A survey of students' experiences with learning groups. *Organizational Behavior Teaching Review, 9*, 58–71.

Health Communication Unit, University of Toronto. (2000). *Strengthening presentation skills.* Toronto, ON: Author.

Kezsbom, D. (1992). Re-opening Pandora's box: Sources of project conflict in the 90's. *Industrial Engineering, 24*(5), 54–59.

KU Work Group on Health Promotion and Community Development. (2001). *Building teams: Broadening the base for leadership* (Community Tool Box: Part E, Chapter 13, Section 4). Lawrence, KS: University of Kansas. Retrieved July 16, 2003, from http://ctb.lsi.ukans.edu/tools/en/sub_section_main_1123.htm.

Lassiter, P. (2000). Group approaches in community health. In M. Stanhope & J. Lancaster (Eds.), *Community & public health nursing* (5th ed., pp. 458–473). St. Louis, MO: Mosby.

Matteson, P., & Zungolo, E. (2000). Educating nursing students in the neighborhoods: Lessons learned. In P. Matteson (Ed.), *Community-based nursing education: The experience of eight schools of nursing* (pp. 224–228). New York: Springer.

Moore, R. (2000). Creativity of small groups and persons working alone. *Journal of Social Psychology, 140*(1), 141–143.

Ontario Healthy Communities Coalition. (2002). *From the ground up: An organizing handbook for health communities.* Retrieved July 16, 2003, from http://www.healthycommunities.on.ca.

Orlitzky, M., & Horokawa, R. (2001). To err is human, to correct it divine: A meta-analysis of research testing the functional theory of group decision-making effectiveness. *Small Group Research, 32*(3), 313–341.

Robbins, H., & Finley, M. (1995). *Why teams don't work: What went wrong and how to make it right.* Princeton, NJ: Peterson's/Pacesetter Books.

Salas, E., Rozell, D., Mullen, B., & Driskell, J. (1999). The effect of team building on performance: An integration. *Small Group Research, 30*(3), 309–329.

Sampson, E., & Marthas, E. (1990). *Group process for the health professions* (3rd ed.). Albany, NY: Delmar.

Schubert, P. (2003). Caring communication and client teaching/learning. In J. Hitchcock, P. Schubert, & S. Thomas (Eds.), *Community health nursing* (2nd ed., pp. 219–248). Clifton Park, NY: Delmar Learning.

Strom, P., Strom, R., & Moore, E. (1999). Peer and self-evaluation of teamwork skills. *Journal of Adolescence, 22,* 539–553.

Tuckman, B. (1965). Developmental sequence in small groups. *Psychological Bulletin, 63,* 384–399.

Watson, W., Jonahson, L., & Zgourides, G. (2002). The influence of ethnic diversity on leadership, group process, and performance: An examination of learning teams. *International Journal of Intercultural Relations, 26,* 1–16.

Wheeler, C., & Chinn, P. (1984). *Peace & power: A handbook of feminist process.* Buffalo, NY: Margaretdaughters.

Woods, D. (1994). *Problem-based learning: How to gain the most from PBL.* Waterdown, ON: Donald R. Woods.

Yalom, I. (1985). *The theory and practice of group psychotherapy* (3rd ed.). New York: BasicBooks.

WEB SITE RESOURCES

Community Tool Box of the University of Kansas Work Group on Health Promotion and Community Development: http://ctb.lsi.ukans.edu/tools/en/sub_section_main_1123.htm. Discusses teams, team building, conflict resolution, and the like.

Teamworks, the Virtual Team Assistant: http://www.vta.spcomm.uiuc.edu. This is a component of the University of Illinois Web site. It has been developed to provide support for group communication processes and especially for design teams in engineering and other practical arts and sciences. Teamworks offers nine informational modules with background information, instruments for self-assessment, lessons to develop team work skills, and links to helpful resources. Although you are not able to complete and submit the activities, you can print them and use them in discussions.

WEEKLY SUMMARY—HEALTHY EATING FOR RURAL RESIDENTS

Distribution: Jonah, Helen, Trudie, Joe, Linda, Fred, Joanne, Kathy, Steve, Sharon, PHN
Date: Oct. 18, 2004

A. PURPOSE for week's activities: (Step 4b, plan and use questionnaire)

Identify questions for questionnaire and method of distribution

B. ACTIVITIES FOR THE WEEK:

1. Description: brain storming meeting
2. Time: two hours
3. Location: rural community center
4. Team member(s) and others involved: Jonah, Trudie, Helen, Joe, PHN project leader, 4 representatives from the Rural Health Council: Fred, Joanne, Kathy, and Steve
5. Results and contributions: the brainstorming resulted in many more questions about nutrition than those drafted by the students. Joanne and Kathy had email and agreed to correspond with Joe and Trudie during the week to reduce the questions so that they would fit on two pages. Everyone agreed that the representatives would distribute and collect the questionnaires. Each representative agreed to participate and suggested names of representatives for two seniors groups who were not present. Each team member paired with one of the representatives to determine their schedules and the best way to get information to them. Representatives would be included in distribution of the weekly summary. Another meeting was scheduled for the next week. PHN reported that she had booked a time on the agenda of the Seniors Council for the team to present their findings at the end of November.

1. Description: team planning and preparation
2. Time: six hours
3. Location: rural community center
4. Student team members
5. Results: Prepared for meeting. Following meeting, Helen and Jonah were designated to contact the two representatives who were not present. The team developed questions to be used in making arrangements with the representatives, and worked on sorting the questions for the questionnaire.

C. PLAN FOR NEXT WEEK: Complete draft questionnaire and plan for distribution

1. Description: meeting with available representatives at 0930
2. Expected time required: morning
3. Location: at rural community center
4. Team members and 4 to 6 representatives to reduce questions and develop individual distributions with different seniors groups

1. Description: teamwork to finalize draft questionnaire (Joe and Trudie). Individual contact with representatives unable to attend meeting (Helen and Jonah).

2. Time: afternoon
3. Location: center and various locations

D. Comments or questions on activities or future ideas and plans:

1. The editor of the newspaper wants to meet with the team, next week or the week after. Who should we invite from the Rural Council? Sharon, how should we prepare for the interview?

E. Team evaluation:

We identified that Jonah was no longer doing all the work. We are still having problems with the weekly summary. We decided to designate tasks this week that required the use of email so members will feel more responsible. When we did that, we found that we were also giving more details. The representatives really want to be involved and provided ideas and suggestions that we would never have considered.

PART 2

The Development of Projects

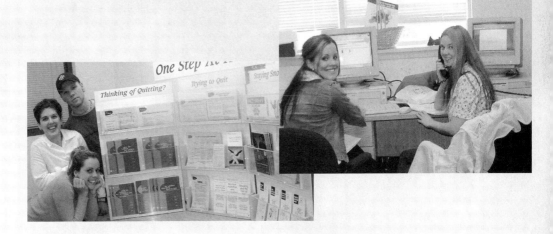

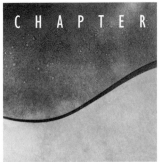

CHAPTER 3

Starting Well: Beginning a Small Scale Project

ALWYN MOYER

SCENARIO · PHYSICAL ACTIVITY AND OLDER ADULTS

Today is the first community project meeting at the Summertown Community Health Center (SCHC). As the lead agency in a community coalition on active living, the SCHC has been asked by the Council on Aging (COA) to provide help with a funding proposal. The instructor has told the students that the proposal is about maintaining the mobility of older adults. The COA has heard of new research that provides evidence of strong links between activity and the prevention of type 2 diabetes. Knowing there is a high prevalence of diabetes in older adults, the COA thinks it will be useful to include diabetes prevention in the proposal to increase the possibility of funding. That is as much as the students know at this point. The student team will report directly to Jeanine, the nurse manager of health promotion services.

When they meet, Jeanine tells them that as well as being the project organizer, she will chair a project steering group of health providers and community members. The steering group includes a member of the SCHC board, two representatives from the COA, a fitness instructor from the City Recreation Department, and the nurse practitioner from the health center. The students learn that during the community clinical placement, their student team will have the task of assembling the existing data on the health issue and the population. The details will be worked out over the next two weeks and agreed upon at the first steering group meeting.

OBJECTIVES   **After reading this chapter and answering the questions throughout the chapter, you should be able to**

1. Appreciate the importance of community assessment.
2. Understand the role and responsibility of the community health nurse to engage communities in health assessment to build capacity.
3. Establish working relationships within a community project.
4. Identify the components of a comprehensive assessment.
5. Identify and locate key policy documents and sociodemographic and epidemiological data.
6. Conduct a document review and organize information according to the community health nursing process.

KEYWORDS   assessment ▪ census data ▪ community ▪ determinants of health ▪ epidemiology ▪ gatekeeper ▪ incidence ▪ morbidity ▪ mortality ▪ prevalence ▪ primary data sources ▪ secondary data sources ▪ sociodemographic data

Collaborative community assessment

Assessment, the first step in the community health nursing process, generates information for health planning. The purpose of the assessment is to obtain information from a variety of sources to define the present situation of a community group and the preferred health situation. The present health situation includes barriers to health and strengths, such as resources that are available and previous experiences working on issues. Health providers often use the term *needs assessment*, but use of this term is seen by some as focusing too much on problems and not enough on community strengths and resources (McKnight & Kretzmann, 1990). Both perspectives are important, however.

As with the assessment of individual and family health status, community assessment is an iterative process, albeit considerably more time consuming and complicated. Communities are complex social systems compared with individuals and families. Communities have many different aspects that need to be considered and many different sources of information to draw upon. Gathering this information provides the opportunity to engage community members in a collaborative process and thereby increase the relevance of health planning. Bracht and Tsouros (1990) commented that even though the principle of community participation is strongly endorsed in the assessment, planning, and evaluation of primary healthcare, the nature and level of involvement can vary widely. It is incumbent on primary healthcare workers to maximize community input and build community capacity for decision making about health (Edwards & Moyer, 2000; Rissel & Bracht, 1999). In this text, collaboration with the community is promoted throughout the process; however, it is acknowledged that the ability to collaborate can vary in different circumstances.

Defining community and community health

Definitions of **community** vary widely, but most contain reference to a group of people who live in a geographical area or who have a common interest and are part of a complex system of networks and associational ties (Buckner, 1988; Israel, Checkoway, Schultz, & Zimmerman, 1994).

Different perspectives of community and community health underpin community health practice (Hawe, 1994). They are not easy to untangle. One view of community is that it is a social setting with a powerful, and incompletely understood, influence on individual and group health and health behavior. Discussing this perspective, Hawe described the community as encouraging or rewarding certain behavior. The implication of this view is that to change behaviors, such as smoking or activity levels, it is not sufficient to promote individual behavior change; rather, it is necessary to change the social and physical environment that supports the behavior. In this way, healthy choices become the easy choices. For example, developing no smoking policies, increasing the price of cigarettes, and restricting the sale of tobacco to adolescents create an environment that discourages initiation of smoking in youth. Community participation is a necessary part of this approach. Health providers use community organizing principles to gain entry to the community, engage residents, and harness community resources to achieve professionally defined health goals such as smoking cessation and active living.

Another perspective, also described by Hawe (1994), is the community as a complex human system in dynamic and mutually influencing interaction with its environment. Community health from this perspective refers to the ability of the community as a social system to take control, solve problems, and adapt to change (Goodman et al., 1998). This ecological model of health (Bronfenbrenner, 1979; McLeroy, Bibeau, Steckler, & Glanz, 1988; Stokols, 1992, 1996) acknowledges that human subsystems—individuals, families, groups, and organizations—form an integral part of the whole, but views the community as greater than the sum of its parts. This is the same as viewing an individual as more than physiological, psychological, social, and spiritual systems and a family as more than the sum of individual family members. The overarching goal of health action from this perspective of community is to strengthen the capacity of the community to function effectively as an integrated whole and be healthy. The health status of individuals, families, and groups is a measure of the health of the community.

Clearly, the way you think about community and community health has implications for what data is collected in the community assessment and how it is collected. In the first model described, the community assessment process is more likely to be professionally driven and focus on identifying the need for specific, evidence-based health promotion and prevention interventions; capacity building is seen as a means to an end. In the second model, the approach is more community driven, and the assessment provides a means to engage the community in a capacity-building or problem-solving process that will identify opportunities for mobilizing resources and building community capacity. Health and social issues provide a vehicle for capacity building. More and more, both approaches are intertwined.

Components of a community assessment

Community health is a multidimensional concept, and therefore a community assessment usually contains the following components: a demographic profile of the population; a description of the patterns and variations in health status; and information on the physical, sociocultural, and political aspects of the community (Anderson & McFarlane, 2000; Rissel & Bracht, 1999; Valanis, 1999). A comprehensive assessment is a large and costly undertaking and usually is facilitated by professional teams. Fortunately, much of the information that is required can be assembled from a range of existing data sources, such as the census. It is expedient to use routinely collected data, sometimes called **secondary data sources,** but because this data was originally collected for other purposes, it may not answer specific questions that are of interest to you. Therefore, it will also be necessary to gather some information directly from **primary data sources**, such as community residents and health service providers.

Gathering secondary information is not unlike the enquiry a community health nurse might undertake when starting a new position or the process that a community group might undertake before developing an agenda for health action. Gathering information is a learning process, and knowledge is power.

Planning the community assessment

In this text, the community assessment is organized into steps of the community health nursing process that build on each other. The establishment of relationships within the project and community precedes the assessment and is the initial step in the process. The second step, which is to assess secondary data, as well as the first are discussed in this chapter. The third and fourth steps involve the assessment of the community and are included in Chapter 4. The fifth step, found in Chapter 5, involves working with the population group to determine action statements. The sixth step, the evaluation of teamwork, occurs concurrently with the previous five steps and is described in Chapter 2. Table 3-1 provides a comprehensive overview of the steps with suggested timelines.

Teams have various options open to them in using the assessment phases of the community health nursing process in this text. If the teams have 90 to 100 hours spread over several weeks and easy access to a population group, all components of the community health nursing process can be addressed by teams of two to four. Table 3-1 depicts the approximate amount of time (shaded areas) based on 7.5 hours per week for 12 weeks that a team would spend on completing the full assessment. The information in the table is based on the team organizing and preparing material with guidance from experienced community health nurses or instructors.

TABLE 3-1 **Community Assessment Timelines**												
	BASED ON 12 WEEKS (90–100 HOURS)											
STEPS IN PROCESS	*1*	*2*	*3*	*4*	*5*	*6*	*7*	*8*	*9*	*10*	*11*	*12*
1. Establish relationships within project and community (Chapter 3)	▓	▓	▓									
2. Assess secondary data: review of population and health issue (Chapter 3)	▓	▓	▓									
3. Initiate assessment of community (Chapter 4)	▓	▓	▓	▓								
4. Conduct specific assessment (Chapter 4)					▓	▓	▓	▓	▓	▓		
5. Determine action statements (Chapter 5)										▓	▓	▓
6. Evaluate teamwork (Chapter 2)	▓	▓	▓	▓	▓	▓	▓	▓	▓	▓	▓	▓

For projects with fewer hours devoted to community assessment or a more compressed timeframe there are other options. Three suggestions are to:

1. Work with a community organization to conduct an extensive review of secondary information on an issue and population, as discussed in this chapter.
2. Review secondary data that has already been assembled and use one or two methods of collecting primary data from the population group, as discussed in Chapter 4.
3. Conduct a component of a larger project such as pilot testing focus group questions or a questionnaire.

Assessment timeline and workplan

A systematic approach is required to successfully conduct a project in the community. A considerable amount of time, resources, and coordination is involved, so it is important to plan ahead. The community health nursing process provides the steps involved in planning and conducting the assessment. These steps are the basis for the assessment timeline and workplan forms given in Appendix C. The assessment timeline is used by the team to plan when activities are expected to start and end. This can also be called a Ghantt chart. The assessment workplan provides the means to document and monitor the assessment. Advance planning provides direction for the project and must be done in collaboration with the project team and preferably with community members. Not only does this allow you to draw on the experiences of others, but it also helps to ensure that the plan will be relevant and supported.

An overview of the steps in the assessment workplan is given in Table 3-2. The detailed assessment workplan is provided in Appendix C. The workplan includes a column for activities related to process and a column for condensing the results from the weekly summaries.

Plans are bound to change given the great many factors that influence them. These changes are much easier to accommodate without losing sight of the goal when activities are planned using the timeline and documented in the workplan.

Step 1: Establish relationships within project and community

The majority of student projects are embedded in broader community health initiatives and relationships that extend beyond the timelines of a student assignment. Usually, health providers or members of a community group or organization have done some preliminary work to identify a need that might be addressed through a student project. Orientation to the project includes reviewing the project proposal, establishing working relations with the project organizers, and confirming with them the details of the project. It may be possible to begin preliminary work based on the original project description; however, both the project organizers and the resources they can direct you to are invaluable in starting the project well.

TABLE 3-2	*Assessment Workplan Steps*

ASSESSMENT WORKPLAN	
Title of project:	Revision date:
STEPS, SUBSTEPS and Activities (list activities under substeps, number and date activities across columns)	**Summary of results with dates**
1. Establish relationships within project and community	
2. Assess secondary data	
3. Initiate assessment of community	
4. Conduct specific assessment	
5. Determine action statements	
6. Evaluate teamwork	

Establish relationships with project organizers

Your student group will be joining the project organizers who have initiated the project. Project organizers include people who will be responsible for the project within a community organization and instructors responsible for the educational requirements of students during the project. These same people will orient your group to the project.

A primary consideration at the first meeting with project organizers is to determine the person or persons who will be responsible for the leadership of the project. You may find that the person orienting you will continue to lead the project because it is part of his or her workload as a public or community health nurse. In other situations, the leadership may come from the instructor because the project is located in a setting where an experienced community health nurse is not available. For example, the instructor would be the project leader if you were working with a class of students learning English or in a factory without an occupational health nurse.

Effective communication is crucial to the success of the project, so start out by scheduling regular meetings throughout the project. More frequent meetings are usually needed initially. Later on, meetings can be more spread out but will be needed to make important decisions. If meetings are not prescheduled, you may find that you lose valuable time trying to have a decision approved. The meetings do not always need to be face-to-face, but initially face-to-face meetings are preferable.

Written communications such as email and faxes are a necessary adjunct to the face-to-face meetings to provide an update and document what has occurred and what is expected to occur. Weekly summary forms are described in Chapter 2. Expectations regarding the communication method and the response time must be determined ahead of time. Regular, timely, and relevant communication is a basic component for maintaining good relationships with everyone on the project team.

Some projects will require you to link with others within the organization. For example, you may be told that any questions used in an assessment must be approved by a manager. This means that questions are to be submitted at least two weeks before they are used. You need to keep track of all the people who are involved in the project and understand your responsibilities to them and theirs to you. At the meetings, record the names and positions of people who are present, or who are identified, by 1) name, 2) contact information, and 3) relationship to the project (see example in Table 3-3). People do not mind signing a sheet or telling you who they are and how you can contact them. Maintain the list. Your project leader can help you determine who is on the project team and who you might contact individually.

Meet community contacts

Although some teams will be working directly with community groups, other projects will be based in an organization such as a public health or community health center and will involve working indirectly with a community group. If the community contacts are not present at the orientation meeting, the team needs to meet with them in the first weeks of the project. A project organizer would usually arrange this first meeting and be present to introduce the team to the community contacts. The meeting could occur as part of a regular meeting or be arranged separately.

The purpose of the early meeting is to assist in the orientation of the team and to initiate a relationship with the community contacts that can develop into collaboration. Often these community contacts are called **gatekeepers** because they control access to the community group. Examples of gatekeepers are principals, teachers, the manager of a business or firm, or the director of a voluntary organization such as a seniors' council.

The preparation for the meeting with community contacts will be similar to that for the meeting with the project organizers. The team will need to determine when the contact person will usually be available, the preferred methods of communication, and the initial expectations. Plan on arranging the next meeting during the initial contact.

Defining the project, population group, and issue

At the orientation meeting with the organizers and community contacts, it is customary to discuss the rationale for the project and to clarify the assessment purpose. Often, this will include a review of the historical perspective and the key events that led to the initiation of the project. For example, you may find that a newly formed coalition of groups has initiated the project based on members' priorities or that an agency has initiated the project on behalf of a community group. Additional background information may be uncovered as the team reviews secondary data sources, such as previous community surveys, and interviews key informants.

Often, the projects are not fully defined at the outset. It is important to ask questions to clarify the purpose. You may be reluctant to do this. When one encounters new people and unfamiliar situations, it is not easy to ask for information. Although this behavior is understandable, it does not give the project organizers or community contact an indication of what you know and what you want to know. One method to get past this awkwardness is for each team member to prepare one question for meetings with different groups. Questions will encourage a discussion and lead to greater understanding.

As well as learning specifically about the project, you need to learn about the community organizations or agencies supporting the project from the organizers and community contacts. The mission statement or mandate of the lead organization and the priority for the project are identified and documented. Although these statements are often quite broad, they provide direction. For example, if the priority is to increase mobility in older adults in the region, then you will have to find ways of reaching all older adults, not just those who attend a particular health center.

PHYSICAL ACTIVITY AND OLDER ADULTS SCENARIO (continued)

The orientation meeting starts promptly, and because this is the first time the group is meeting, Jeanine asks everyone to introduce themselves. There is a printed agenda, and the nurse practitioner volunteers to record the minutes. Jeanine provides a brief overview of the coalition for the students' benefit, and then the COA members talk about their organization and the importance of mobility for healthy aging. Clearly they are very excited about the project. They invite questions and provide four copies of a bulletin called "Let's Get Moving" (National Advisory Council on Aging, Winter 2002–03) for the students to take away and read.

Jeanine leads a discussion on roles and responsibilities. She explains that the students will be responsible for putting together demographic data and existing information on the health status of older adults in the community under her guidance and asks other members how they would like to be involved. Most agree that they have limited time to comment on weekly summaries, but everyone can attend meetings every other week to discuss progress and participate in decisions.

The COA members would like to include some findings in the first draft of their proposal, which is due in four weeks. This draft will be discussed at a coalition meeting, to which the students are invited. Because the clinical experience is 12 days over a 4-week period, the students agree that there is probably time to produce some of the necessary information. Acting on a recommendation from the SCHC board member, the group agrees on the dates for the steering group meetings before the meeting is adjourned. After the meeting, the students set weekly meeting times with Jeanine and start to put together the contact list, which is shown in Table 3-3.

On the way to the bus, the students agree that Jeanine is very well organized, and they feel confident in her ability to manage the project. Darren says: "I can't believe it, they really were pleased to have us helping." Lise slowly agrees, saying, "This increases the pressure to do well. I know I will feel better once we get started, but right now I wish I felt more certain about what to do. What if we gather the wrong information?"

DISCUSSION QUESTIONS

1. To what extent do you think community members can and should be involved in the process of gathering data on priority health problems?
2. How might the students draw on the expertise of the steering group members to guide their search for information?
3. Discuss the implications for students of the request to provide findings for the draft document to be presented at the coalition meeting.

TABLE 3-3	Project Contact List

PROJECT CONTACT LIST

Name	Position	Email/Phone/Reporting Frequency	Relationship to Project
Jeanine Roger	Community health nurse, seniors' health program	jroger@work 555-6666 ext. 226 Include in weekly summary	Project leader Provides direction for project (in person or by email)
Jan Surrey	Instructor	jsurrey@university 444-3333 ext. 123 Include in weekly summary	Academic advisor for project Provides direction for educational objectives in person or by email
Jean Morrow	Manager of community programs	jmorrow@work 444-3333 ext. 345 (Exec. assist: Simon Fannsfann@work ext. 346; fax: 333-4444) Include in summary as needed	Approves staff time to work on project Reports to executive on project Approves any questionnaires
Kerri Czabo	Fitness instructor, Recreation Department	kczabo@city	Director of fitness programs in seniors' apartment buildings Developed chair exercises for less active seniors
Rita Valli	Nurse practitioner	rvalli@work 555-6666 ext. 543 Works 2 PM to 8 PM Include in weekly summary	Runs falls clinics (fall prevention and injury management) Knowledgeable about activity in older adults
Ruth Hemliner	Executive Director, Council on Aging	rhemliner@agency 456-7890 ext. 456 Works Monday–Thursday Steering group only	Identified the original concern with the community Knows most people in the community and how they like to work Contact to obtain coalition meeting date
Ed Jones	Member of SCHC Board	ejones@home Steering group only	Retired city planner Chair of SCHC planning committee Contact to obtain copy of last SCHC needs assessment

Step 2: Assess secondary data

The purpose of assessing secondary data is to identify characteristics of the population and health issue in the literature. The six substeps of this component of the community assessment are the following:

- Review national and local policy documents.
- Review sociodemographic data.
- Review epidemiological data.
- Review previously conducted community surveys and program statistics.
- Review literature and best practice guidelines.
- Secondary data.

Many sources of routinely collected health-related information exist. They include census data, vital statistics, disease registries, communicable disease reports, and hospitalization data. The main sources and types of data are summarized in Table 3-4. Additional

TABLE 3-4	Sources and Types of Readily Available Health Data	
DATA SOURCE	**TYPE OF DATA**	**COMMENTS**
Census data	Sociodemographic variables (e.g., age, gender, income, geographical area) Some information on determinants of health	Standard questions, available for the whole population
Vital statistics (e.g., registry of births and deaths)	Mortality by cause of death, age, and gender	Comprehensive Not a sensitive measure of health because it is a relatively infrequent event
Notifiable disease reports Registers (e.g., cancer)	Morbidity data Incidence and prevalence of specific conditions	Limited to a few conditions
Hospital discharge data Drug utilization data Workplace injuries	Used as a proxy measure of morbidity	Emphasis on conditions requiring medical treatment
National or regional health and social surveys	Morbidity Health behavior and practices (e.g., type and level of exercise and activity; patterns of mammography)	Sample size may not be large enough for a specific area
Air pollution index Crime statistics	Physical, social, and environmental determinants of health	Relevant to community as a whole
Local surveys and research reports	Needs assessments of communities and population groups	Specific focus Data may not be comparable

sources of secondary data (existing data or data collected by others) are national, regional, and local health surveys; health agency reports; and policy documents. It is wise to systematically review the existing data before initiating any costly data collection process. Not only does it save time and avoid duplication of effort, but it also helps to focus the enquiry. Some resources, such as *Community Nursing: Promoting Canadians' Health,* 2nd ed. (Edwards & Moyer, 2000) provide a detailed review of the sources of national health statistics and public health information.

Because the data was collected for other reasons, it will be necessary to think carefully about what information you need, identify and locate the data sources, extract pertinent information, and assemble it in such a way as to tell a story. The "story" you want to tell will comprise the summary of secondary data in the workplan. Think of it as building a jigsaw puzzle. The order in which you retrieve the information is not crucial; you can start at any point and gradually fill in the pieces until at the end of this exercise you have a complete picture and can understand how the pieces fit together. A thorough examination of existing data will help you to understand the patterns of health and illness in your community or population. A review of strategy documents helps to situate your project in relation to what is currently happening in the community. The following sections discuss policy documents, sociodemographic data, and health status information in more depth.

Policy documents

National and regional governments provide broad direction for health through public policy documents and strategic plans. It is important to be familiar with these documents, particularly as they pertain to your population of interest. In the last 20 years, the World Health Organization's *Health for All by Year 2000* with its emphasis on health promotion has helped to shift the emphasis of health planning from the provision of health services to the health of populations. Within this new framework for health, the role of government is to develop what has been described as healthy public policy (Glass & Hicks, 2000). Such policy, which is grounded in the values of the people, guides decision making about health across different sectors. Policy frameworks ensure a common understanding and promote consistent approaches toward a common goal of health for all.

Governments in Western countries have produced a number of policy documents that identify the health of the population as a priority. These documents signal the intent to use comprehensive and collaborative approaches to improve the health of their people. For example, the government of Canada, in collaboration with the provincial and territorial governments, produced a population health strategy (Federal Provincial and Territorial Advisory Committee on Population Health [FPTACPH], 1999b) together with a population health framework and action guidelines (Health Canada, 2001). The strategy seeks to reduce inequalities in the factors that determine health that place some Canadians at disadvantage. Three priorities for action are identified:

1. Renewing and reorienting the health sector
2. Investing in the health and well-being of key population groups
3. Improving health by reducing inequities in literacy, education, and the distribution of incomes in Canada (FPTACPH, 1999b)

The United States and England have taken this a step farther and articulated national health strategies, identified priority areas, and set national goals or targets with timelines for achievement. Recent revisions of these strategies are in line with the population health approach identified by Health Canada. For example, the United States identified two goals in *Healthy People 2010* (U.S. Department of Health and Human Services [USDHHS], November 2000):

Goal 1: Increase quality and years of healthy life.
Goal 2: Eliminate health disparities.

Ewles and Simnett (1999, p. 116) described the development of similar strategy documents in England. The 1999 version, referred to as *Our Healthier Nation*, sets out two key aims (Secretary of State for Health, United Kingdom, 1999):

To improve the health of the population as a whole by increasing the length of people's lives and the number of years people spend free of illness
To improve the health of the worst off in society and to narrow the health gap

In turn, the national goals provide direction for regional planning authorities. For example, the Canadian province of British Columbia set more specific provincial health goals, which reflect the population health approach (Office of the Provincial Health Officer, Government of British Columbia, 2004):

Goal 1: Positive and supportive living and working conditions in all our communities
Goal 2: Opportunities for all individuals to develop and maintain the capacities and skills needed to thrive and meet life's challenges and to make choices that enhance health
Goal 3: A diverse and sustainable physical environment with clean, healthy, and safe air, water, and land
Goal 4: An effective and efficient health service system that provides equitable access to appropriate services
Goal 5: Improved health for Aboriginal peoples
Goal 6: Reduction of preventable illness, injuries, disabilities, and premature death

Other useful sources of health policy documents are the World Health Organization (WHO) and the Pan American Health Organization (PAHO), an arm of the WHO. Voluntary and nongovernment organizations, special interest groups, and professional organizations also produce health policy documents for their own ends and to influence government policy. Nowadays, many of these documents are available on the Internet. At the local level, most organizations have policy documents and strategic and operational plans that guide planning decisions. It is not realistic to try to provide a comprehensive list of data sources because the production of health information is an iterative process. At the end of this chapter you will find a list of key national Web sites, which will provide an entry point to regional resources.

Population health strategy documents and action plans provide direction and are a valuable resource. They not only articulate the conceptual models of health that guide decision making, but also present the analyses of epidemiological and experimental evidence on which needs and priorities are based. Considerable work has been done to put together this evidence base. In addition to identifying priorities and providing detailed and specific direction on effective interventions, the documents also guide funding allocations.

Understanding policy frameworks and aligning new programs with priority areas increase the probability of gaining project support.

Population-based or issue-based?

At this point it is useful to reflect on the many different starting points for community health projects. Sometimes a project starts with questions about a geographically defined population, for example, the residents of a rural community, perhaps further defined by age (e.g., all adults older than age 65 living in the community) or by developmental stage (e.g., adolescents or pregnant women and their families). A variation of this approach is to focus on community settings such as workplaces and schools that provide access to certain populations and that, like communities, provide an environment that influences health and well-being. Alternatively, projects might take as their starting point a population group like single parents or Aboriginal men thought to be at high risk with unmet needs.

Other starting points are a health issue or concern such as homelessness, a disease or condition such as diabetes, or health-related practices such as the use of family planning methods. Within these categories, the population may also be defined by age, as in teenage smokers. Regardless of whether your project starts with a people-based or issue-based question, you will need to clarify the geographical boundaries of your population and its defining characteristics, such as age or gender, to focus your enquiry.

Sociodemographic data

Information on social and demographic patterns yields **sociodemographic data**—especially age structure—which is crucial for health planning at national, regional, or provincial and local levels, regardless of which perspective of community you hold. The census, which is conducted on a regular basis, is the main source of demographic data. Collected by household, **census data** includes the number of people in the household by age, sex, marital status, occupation, and ethnicity. The census reports provide a profile of the population as a whole at one point and allow comparison between and within different regions of the country. The census can also be used to identify trends and make projections about what the population will look like in the near future. Remember that some groups, for example, the homeless, and in Canada, Aboriginal peoples living off a reserve, are not well represented in the census. It is difficult to obtain accurate numbers for these populations for health planning.

It is much easier to assemble sociodemographic information when the community is defined geographically using the commonly accepted boundaries defined by the census. Census information is aggregated from the census divisions to provide community-level data. Usually these boundaries correspond to recognizable neighborhoods, but it is essential to check. Knowing the boundaries of your community is important.

Regional and local data

Although it is now possible to gain access to aggregated census data for cities and planning regions in Canada and the United States, it is not necessary to do this. Usually public health

BOX 3-1	Sample questions on the community and population

- What are the boundaries of my community?
- What proportion of the community is in my target group (e.g., men and women aged 65 years and older; Somali immigrants)?
- What is the profile of this population (e.g., by gender, language, education, income, housing, and living conditions)? How does it compare with the community as a whole?
- How will the size of this population change in the next 10 years—is it likely to increase or decrease?
- Where does this population live in the community? Are members spread evenly throughout the community, or do some areas have larger numbers than others?

departments or health intelligence agencies have responsibility for assembling health information to guide health decision making. For example, the Eastern Ontario Health Information Partnership compiles demographic profiles of public health department planning regions and counties in its area and displays them on its Web site (Bains, 1998). Furthermore, a variety of health and social service agencies and other organizations assemble and publish detailed local reports to meet their own planning needs.

Planning your search strategy and documenting it accurately the first time will save time in the long run. You need to identify what data will be useful to your project and where it is likely to be found. You will find it useful to develop a set of questions to guide your search. Box 3-1 provides a sample set of questions that can help to structure your search and provide a framework for collating the information that you find.

PHYSICAL ACTIVITY AND OLDER ADULTS SCENARIO (continued)

The students prepared their assessment timeline following the steering group meeting. They wanted to have it ready for discussion at the next meeting.

After consultation with Jeanine, they decide to gather demographic data on adults 65 years and older for the health region, which includes the city where the SCHC is located and the surrounding rural area. This will provide a sufficiently large population for obtaining meaningful health statistics.

After a lively discussion on the best way to proceed, the students start out by developing the questions to guide their search together and then split up to work in pairs. Robin and Darren chose to gather the demographic information, which left the search for policy documents to Lise and Mika. Jeanine suggests they look at the Health Canada Web site for policy documents related to older adults and active living. The beginning of their workplan is given in Table 3-5.

Lise and Mika find that their search took them longer than they had anticipated and was not as productive as they had hoped. Visiting the Web site of the Division of Aging and Seniors, they found a National Framework on Aging, designed to guide current and future policy development (Health Canada, 2002) and links to many other sites including the National Council on Aging. The National Council site contained a physical activity guide for older adults embedded in a broader policy on active living; otherwise there was no relevant information on activity for seniors. The main result of the search was a detailed report on Canada's aging population, which included a demographic profile and health assessment complete with tables and graphs (National Advisory Council on Aging, 2001). This they forward to their colleagues. Says Mika, "At least we know how to navigate the site now and have identified some keywords such as physical activity, diabetes, and seniors." Lise and Mika arrange to develop the questions for the health status assessment.

TABLE 3-5	*Beginning Workplan*

ASSESSMENT WORKPLAN

Title of Project: *Physical Activity and Older Adults*	Revision Date: *10/09/05*
STEPS, SUBSTEPS and Activities (list activities under substeps, number and date activities across columns)	**Summary of results with dates**
1. Establish relationships within project and community, *Sept. 8–Sept. 21*	*[complete on Sept. 21]*
a. Establish relationship with project organizers, *Sept. 8*	*Met Jeanine, the project leader, and reviewed the project proposal. Roles and responsibilities were discussed and agreed upon. Agreed to meet face-to-face every second week and by email weekly.*
b. Meet community contacts, *Sept. 8*	*Met contacts from the coalition and SCHC at orientation. Next meeting and communication determined.*
c. Define the project, population group, and purpose, *Sept. 8–16*	*Sept. 8 and 9. Reviewed background document provided by SCHC and COA. Drafted assessment timeline. Drafted assessment goal with Jeanine.*
2. Assess secondary data,* *Sept. 8–Oct. 10*	*[insert summary on Oct. 10]*

a. Review national, regional, and local policy documents, *Sept. 8–16: Elise and Mika*
    1) identify and locate sources
    2) review sources
    3) extract information
	1) Sept. 9 On hold until after the review of health status

b. Review sociodemographic data, *Sept. 8–16: Robin and Darren*
    1) develop guiding questions
    2) locate sources
    3) extract information	

*The substeps for Step 2 in the workplan are to be attached in a separate document. Two substeps are displayed here to indicate the activities that can be used to obtain the data.

DISCUSSION QUESTIONS

1. Identify your community. With two or three other students, discuss the boundaries and explain what community means to you.
2. Using your own community as an example, identify ways in which the community reinforces healthy or unhealthy behavior.
3. Goodman et al. (1998, p. 258) used the following definition of community capacity to guide their work: "the characteristics of communities that affect their ability to identify, mobilize, and address social and public health problems." With two or three other students, compare two communities using this definition.

Health status and the determinants

Gathering information on the health status of your target population and on the **determinants of health** is the next part of the community assessment. You will need to understand epidemiological concepts and methods to interpret health surveys and reports, so you may find it useful to refer to a basic epidemiology text. **Epidemiology** is the science concerned with the patterns of health and illness in the population and in understanding "what environmental conditions, lifestyles, or other circumstances are associated with the presence or absence of disease" (Valanis, 1999).

The basic methods of epidemiology are to count the frequency of events such as stillbirths and to estimate proportions or rates in populations. Then comparisons are made between different people, places, and times to understand the patterns of health and illness and trends. The two most commonly used rates, which all nurses should understand, are the prevalence rate and the incidence rate.

The **prevalence** rate measures the number of persons with a condition in a group or population at a given time. It is expressed as a rate per unit of population (such as per 100,000):

$$\text{Prevalence} = \frac{\text{Number of existing cases in place at point in time}}{\text{Number of persons in place at midpoint of year}} \times K$$

Prevalence rates provide a snapshot at a particular point and are useful for making decisions about diseases of a chronic nature that will require long-term care. For example, data gathered in 1996 to 1997 showed that the prevalence of diagnosed diabetes in Canada was 0.5% in persons aged 12 to 34, 3.2% in persons aged 35 to 64, and 10.4% in persons older than age 65 (Health Canada, 1999b, p. 13). With the aging of the population, the burden of diabetes on the healthcare system is likely to increase because the prevalence rates increase with age.

The **incidence** rate measures all new cases arising in a population at risk during a defined period, usually one year:

$$\text{Incidence} = \frac{\text{Number of new cases in place during time of observation}}{\text{Population in place at midpoint of time}} \times K$$

Incidence rates provide information about the rate of development of a condition. Using calculations from the same data set as the prevalence rates, an estimated 2.6 new cases of diabetes were being diagnosed for every 1000 persons in Canada older than age 12 (Health Canada, 1999b). The Health Canada report notes that the incidence of diabetes appears to be increasing outside of North America. However, an Ontario study found that even though the number of persons with diabetes is growing, the incidence has not increased; rather, the prevalence is increasing because people with diabetes are living longer (Hux & Tang, 2002). Birth rates and death rates are special cases of incidence referring to the number of people being born or dying in a specific place and at a specific time.

Measures of morbidity, mortality, and well-being provide a snapshot of the health status of the population. **Mortality** data are compiled from death certificates and has long been used as a proxy measure of health or life expectancy. Age-standardized data pinpoint the primary causes of death by life stages. Other measures such as untimely death or potential years of life lost (PYLL) are calculated from mortality data. PYLL can be used to compare the benefits of different types of intervention in extending life. **Morbidity** data provide information on the major burden of illness in the population. The various measures include prevalence data on conditions such as sexually transmitted disease, symptoms of ill health, and risk behaviors (such as engaging in unprotected sex), together with indirect measures of ill health such as days of work lost.

The collection of morbidity and mortality data presents many methodological difficulties. For instance, a medical assessment or laboratory tests are required to accurately determine the presence or absence of illness. Much of the data is obtained through self-report and may contain inaccuracies. People tend to overestimate or underestimate amounts because of the desire to present a good picture or because it is difficult to remember accurately. For these reasons, well-designed national and regional surveys with large samples and standardized approaches help to ensure reliable and valid data. Smaller-scale surveys may provide equally valid and reliable data, but often the measures may not be comparable to those used in other regions. That is why it is important to review a survey's study methods and to know what questions were asked and how the data were handled.

National, regional, and local health surveys collect information on self-reported health and on a broad range of risk and protective health behaviors and other health determinants. For example, the Statistical Report on the Health of Canadians (FPTACPH, 1999a) provides detailed information on self-reported health, positive mental health, job satisfaction, and lifestyle behaviors (e.g., physical activity, dietary practices, and seatbelt use) that contribute to the risk of injury and disease. In addition, the report includes measures of the social, economic, and physical environment; health services; personal resources and coping; and health knowledge. In the United States, some state and local health departments provide access to similar reports based on routinely collected data. For example, the Illinois Project for Local Assessment of Needs (IPLAN) provides reports based on a community health assessment and planning process that is conducted every five years by local health jurisdictions (Illinois Department of Public Health, 2002).

Review of literature

It is not necessary to conduct an exhaustive review of the literature as part of a community assessment, other than to fill in any gaps in knowledge. However, to appreciate the importance of health data and interpret what it means, it is necessary to understand the complex relationships that contribute to wellness and illness. Epidemiologists have long used a model of agent, host, and environment factors to understand the natural history of a

BOX 3-2	Sample questions on health and the determinants

- What are the indicators of wellness in the population?
- What are the prevalence and incidence of preventable ill health and disability in the community? How does this community compare with other like communities? With the nation?
- Are some population groups affected more than others?
- How does this community compare with other communities on factors that have an impact on health?
- How does the health problem or issue impact on other problems identified as a priority in the community?

disease. A more complex view of the dynamic interplay of multiple factors that influence health and wellness is referred to as a *web of causation* (Brunt & Sheilds, 2000; Valanis, 1999). To be fully informed about these causal links you will need to become familiar with the models and review the medical and nursing evidence, including best practice guidelines (see Chapter 7). Sometimes you will find that the information on a particular health topic has been critically reviewed in national and regional strategy documents. The questions listed in Box 3-2 can be used to guide your enquiry.

Table 3-6 lists key determinants of health and explains the premises underlying the relationship between the determinant and health. A summary of the supporting evidence can be found on the Health Canada (2004) Web site. A cogent discussion of the social determinants of health and the underlying premises regarding their impact on health can also be found on the WHO Web site (WHO, 1998). A third column can be added to the table to record population or health issue–specific information, pertinent to the determinant.

PHYSICAL ACTIVITY AND OLDER ADULTS SCENARIO (continued)

After two weeks, the students meet to review their progress. Darren and Robin report that there are 73,520 adults older than age 65 in the region and provide an illustration of the population pyramid together with numerous tables showing a breakdown of the population by ten-year intervals, gender, living arrangements, and other characteristics. Robin says he has found some statistics that confirm what the COA members had told them—the population is aging. Robin explains Table 3-7, which compares the age dependency ratio in the province and local region. This ratio is calculated by dividing the number of persons aged 65 years and older by the total population aged 15 to 64. Table 3-7 shows that the ratio has risen in the East from 15.3 to 16.5 persons older than age 65 for every 100 persons aged 15 to 64. However, the rate remains lower than in the province as a whole. The change reflects an aging population, which has implications for home care and chronic disease services. Mika suggests they work out whether the rate is increasing faster in the East than in the province.

Mika and Lise share a table on the different patterns of physical activity with aging, shown in Table 3-8. The table generates a lot of discussion on the reasons for the large drop in physical activity at the end of the teenage years. Kerri, the seniors' fitness instructor, comments that the decrease after age 75 fit with her experience with exercise groups in the seniors' apartment buildings. She notes that it would be useful to look more closely at the 65- to 74-year-old age groupings to see whether the decline in intensity of physical activity happened gradually over the 10-year period.

TABLE 3-6	Key Determinants of Health
KEY DETERMINANT	**RATIONALE**
Income/social status	Health status improves at each step up the income and social hierarchy. High income determines living conditions such as safe housing and the ability to buy sufficient good food. The healthiest populations are those in societies that are prosperous and have an equitable distribution of wealth.
Social support network	Support from families, friends, and communities is associated with better health. Such social support networks could be very important in helping people solve problems, deal with adversity, and maintain a sense of mastery and control over life circumstances. The caring and respect that occur in social relationships and the resulting sense of satisfaction and well-being seem to act as a buffer against health problems.
Education and literacy	Health status improves with level of education. Education is closely tied to socioeconomic status, and effective education for children and lifelong learning for adults are key contributors to health and prosperity for individuals and for the country. Education contributes to health and prosperity by equipping people with knowledge and skills for problem solving, and helps provide a sense of control and mastery over life circumstances. It increases opportunities for job and income security and job satisfaction, and improves people's ability to access and understand information that will help keep them healthy.
Employment/working conditions	Unemployment, underemployment, and stressful work are associated with poorer health. People who have more control over their work circumstances and fewer stress-related demands of the job are healthier and often live longer than those in more stressful or riskier work and activities.
Social environments	The importance of social support also extends to the broader community. Civic vitality refers to the strength of social networks within a community, region, province, or country. It is reflected in the institutions, organizations, and informal giving practices that people create to share resources and build attachments with others. The array of values and norms of a society influence in varying ways the health and well-being of individuals and populations. In addition, social stability, recognition of diversity, safety, good working relationships, and cohesive communities provide a supportive society that reduces or avoids many potential risks to good health. A healthy lifestyle can be thought of as a broad description of people's behaviour in three inter-related dimensions: individuals, individuals within their social environments (e.g., family, peers, community, workplace), and the relation between individuals and their social environment. Interventions to improve health through lifestyle choices can use comprehensive approaches that address health as a social or community (i.e., shared) issue. Social or community responses can add resources to an individual's repertoire of strategies to cope with changes and foster health.
Physical environments	The physical environment is an important determinant of health. At certain levels of exposure, contaminants in our air, water, food, and soil can cause a variety of adverse health effects, including cancer, birth defects, respiratory illness, and gastrointestinal ailments. In the built environment, factors related to housing, indoor air quality, and the design of communities and transportation systems can significantly influence our physical and psychological well-being. *(continued)*

TABLE 3-6	*Key Determinants of Health* (Continued)
KEY DETERMINANT	**RATIONALE**
Personal health practices and coping skills	Personal health practices and coping skills refer to those actions by which individuals can prevent diseases and promote self-care, cope with challenges, develop self-reliance, solve problems, and make choices that enhance health. Definitions of lifestyle include not only individual choices, but also the influence of social, economic, and environmental factors on the decisions people make about their health. There is a growing recognition that personal life "choices" are greatly influenced by the socioeconomic environments in which people live, learn, work, and play. These influences impact lifestyle choice through at least five areas: personal life skills, stress, culture, social relationships and belonging, and a sense of control. Interventions that support the creation of supportive environments will enhance the capacity of individuals to make healthy lifestyle choices in a world where many choices are possible.
Healthy child development	New evidence on the effects of early experiences on brain development, school readiness, and health in later life has sparked a growing consensus about early child development as a powerful determinant of health in its own right. At the same time, we have been learning more about how all of the other determinants of health affect the physical, social, mental, emotional, and spiritual development of children and youth. For example, a young person's development is greatly affected by his or her housing and neighborhood, family income and level of parents' education, access to nutritious foods and physical recreation, genetic makeup, and access to dental and medical care.
Biology and genetic endowment	The basic biology and organic make-up of the human body are a fundamental determinant of health. Genetic endowment provides an inherited predisposition to a wide range of individual responses that affect health status. Although socioeconomic and environmental factors are important determinants of overall health, in some circumstances genetic endowment appears to predispose certain individuals to particular diseases or health problems.
Health services	Health services, particularly those designed to maintain and promote health, to prevent disease, and to restore health and function, contribute to population health. The health services continuum of care includes treatment and secondary prevention.
Gender	Gender refers to the array of society-determined roles, personality traits, attitudes, behaviors, values, relative power, and influence that society ascribes to the two sexes on a differential basis. "Gendered" norms influence the health system's practices and priorities. Many health issues are a function of gender-based social status or roles. Women, for example, are more vulnerable to gender-based sexual or physical violence, low income, lone parenthood, gender-based causes of exposure to health risks and threats (e.g., accidents, sexually transmitted diseases, suicide, smoking, substance abuse, prescription drugs, and physical inactivity). Measures to address gender inequality and gender bias within and beyond the health system will improve population health. *(continued)*

TABLE 3-6	Key Determinants of Health (Continued)
KEY DETERMINANT	**RATIONALE**
Culture	Some persons or groups may face additional health risks due to a socioeconomic environment, which is largely determined by dominant cultural values that contribute to the perpetuation of conditions such as marginalization, stigmatization, loss or devaluation of language and culture, and lack of access to culturally appropriate healthcare and services.

Source: What determines health? Key Determinants, Health Canada (2004). © Reproduced with the permission of the Minister of Public Works and Government Services Canada, 2004.

TABLE 3-7	Dependency Ratio for the Province and Health Region	
REGION	**1991**	**1996**
Ontario	17.3	18.5
East	15.3	16.5

TABLE 3-8	Intensity of Physical Activity by Age, Ontario, 1996-1997				
	12–19	**20–24**	**45–64**	**65–74**	**75+**
Active	39%	20%	16%	18%	11%
Moderate	25%	24%	23%	23%	16%
Inactive	37%	57%	61%	59%	73%

Source: Public Health Research, Education and Development Program (PHRED), 2000, p. 112.

Mike and Lise quickly scan the Web sites and locate the Statistical Report on the Health of Canadians (FPTACPH, 1999a), as well as a number of policy documents on diabetes prevention. The most comprehensive is the Canadian Diabetes Strategy (Health Canada, 1999a), which identified prevention and promotion as major elements of the strategy. Looking at their results, Jeanine mentions that interest in diabetes prevention has increased rapidly since the presentation of the results of two intervention projects, which provided strong evidence that type 2 diabetes could be prevented through lifestyle interventions that included physical activity. Mika had seen the references in one of the policy documents and agrees to locate the papers at the university library. The group is pleased to find that so much information is available. They discuss how the situation would be quite different in the case of newly emerging health issues, such as the onset of the acquired immunodeficiency syndrome (AIDS) epidemic or more recently severe acute *respiratory syndrome (SARS), when the evidence base was lacking and few policy documents were in place.*

In their search of Web sites, Lise locates a diabetes atlas, which provided data on the prevalence and incidence of diabetes in Ontario. From this document they learn that the incidence of diabetes in the province had not changed in the past five years, but the prevalence was increasing steadily because of the aging population (Hux & Tang, 2002).

After reviewing the information, they identify gaps in the data and additional questions about the ethnic composition of their population and the number of Aboriginal people living in the area. These questions were generated from the policy documents, which reported high levels of type 2 diabetes in Aboriginal people and certain ethnic groups. Robin and Darren agree to locate figures on Aboriginal peoples and other ethnic groups in the population.

The group members agree that efforts have been successful beyond their wildest dreams. "Maybe we have been too successful," says Darren. "How are we going to keep track of this information?"

Local surveys and program statistics

Public health units, community health agencies, and health and social planning departments are rich repositories of up-to-date health information on the community. These agencies conduct needs assessments periodically for strategic planning or to assess specific health needs in a community. The periodic reports and planning surveys can provide more detailed information on a community, or particular segments of it, than are available through national reports.

Routinely gathered data on the utilization of health services and program evaluations are another valuable source of community data. A potential drawback is that the program statistics may be coded differently from one agency to another and so will not be comparable. Table 3-9 provides an example. The table compares the number of clients using diabetes services located in a hospital with those using similar services in a community health center (CHC). At first glance it looks as though more clients use the hospital services, but CHC clients have more visits. On further examination, it turned out that clients might see any combination of doctor, nurse, and dietitian at each visit. The CHC coded each consultation as a separate visit, whereas the hospital just coded the visit.

TABLE 3-9   Utilization of Diabetes Services, 2002–2003

CLIENT DATA	HOSPITAL	CHC
Total clients served	3197	1352
Total new clients	920	1352
Total visits	2695	4716
Total visits: one-on-one	1639	3881
Total visits: group	1056	835
Total visits: telephone	2712	2427

Managing the information and references

A systematic process will facilitate the review of existing information. As you locate and read the numerous documents, reports, and Web-based materials, you will accumulate a lot of information. It will be easier to put together a report of your findings if you keep a complete record of all the written and Web-based resources you consult, with notes. Any photocopies or printed material should be clearly marked with full reference information in case you need to return to the source. Similar to any academic paper, information given must be referenced. This is not any different from keeping study notes or conducting a review of the literature. However, because this is a group effort, it will be necessary to agree to a process that works for all members of the group and that avoids unnecessary duplication.

Table 3-10 shows how to keep track of information sources, including the reference information and a summary of key findings.

Time management is important to consider when seeking and reviewing secondary data. For some issues, such as smoking, there will be an overwhelming number of studies and reports. In those cases look for a review of studies or best practice guidelines (see Chapter 7). For other issues, a considerable amount of time can be spent with few results. To use time efficiently, seek advice from the project organizers on key words, data sources, and approximate amount of time to spend searching.

DISCUSSION QUESTIONS

1. Compare the services described in Table 3-9, and then identify the similarities and differences in the hospital and community health services.
2. Give an example of an age-specific mortality rate and a cause-specific mortality rate. How do you know what constant to use when calculating a mortality rate?
3. How would you interpret the different levels of intensity of exercise found in Table 3-8? Explain how you might ensure that the responses to this question were comparable?

Summary

Community assessment is the first step toward understanding community needs and resources and is an essential component of community health planning. The assessment also serves other, less tangible, purposes that are thought to build community participation. The community assessment presents an entry point for citizen involvement and can be used to raise awareness about health issues. The examination of existing data is a key component of the assessment. The information gathered from policy documents, sociodemographic data, and health status data provides the basis for a shared understanding of community health issues. Achieving this shared understanding is a good start to the project.

PRACTICE AND APPLICATION

1. Obtain a health policy or strategy document from a community clinic or public health department and compare it with national documents such as "Toward a Healthy Future"

TABLE 3-10	Tracking Information	

TOPIC	REFERENCE	KEY IDEAS
Canadian Diabetes Prevention Strategy	Health Canada. (1999a, 2002-11-19). *Canadian diabetes strategy.* Retrieved July 10, 2003, from http://www.hc-sc.gc.ca/ pphb-dgspsp/ccdpc-cpcmc/diabetes-diabete/english/strategy/index.html Or: http://www.hc-sc.gc.ca –Diseases and Conditions –Diabetes	Prevention of diabetes and health promotion for the entire Canadian population with special funds allocated to Aboriginal peoples. Promotion of physical activity and healthy eating. Support for community-based projects. Focus on partnerships; increasing awareness and education of diabetes, its complications and major risk factors; sharing best practices; coordinating and leading diabetes efforts nationally
Ontario Diabetes Strategy for Prevention	Ontario Ministry of Health and Long-Term Care. (1999). *Ontario Diabetes Strategy for Prevention: Report of the Chief Medical Officer of Health.* Retrieved June 2, 2004, from http://www.health. gov.on.ca/english/public/pub/ ministry_reports/diabetes/diabetes.html	Identifies priority populations, settings, and approaches toward preventing type 2 diabetes. Framework for action includes investing health dollars in strategies for seniors.
Ontario Diabetes Atlas, Patterns and Prevalence	Hux, J. E., & Tang, M (2002). Patterns and prevalence and incidence of diabetes. In J. E. Hux, G. Booth & A. Laupacis (Eds.), *Diabetes in Ontario, An ICES Practice Atlas.* (pp. 1.1-1.18). Toronto: Institute for Clinical Evaluative Sciences Or: http://www.ices.on.ca	Maps and tables comparing prevalence and incidence of diabetes and use of specific health services across health planning regions.
Cooperative survey of diabetes education centres	Local surveys	Utilization of diabetes clinics by city

(FTPACPH, 1999b) or "Healthy People in Healthy Communities" (USDHHS, 2001). Trace one initiative and show the links to the national strategy. Identify discrepancies.

2. Prepare a web of causation to show the connections between active living and type 2 diabetes.

3. You have been selected to present findings to the steering group. From the data presented in this chapter, prepare key messages for three overheads.

REFERENCES

Anderson, E. T., & McFarlane, J. (2000). *Community as partner: Theory and practice in nursing* (3rd ed.). Philadelphia: Lippincott Williams & Wilkins.

Bains, N. (1998). *Demographic profile of Eastern Ontario—1996 census.* Kingston, ON: Health Information Partnership, Eastern Ontario Region.

Bracht, N., & Tsouros, A. (1990). Principles and strategies of effective community participation. *Health Promotion International, 5*(3), 199–208.

Bronfenbrenner, U. (1979). *The ecology of human development.* Cambridge, MA: Oxford University Press.

Brunt, J. H., & Sheilds, L. E. (2000). Epidemiology in community health nursing: Principles and application for primary health care. In M. J. Stewart (Ed.), *Community nursing: Promoting Canadians' health* (2nd ed., pp. 564–583). Toronto, ON: Saunders Canada.

Buckner, J. C. (1988). The development of an instrument to measure neighborhood cohesion. *American Journal of Community Psychology, 16*(6), 771–791.

Edwards, N. C., & Moyer, A. (2000). Community needs and capacity assessment: Critical components of program planning. In M. J. Stewart (Ed.), *Community nursing: Promoting Canadians' health* (2nd. ed., pp. 420–442). Toronto, ON: Saunders Canada.

Ewles, L., & Simnett, I. (1999). *Promoting health: A practical guide* (4th ed.). Edinburgh: Baillière Tindall.

Federal Provincial and Territorial Advisory Committee on Population Health (FPTACPH). (1999a). *Statistical report on the health of Canadians, 1999. Prepared for the meeting of Ministers of Health, Charlottetown, P.E.I. September 16–17, 1999.* Ottawa, ON: Ministry of Supply and Services.

Federal Provincial and Territorial Advisory Committee on Population Health (FPTACPH). (1999b). *Toward a healthy future: Second report on the health of Canadians. Prepared for the meeting of Ministers of Health, Charlottetown, P.E.I., September 16–17, 1999.* Ottawa, ON: Ministry of Supply and Services.

Glass, H., & Hicks, S. (2000). Healthy public policy in health system reform. In M. J. Stewart (Ed.), *Community nursing: Promoting Canadians' health* (2nd ed., pp. 156–170). Toronto, ON: Saunders Canada.

Goodman, R. M., Speers, M. A., McLeroy, K., Fawcett, S., Kegler, M., Parker, E., et al. (1998). Identifying and defining the dimensions of community capacity to provide a basis for measurement. *Health Education and Behaviour, 25*(3), 258–278.

Hawe, P. (1994). Capturing the meaning of "community" in community intervention evaluation. *Health Promotion International, 9*(3), 199–210.

Health Canada. (1999a). *Canadian diabetes strategy.* Retrieved July 10, 2003, from http://www.hc-sc.gc.ca/pphb-dgspsp/ccdpc-cpcmc/diabetes-diabete/english/strategy/index.html.

Health Canada. (1999b). *Diabetes in Canada: National statistics and opportunities for improved surveillance, prevention and control.* Ottawa, ON: Minister of Public Works and Government Services.

Health Canada. (2000). *Key determinants of health.* Retrieved February 12, 2003, from http://www.hc-sc.gc.ca/hppb/phdd/docs/common/appendix_c.html.

Health Canada. (2001). *The population health template: Key elements and actions that define a population health approach.* Retrieved July 10, 2003, from http://www.hc-sc.gc.ca/hppb/phdd/resources/subject_approach.html.

Health Canada. (2002). *National framework on aging.* Retrieved July 10, 2003, from http://www.hc-sc.gc.ca/seniors-aines/nfa-cnv/index_e.htm.

Hux, J. E., & Tang, M. (2002). Patterns and prevalence and incidence of diabetes. In J. E. Hux, G. Booth, & A. Laupacis (Eds.), *Diabetes in Ontario: An ICES practice atlas* (pp. 1.1–1.18). Toronto, ON: Institute for Clinical Evaluative Sciences.

Illinois Department of Public Health. (2002). *Health statistics.* Retrieved July 10, 2003, from http://www.idph.state.il.us/health/statshome.htm.

Israel, B. A., Checkoway, B., Schultz, A., & Zimmerman, M. (1994). Health education and community empowerment: Conceptualizing and measuring perceptions of individual, organizational and community control. *Health Education Quarterly, 21*(2), 149–170.

McKnight, J. L., & Kretzmann, J. P. (1990). *Mapping community capacity.* Evanston, IL: Center for Urban Affairs and Policy Research, Northwestern University.

McLeroy, K. R., Bibeau, D., Steckler, A., & Glanz, K. (1988). An ecological perspective on health promotion programs. *Health Education Quarterly, 15*(4), 351–377.

National Advisory Council on Aging. (Winter 2002–03). "Let's get moving." *Expressions: NACA Bulletin, 16.*

National Advisory Council on Aging. (2003). *Interim report card: Seniors in Canada,* (2003). Retrieved May 25, 2004, from http://www.hc-sc.gc.ca/seniors-aines/naca/report_card2003/rptcard2003_toc_e.htm

Office of the Provincial Health Officer, Government of British Columbia. (2004). *Health goals for British Columbia.* Retrieved June 2, 2004, from http://www.healthservices.gov.bc.ca/pho/hlthgoals/goals.html.

Ontario Ministry of Health and Long-Term Care. (1999). Ontario diabetes strategy for prevention: Report of the Chief Medical Officer of Health. Retrieved June 2, 2004, from http://www.health.gov.on.ca/english/public/pub/ministry_reports/diabetes/diabetes.html.

Public Health Research Education & Development Program (PHRED). (2000). *Report on the health status of the residents of Ontario.* Toronto, ON: Author.

Rissel, C., & Bracht, N. (1999). Assessing community needs, resources and readiness. In N. Bracht (Ed.), *Health promotion at the community level: New advances* (2nd ed., pp. 59–71). Thousand Oaks, CA: Sage.

Secretary of State for Health, United Kingdom. (July 9, 1999). *Saving lives: Our healthier nation.* Retrieved July 10, 2003, from http://www.archive.official-documents.co.uk/document/cm43/4386/4386-01.htm.

Stokols, D. (1992). Establishing and maintaining healthy environments: Toward a social ecology of health promotion. *American Psychologist, 47*(1), 6–22.

Stokols, D. (1996). Translating social ecological theory into guidelines for community health promotion. *American Journal of Health Promotion, 10*(4), 282–298.

U.S. Department of Health and Human Services. (November 2000). *Healthy People 2010: Understanding and improving health* (2nd ed.). Retrieved July 10, 2003, from http://www.healthypeople.gov/Publications.

Valanis, B. (1999). *Epidemiology in health care* (3rd ed.). Stamford, CT: Appleton & Lange.

World Health Organization. (1998). *Social determinants of health: The solid facts.* Retrieved July 10, 2003, from http://www.who.dk/InformationSources/Publications/Catalogue/20020808_2.

WEB SITE RESOURCES

There are many useful Web resources for health data. A few key sites are listed in this section. If you are unable to gain access to specific pages within a Web site, go to the main site and either follow the links or try to locate the information using the appropriate keywords in the search engine. The Centers for Disease Control and Prevention (CDC) Web site provides access to health data organized by the focus areas outlined in *Healthy People 2010.*

Health Canada: www.hc-sc.gc.ca
Centers for Disease Control and Prevention: www.cdc.gov
National Center for Health Statistics: www.cdc.gov/nchs/

Canadian provincial ministries of health or U.S. state departments of public health can be reached through the national Web site links.

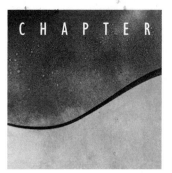

CHAPTER 4

Collaborative Assessment

ELIZABETH DIEM

PRENATAL AND POSTNATAL HEALTH

The Public Health Department in a city of almost 1 million people felt that it was time to review its prenatal and postnatal program. The staff realized from the statistics that services were reaching predominantly middle-income people. The profile of the people living in the city was also changing. Two groups were underserved by the programs: relatively poor women and immigrants from China.

Women and families living below the poverty line were located throughout the city in low-cost housing units and in relatively inexpensive apartments. One specific area, called Fairway, had a high percentage of families living in poverty. The great majority were English speaking. Many of the infants born in the area had a low birth weight, were not breast fed, and were often taken to the nearby emergency department for various illnesses and injuries.

The number of immigrants from Asia, with the largest portion from China, had recently outnumbered immigrants from all other areas including Europe. The Chinese immigrants spoke either Cantonese or Mandarin and were attracted by jobs in the high-technology sector or by family and friends living in the city. Most of the Cantonese immigrants lived in a 10-block area known as "Chinatown" that had numerous Chinese shops and restaurants. Those speaking Mandarin largely worked in the high-technology industry and lived in the suburban areas where the businesses were located.

The Public Health Department decided to offer two projects on prenatal and postnatal programming to nursing students for their community assessment placement through its Child-Bearing Families Program. The two project teams each had four students, a public health nurse who was the project leader, and a community health nurse instructor from the educational institution. The community placement was one day a week for 12 weeks.

The orientation of the students in the low-income and Chinese projects started with an explanation of the Public Health Department and then included a description of the project and the project team. After the first day, the students were uncertain of their roles and what they would be able to accomplish but felt that the project would come together as they learned more.

CHINESE PROJECT: The students working with the Chinese immigrants felt especially anxious about working with people who barely spoke English and had an entirely different culture. They were determined to obtain all the information they could from the rest of the project team. They booked a project team meeting every week for the first month and every two weeks after that. They kept asking questions about who could tell them more about the community and what methods had worked well in the past. At the meeting in the second week, they reviewed the original assessment goal of "assess the prenatal and postnatal needs of Chinese women." The team decided to change the goal to "assess the prenatal and *postnatal health of Cantonese women living in Chinatown and Mandarin women living in the high-technology suburb." The new goal was more specific about the community group and allowed an assessment of strengths and assets as well as needs. At the end of the second meeting, they had five people on their contact list.*

LOW-INCOME PROJECT: *The students working with the low-income women in Fairway felt that their job would be somewhat easier than that of the other student group because the women spoke English. They decided that they really wanted to learn how to conduct focused discussions. They felt that they had some preparation because one member of the team had previously worked with street youth and another had worked for a summer doing door-to-door interviews for a research project. They decided that they did not need to meet with the project team right away after the orientation and were not sure when they would meet with them. Some began reviewing secondary census tract data on Fairway, and others looked for more information on focused discussions.*

BOTH TEAMS: *At the same time as they were planning their specific assessment, the teams sought and reviewed the secondary data on prenatal and postnatal health (step 2 in the assessment) and the use of local services. The information reviewed appears in Application 4-1.*

OBJECTIVES   **After reading this chapter and answering the questions throughout the chapter, you should be able to**

1. Collaboratively plan and collect primary assessment data from the community group within timelines.
2. Determine the assessment methods that are appropriate for the community group and situation.
3. Consider the implications for teams during assessment.
4. Document and communicate the assessment plan and the data collected.

KEYWORDS   **community mapping** ▪ **community meetings** ▪ **focused discussions** ▪ **key informants** ▪ **planning the assessment** ▪ **primary sources** ▪ **progressive inquiry** ▪ **questionnaires** ▪ **sustainability**

Collaborating with the community: Planning the assessment

People in the community are the first and main source of your data. As **primary sources,** they are also your actual or potential partners on the project. The purpose of **planning the assessment** is to identify with them core themes or issues that elicit their social and emotional involvement (Minkler & Wallerstein, 1997). The community health nursing process is used to reach the full range of people in the community group, not just those who are vocal.

The active involvement of the people in the community is important not only to encourage **sustainability** to ensure that the project will be viable and continuing but also to increase the community's capacity for the project. When you approach people with a "listen to learn" attitude and are prepared to start where the people are (Nyswander, 1956), they are reassured that their views and involvement are important. The purpose of the assessment is to obtain information from a variety of sources to define the present health situation of a community group and the preferred health situation. The present situation includes barriers to health and strengths, such as resources that are available and previous experiences working on issues.

In this book, collaborative assessment in the community health nursing process is presented in steps that build on each other. In step 1 in Chapter 3, the preparation for assessment includes an orientation to the assessment project and project organizers and a review of the issues, population, and situation. The secondary data collection methods identified in step 2 in Chapter 3 could be used before or have some overlap with step 3, which is to initiate community assessment, as identified in the first part of this chapter. Once steps 1 and 2 have been fairly well completed, steps 3 and 4 can follow. The organizers, team, and community members need to consider and use specific assessment methods. Step 5 is provided in Chapter 5 and covers working with the community group to determine draft action statements.

Project teams have various options open to them in working with community groups to collect primary data. If the project team has 100 to 120 hours spread over several weeks and easy access to a community group, teams of two to four can complete the general assessment of the community and setting and conduct a specific assessment using one or two specific assessment methods. For projects with fewer hours, more compressed time, or fewer people other options are available. The priority should be given to methods that foster a good exchange of ideas between the project team members and the community group.

Some suggestions are to

1. Use the full process, but reduce the time spent according to the suggestions given with each method.
2. Include only key informant interviews and one of the specific assessment methods.
3. Use progressive inquiry with people in the community to identify their major issues, their ability to communicate, and their comfort speaking in public.

From that information, determine which would be more appropriate: focused discussions or a type of **questionnaire** (a data gathering device composed of a variety of questions). Questionnaires would need to be quite short or revised from previous work on the same issue or with a similar community group.

The amount of time required for the assessment with community groups also depends on the number of members and characteristics of the community group and the previous preparation done by the project organizers. The process for the assessment is based on nursing students or new practitioners working with an experienced leader, such as a community nursing instructor or a community health nurse, on a project team. Project teams or individuals who start at different points in the community health nursing process—such as planning, discussed in Chapter 6—can use the information in this chapter to determine the quality of the data they have been given to plan their project.

Using the assessment timeline and workplan

The assessment timeline and workplan (Appendix C) serve as a guide for the community health nursing process. The timeline shows when an activity starts and is expected to end. The workplan documents the activities and summarizes the results.

Planning the steps of the assessment project is crucial to ensuring success. Projects in the community often must change to take advantage of new opportunities or to deal with a series of problems or barriers. Changes are much easier to accommodate without losing sight of the assessment goal when a plan is in place.

Planning begins with step 1 as discussed in Chapter 3. During the substep to define the project (step 1c), the project team needs to plot out approximate times for all the steps and substeps in the assessment timeline. Although some adjustments may be necessary as the assessment progresses, the team is expected to use the times to determine their activities each week.

The timelines need to be considered in terms of the assessment goal. An assessment goal might be to conduct a thorough literature search in collaboration with a community organization, as exemplified in the scenario in Chapter 3. In that case, most of the time will be spent on completing step 2. In contrast, projects that involve both secondary and primary data will have limited time (see Table 4-1) to spend on secondary data. The emphasis for those projects is to find the most recent, relevant source for each type of data in a short time period.

This chapter addresses steps 3 and 4 in the assessment workplan. The following list provides the substeps to steps 3 and 4.

Step 3. Initiate assessment of the community
  a. Observe and map (if geographical) the community, setting, and/or resources.
  b. Interview key informants (individuals or groups who know the community and/or who have information on the issue of interest at the beginning of a project).

Step 4. Conduct the specific assessment
  a. Determine specific assessment methods from progressive inquiry, community/group meetings, focused discussions, and questionnaires.
  b. Plan and use the first selected assessment method.
  c. Plan and use the second selected assessment method.
  d. (Plan and use another assessment method as needed.)

Steps 3 and 4 build on each other to ensure that there is adequate knowledge about the community and the issue before the specific assessment is conducted. The approximate relationship of the steps and substeps to complete the assessment is displayed in Table 4-1 using the example of an assessment project of 90–100 hours over 12 weeks. The shaded weeks in Table 4-1 indicate when most of the activities of a step and related substeps are expected to occur. Teams can use Table 4-1 as a guide to plot their own timelines for their projects.

Criteria for selecting assessment methods

Teams working in the community need to have some understanding of the community group that they will be working with before they can decide which assessment methods are appropriate and in which order they should be used. For example, methods that assist in the development of a relationship with members of the community are important to use before those that convey a professionally driven agenda. Specifically, many community groups that are somewhat isolated from society, such as those who do not speak the

TABLE 4-1 Timelines for Assessment of Primary Data

STEPS IN PROCESS*	WEEK OR NUMBER OF CLINICAL DAYS (90–100 HOURS)											
	1	2	3	4	5	6	7	8	9	10	11	12
1. Establish relationships within project and community	■	■	■									
a. Establish relationship and responsibilities with project organizers	■	■										
b. Meet community contact(s)	■											
c. Define project, population, issue	■	■	■									
2. Assess secondary data	■	■	■	■								
a. Review national and local policy documents	■	■	■	■								
b. Review sociodemographic data	■	■	■	■								
c. Review epidemiological data	■	■	■	■								
d. Review previous community surveys and program statistics	■	■	■	■								
e. Review literature and best practice guidelines	■	■	■	■								
f. Summarize secondary data	■	■	■	■								
3. Initiate assessment of community	■	■	■	■								
a. Observe and map area, setting, or resources	■	■	■	■	■							
b. Interview key informants	■	■	■									
4. Conduct specific assessment						■	■	■	■			
a. Determine specific assessment methods						■	■	■	■	■	■	
b. Plan and use first selected method							■	■	■			
c. Plan and use second selected method								■	■	■		
d. Plan and use additional methods (as needed)									■	■		
5. Determine action statements										■	■	■
a. Analyze data and prepare presentation on findings, issues, and possible action statements										■	■	
b. Validate findings and devise 3 action statements with community members and stakeholders											■	■
c. Prepare assessment report											■	■
6. Evaluate teamwork	■		■								■	■

*Steps 1 and 2 appear in previous chapters; steps 5 and 6 appear in subsequent chapters.

BOX 4-1	Criteria used to select assessment methods for specific community groups

1. Does the method assist in building relationships?
2. Does the method accommodate people who have difficulty with communication?
3. Does the method accommodate people who have discomfort speaking in public (or a group)?
4. How much advance planning is required to appropriately use the method?
5. Does the method provide numbers?

dominant language or whose mobility is reduced, could feel threatened if they are asked to complete a questionnaire before they know who is asking the questions and why the questions are being asked. Providing appropriate information so that people can make an informed decision on whether or not to participate is a part of ethical practice for all nurses (Canadian Nurses Association, 2002). Establishing a relationship first also increases the chances of asking the right questions of the right people at the right time and location, using the right approach.

Five criteria for selecting assessment methods are given in Box 4-1. These criteria take into account both the characteristics of the community and the purpose of the assessment.

Building relationships

Some assessment methods, such as key informant interviews, help initiate the building of relationships. Once relationships with community members have been initiated, those community members can assist in the selection of the more specific assessment methods by identifying the characteristics of the community group. For some projects involving a large number of people, further development of relationships is not expected. For smaller projects, especially with vulnerable people, methods that maintain a relationship are important.

Accommodating difficulty with communication

The team needs to determine whether the community group has difficulty with either verbal or written communication. For example, people speaking a language different from that used by the team will require assessment methods in which questions can be asked slowly and in which pictures can be included. People who have difficulty hearing or seeing also have difficulty with communication and would require the use of certain assessment methods. Often methods that build a relationship also accommodate communication difficulties.

Accommodating discomfort with speaking in public

Many people in the community are not comfortable speaking in public or may even rarely go out in public. These people range from those who are simply shy to those who have been isolated from other people for a variety of reasons. The assessment methods that accommodate shyness and isolation also need to foster a relationship or build on methods that have already initiated a relationship. The collaborative assessment used in this text emphasizes inclusive approaches to accommodate people who are normally not heard or who do not usually participate in community activities.

Time required for advance planning

Time is an important factor when selecting assessment methods. Some methods can be used quickly, whereas others require more preparation or must be preceded by methods that foster a relationship. To encourage efficient use of time in short-term projects, the two methods used to initiate assessment of the community—observation and mapping and key informant interviews—are expected to be used first and used in every assessment. The three methods that require the most time in preparation are focused discussions, structured questionnaires, and community forums. Allowing enough preparation time for these three methods is important to ensure that the results will be useful.

Requirements for numbers or statistics

In some assessments, you will need to obtain numbers to provide an argument for changing or implementing new programs or services. Numbers can be obtained through structured questionnaires that are written or answered by telephone or face-to-face. Those questionnaires, however, are most effective when either a relationship has been developed or the questionnaire assesses issues that interest the population. Because funds to encourage people to participate in surveys in small-scale projects are usually limited, their involvement in the assessment project or interest in the results will need to serve as the motivation for their participation.

Step 3: Initiate assessment of the community

Teams need to have an understanding of the community (geography, history, and methods of interaction) to determine how best to conduct a community health assessment. This is the team's introduction to the community and the community's introduction to the team. An important part of the introduction is for the team to work on **community mapping**. This involves getting a picture of the geography of the community, some sense of what it would be like to live there, and the resources that are available to the community. For the other part of the introduction, the team needs to talk to people who know or live in the community and have an interest in the project. The team will want to hear the stories about people and events in the community so they can both understand what is important to community members and consider how the team can work with the community to build on past successes. The key informants from the community can serve as the guides to understand how the community functions.

For this step in the workplan, community members, such as key informants, need to be included to ensure that a collaborative process has been initiated. When the step is completed in about three weeks, the feedback from the community on the important issues and approaches are summarized in the final column of the workplan.

Two basic methods are used to initiate the assessment of the community: 1) *observation and mapping of the area, setting, and/or resources* (community mapping) and 2) *key informant interviews*. Both provide pertinent information to assist in avoiding costly mistakes and building your relationship with the community group. Both also provide the basis for the selection of specific assessment methods and are therefore required for every assessment project. Because mapping is quicker to arrange, it is described first.

Observation and mapping of an area, setting, or resources

A systematic recording of observations provides an overview of the features and functioning of an area from the perspective of a specific group or issue. If the assessment project deals with a population living in a defined geographical area, you would be observing and mapping the geographical area. If the assessment project deals with an issue that concerns people in scattered areas, you would identify a setting where behavior related to the issue could be observed. If the issue deals with services for a particular community group living throughout a community, such as adults with a disability or those living with human immunodeficiency virus (HIV) infection or acquired immunodeficiency syndrome (AIDS), you would map the services and resources that are available for that group. The purpose of observation and mapping is to provide the team with the context for the project, the project organizers with a fresh view of the community and situation, and an initial set of possible issues or factors that affect the specific group. Features of observation and mapping:

- Is part of the beginning assessment for every assessment project
- Is conducted according to the specific type of mapping and the perspective of the community group needing services
- Is quickly arranged after the population and issue are determined
- Can begin as soon as a checklist is created and resources are obtained
- Is informal
- Helps to orient the team and indicates their interest in the community

Figure 4-1 shows an example of a community map relevant for families with children.

Process

A community survey can be used to describe the characteristics of an area. The survey can be obtained by car, by bus, or on foot. A survey obtained by motor vehicle is called a *windshield survey*. The team needs to first define the area on a map and determine which features are important and the symbols that will be used to indicate the features. The features must be particular to the people in the specific community group. For example, if you were working with disabled people, you would be looking for wheelchair accessibility. If you were working with mothers with toddlers, you would look for playgrounds. Both groups would be interested in reasonably priced groceries.

Enlarged street maps of the area are needed to record the data. Along with the features, general impressions of the conditions of buildings, roads, vehicles, people, and services are included. All symbols, such as those for churches, schools, grocery stores, transportation services, and recreation areas, are listed in a legend for the map. In comments to the symbols, consider how easy or difficult it would be for specific community members to use

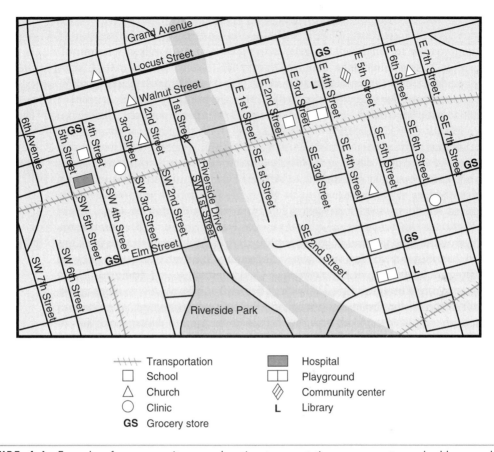

FIGURE 4-1. Example of a community map denoting transportation, grocery stores, healthcare, schools, churches, and other facilities.

the service. The availability of health services and products such as community health centers, physicians, dentists, public health nurses, hospitals, and pharmacies also needs to be included.

Along with the structures, mapping includes identifying the places where people gather. The team should also look for something in the area that they admire. This does not need to be a structure but could include observations about the cleanliness of the area, the number of people out walking, or the friendliness of people. This type of information is useful to discuss with the key informants. Systematic documentation of the information is a key part of the process. A checklist for the geographical assessment can be devised from a brainstorming session or other sources (Anderson & McFarlane, 2000, pp. 168–171) and can be used as a guide.

To continue with general impressions of a community, community observation includes interacting with members of the community in an informal way to determine how the community functions. View the interactions through the lens of a person in the specific group, for example, a mother with young children. Consider what that person would do if she were thinking of moving to the area. She would want to know where to shop, what the transportation service was like, and how safe the neighborhood was. Community observation is an attempt to find out what it is like to walk in the shoes of the people who are living in the situation.

For some projects, the team may need to observe the behavior of a particular group of people. For example, if you were interested in the smoking behavior of youth, the team would probably decide to spend time at a school or a popular shopping center. The time of day that would be most appropriate also needs to be considered. At shopping centers, for example, greater numbers of older people would probably be present during the day and greater numbers of younger people in the evening. Before starting, your team would make up a list of items related to the behavior. After spending time observing, team members will probably revise the list.

To map the services available for a particular group, such as people with a disability or people who do not speak the dominant language, the team needs to first determine whether there are local associations for the group and whether there is a listing of community services for the municipality or county that are relevant to them. By looking for information that has already been collected, the team will not recreate what already has been done, but can determine whether the information is current and can add more detailed information.

More specific observation is used to gain information about a particular group or situation with minimal disturbance of usual activity. Usually when you are new to a situation, you do not say a lot in the beginning because you are observing how people function. When you record those observations, you are taking field notes. In a new situation, such as in a classroom, at a manufacturing plant, or at a coalition meeting, your presence would be explained, and then normal activities would continue. If, for example, there have been traffic accidents at a school crossing or back injuries from lifting, you would want to observe the situation in those locations and record your findings. You may ask questions to clarify your understanding, but you would strive to be as unobtrusive as possible. Because you are new, your observations can provide a needed insight that may be missed by people who are familiar with the situation.

Time considerations

Community observation and mapping of a geographical area can start at the very preliminary stage, even before you meet with the project team. When time is short, first complete a windshield survey and then make decisions about what information is necessary and what is nice to know. Documenting the physical and social components can take months, days, or hours depending on the size of the area and the amount of detail required. The observations can be staged, moving from a broad overview to specific interactions within one setting or vice versa. A good use of time is to plot out the area on a map, expand and print the map to ensure that all important areas are covered and not duplicated, and distribute copies to team members. For observations of settings, choose easily accessible locations and a time and day of the week when the behavior will be most likely to occur. Since you only have one or two days to complete the observations, ask for advice on how to do this efficiently.

TABLE 4-2	*Illustration of Beginning of Step 3*

ASSESSMENT WORKPLAN   Revision date: *Sept. 21, 2004*

Title of Project: *Pre- and Postnatal Health of Cantonese and Mandarin Speaking Women*

STEPS, SUBSTEPS AND ACTIVITIES (LIST ACTIVITIES UNDER SUBSTEPS, NUMBER AND DATE ACTIVITIES ACROSS COLUMNS	SUMMARY OF RESULTS WITH DATES
1.	
2.	
3. Initiate assessment of community *Sept. 21–Oct. 5*	
a. Observe and map area (if geographical), setting, or resources 1) Preliminary view of community, Sept. 7 2) Plan mapping of Chinatown, Sept. 14 3) Conduct mapping, Sept. 21 4) Compile map, Sept. 28	1) *Chinese church frequented by mothers with infants.* 2) *Determined where to obtain maps and divided up area for next week. Features to look for: areas used by mothers with infants, grocery stores, clinics, pharmacy, playgrounds, laundry.* 3) *Used checklist to identify features and locations.*
b. Interview key informants.	

PRENATAL AND POSTNATAL HEALTH SCENARIO (continued)

CHINESE PROJECT: *After their orientation meeting, the students working with the Chinese communities went as a group to see where the Cantonese people lived in Chinatown. Sidewalks overflowed with people and produce. A Chinese church in the area had many cars in the parking lot, and several women with young children were going in and out. The small stores, restaurants, and the three laundromats were quite busy. After their initial visit, the students prepared a list of features and services that they wanted to check. They obtained enlarged street maps of the area and divided the maps among the team members. Two weeks later they attended an event at the church to observe how people interacted and were introduced to the two community key informants. They showed the two women the community map that they had put together. The women were very excited by the map and called others over to look at it because they could pick out familiar places by the symbols. They seemed really pleased that the students took such an interest in their community. In the discussion about the project and the map, the students learned that the church had an English as a second language (ESL) class that consisted almost entirely of young women who spoke Cantonese and Mandarin.*

Table 4-2 illustrates how the information from the three weeks of working on mapping would be recorded in the assessment workplan. Note that the date is not repeated in the summary column because the activity was completed on the planned date.

LOW-INCOME PROJECT: *The students working with low-income women took a bus to look at the Fairway area. Several high-rise apartment buildings crowded each other and litter was blowing around. They were surprised to find a busy and attractive playground for young children. Several young women were sitting on the benches watching their children. A sign beside the playground stated that the playground had been completed that year by the tenant association.*

DISCUSSION QUESTIONS

1. What features would be important for prenatal Cantonese women, and what symbols could be used on a map to depict them?
2. What assets or strengths of the Chinese and low-income communities were apparent from the community observation and mapping?
3. What opportunities might be available to meet with young women in Fairway?

Key informant interviews

Key informant interviews are short, semistructured discussions with individuals or groups who know the community and/or have information on the issue at the beginning of the project. The purpose of the key informant interviews is for the team to learn more about the community and the issues. If the community and issue have already been defined, the key informant interviews can be more specific and include questions about assessment methods and the effectiveness of using different approaches. Although these same people or others who they have identified may continue to be involved in the project, at later stages the type of information they provide will be different. Features of key informant interviews:

- Are part of the beginning of every assessment.
- Are conducted individually or with an established group.
- Are quickly arranged either with an individual or by being put on the agenda of a group meeting.
- Can begin as soon as people are identified and questions are determined.
- Are informal with a person, but more formal with a group.
- Can be conducted in person, by phone, or by e-mail.
- Initiate relationship building.
- Provide the means to recruit people as collaborators or advisors.

Process

Key informants are identified through a widening network, beginning with people or groups mentioned by the project organizers and community contacts, and then expanded by the people who are mentioned in those interviews. The project organizers and community contacts can greatly assist the team by identifying the initial people for the key informant interviews and hopefully informing them that they will be contacted by the team members. This preparation of the key informants will assist the team in the preliminary stages and increase their confidence in initiating contact with others that they learn about.

Some key informants will have formal positions and responsibilities relevant to the community or issue; others will have an informal leadership role or have particular knowledge of the community or of the issue and have different perspectives. Both need to be interviewed in person or on the phone before plans are confirmed.

For example, if the project was dealing with vulnerable seniors living in a certain area, the formal key informants could be the people on a seniors' council or association, church leaders, and the home health nurses working in the area. The informal key informants could be an elderly man or woman who has lived in the area for years and is known by everyone. Key informants with particular knowledge of seniors in the area would include people working in the corner stores, pharmacists, and postmen. The questions for each type of key informant group would vary according to the type of knowledge that they would be expected to have and whether they are likely to become collaborators. In this situation, the formal and informal key informants would probably be considered as potential collaborators in the project.

When meeting each time with the project organizers and community contacts, the team needs to ask who should be contacted for key informant interviews and follow through with the advice. By using this approach, the team can feel assured that the most prominent informants will be included. The project contact list provided in Chapter 3 will assist the team in keeping track of key informants.

Key informant interviews provide recognition for the people and groups who already have some involvement with the community and issue and can either bring them "on board" or support the efforts that have already been started. If a person or group has been active in the area of the assessment project and is missed in the key informant interviews, they can create difficulties that could have been avoided.

Meeting or talking with certain individuals in the community requires some advance preparation to determine a mutually appropriate time and method of contact. These arrangements are necessary so people will have time available even if the team has not yet prepared the questions that they will ask. Once some arrangements have been made, the next priority is for the team to determine what questions will be asked and the means (telephone, face-to-face, email, or group presentation) that are available to them. Develop the questions and script and ask pertinent people to review it and the format for collecting the responses before you start. By practicing the interview with each other or the project organizers beforehand, the team members are likely to feel more relaxed when they actually conduct the interview.

Either when setting up the appointment or at the beginning of the interview, the team must indicate the purpose of the interview and how the information will be used. The team will then want to obtain some idea of what the person thinks generally about the community and issue. For example, the team can ask how the community has come together in the past, and the people and issues that brought them together. Questionnaires that begin "What do you think about _____ community" or "What do you think about _____ issue?" can provide a considerable amount of information. Further questions can become more specific, based on the initial response. If the community and issues have already been clearly defined or if the key informant is in a formal position with responsibilities related to the community or issue, the interview can also include questions that are more specific, such as how, when, and where to conduct the specific assessment. The key informant interviews need to include a question for identifying who else to contact for information on the community. The team should also ask whether the key informants would be able to provide some further assistance on certain areas of the assessment or whether they could be called again in the future. The same questions can be presented at a group meeting.

When approaching people, team members need to indicate that they are in the assessment phase and are open to advice from a variety of people. Adopt a "listen to learn" approach. Team members should finish the interview by thanking the participants for their information and time.

To collect relevant data from the community in a systematic way, the team needs to talk to the right community people and ask them the appropriate questions. If insufficient time is allowed for preparation, interviews, or presentations to groups, the quality or quantity of the data and the relationship with participants can be compromised.

Time considerations

Key informant interviews should begin after you have spent a few days with the project team and have met the community contacts. When time is short, the number of people interviewed could be reduced by setting up a priority list and ranking people according to how many people identified each person as important to the overall project. Team members should then start contacting and setting up meetings with those at the top of the list if they are available within a prescribed time period. Face-to-face meetings are preferable, but interviews by phone or through email are also possible. After a few people have been contacted, the team should review and readjust the priority list based on the information received. Continue contacting the remaining and newly identified people by phone or in person if they are available within the time you have.

PRENATAL AND POSTNATAL HEALTH SCENARIO (continued)

CHINESE PROJECT: In the second week of working with the project organizers, the students working with the Chinese communities identified two key informants who they wanted to interview in the third week and drafted a list of questions for the key informant interviews. The project leader made some suggestions, and the questions were revised before the interviews.

The first key informant on their list was the multicultural worker from the Public Health Department. The second person was the director of an agency who worked with most of the multicultural groups in the city. The multicultural worker who worked with the Cantonese community agreed to meet them the next week. They had a difficult time getting in touch with the director and eventually talked to her assistant. The assistant suggested that they send the director an email requesting the information. When they sent the email, they received a prompt reply.

Table 4-3 illustrates how the information from step 3, both the mapping and the key informant interviews, would be recorded on the workplan once the step is completed.

LOW-INCOME PROJECT: The students working with the low-income women did not feel much further ahead at the third week. They had collected some census tract data and confirmed that Fairway had the third highest proportion of low-income families and single mothers in the city. Each of the team members had been talking to different people independently and getting mixed messages. The project leader introduced them to a public health nurse (PHN) who organized the prenatal classes in Fairway. They learned from her that several PHNs were visiting new mothers in Fairway.

DISCUSSION QUESTIONS

1. How much time would you expect to need to draft key informant interview questions, have them reviewed by a supervisor, and revise them again?
2. What did the Fairway team lose by not having scheduled regular meetings?

Step 4: Conduct the specific assessment

Up to this point in the assessment, the team has been collecting data from various available sources. The purpose has been to learn about the issues, the project, and the area in the initial steps of the assessment process to determine the following:

1. The issues that are important to the community
2. The people who need to be asked questions about the issues
3. How, when, and where to ask the questions
4. The features and resources of the community or setting
5. Possibly, the community members willing to work with the team in collecting the information

TABLE 4-3	The Completed Step 3 in the Assessment Workplan

ASSESSMENT WORKPLAN   Revision date: *Oct. 5, 2004*

Title of Project: *Pre- and Postnatal Health of Cantonese and Mandarin Speaking Women*

STEPS, SUBSTEPS and ACTIVITIES (list activities under substeps, number and date activities across columns)	Summary of results with dates
1.	
2.	
3. Initiate assessment of community *Sept. 7–Oct. 5*	*Multicultural worker and Director identify child-bearing families as needing services. All helped identify major features of map. Have contacts within Cantonese community. Will meet people at high tech firm to explore assessment of Mandarin women.*

a. Observe and map area (if geographical), setting, or resources
    1) Preliminary view of community, Sept. 7
    2) Plan mapping of Chinatown, Sept. 14
    3) Conduct mapping, Sept. 21
    4) Compile map, Sept. 28
	1) Chinese church frequented by mothers with infants.
	2) Determined where to obtain maps and divided up area for next week. Features to look for: areas used by mothers with infants, grocery stores, clinics, pharmacies, playgrounds, laundries.
	3) Used checklist to identify features and locations.
	4) Symbols used to indicate resources on map. Many resources within walking distance. No play areas. Church remains most active center for mothers.

b. Interview key informants
    1) Interview with multicultural worker, Sheila and Lee, Sept. 21
    2) Interview with Director of Multicultural Association, Jan and Jeff, Sept. 21
	1) Very interested and willing to be involved.
	—Worked for 14 years with community.
	—Most recent immigrants are younger, are having more children, and have the most difficulties.
	—Two older Chinese women identified as contacts.
	—Event next week at a community church where she would introduce us to the women and the community leaders.
	2) Sept. 28. Unable to contact by phone. Sent email. Response to email: many of the Mandarin immigrants are young and had just recently arrived. They work for a large high technology firm in the city. See contact list for names of people within the firm.

The initial three steps are very important in ensuring that you will be able to collect information that is important to the community.

Once the team has gained some understanding of the project, issue, and community, the project working group, and hopefully some people from the community, are ready to determine how to collect the specific information from the people directly involved in the situation. Different specific assessment methods are available: progressive inquiry, community meetings, focused discussions, and questionnaires. The project team must decide which method or methods will work the best with their particular community and could be completed in the time available. Although the methods are presented individually, they are interrelated and can build on the work done with previous methods. For example, progressive inquiry and/or community meetings are necessary before focused discussions or questionnaires are considered.

Although the methods used in the specific assessment may appear to be similar to those used in research, the specific methods described in this text are not research methods. The methods are used to define the present health situation and preferred health situation of a defined group in terms of program development or evaluation, not to generalize the results to others. Frequently, because of time constraints, only a small number of people who are readily available can be assessed, and the tools, such as questionnaires, are not tested for reliability or validity. Despite those limitations, the assessment provides useful information for planning services or resources relevant to some community members.

Throughout the collection of data, results are summarized in the final column of the workplan. The actual numbers, if more than 5, and the effectiveness of using each method are to be included. For difficult-to-reach community groups, it is particularly important to identify the methods that did not work as well as those that did.

Because the methods have different advantages and disadvantages, the best choice in a short-term comprehensive study would be to combine the methods. This is called *methodological triangulation* (Janesick, 1997).

Each method can cover the biases of another, but analyzing the results from all methods can be more difficult. When teams are working with "difficult to reach" community groups, the emphasis of the assessment may be more on including those who are the most isolated rather than obtaining information from a great number of people.

Once the methods are selected and recorded in step 4a, the timing for remaining steps must be reassessed in the assessment timeline. For example, if the decision is made to hold two focused discussions, the dates must be booked so that there is sufficient time to notify people and to analyze the data before the end of the assessment. When the dates for the focused discussions are determined, you work backward to create the due dates for when the focused discussion questions must be approved, pilot tested, and drafted.

In most cases, the work done in projects is small-scale program development or quality assurance, not research. However, community members must be made aware of who you are, of what you are planning to do with the information they provide, and of the fact that they have a right not to contribute. For the informal methods of progressive inquiry and community meetings, you and the assessment project can be introduced in the initial part of the encounter when meeting new people. For the more formal methods of focused discussions and questionnaires, prepare a short letter explaining who you are, who you are working with, why you are collecting the information, and how the information will be used in planning or evaluating programs. Before you ask people to participate, provide them with a copy of the letter. These actions are a necessary part of obtaining informed consent.

The next sections describe each method in detail. The assessment methods are presented from the quickest to arrange to the longest and from most supportive in developing relationships to least supportive.

Progressive inquiry

Progressive inquiry is an informal, systematic way for team members to collect and refine information from people on their present and preferred situations. It can be used in the same setting over time or in a variety of settings. Progressive inquiry follows a cycle from general to continually more specific questions on similar topics and attempts to clarify issues and reach the people who could be affected by the results. Only one to three simple questions would be used for each encounter so that people do not feel threatened. You want to identify their own and the community group's assets, strengths, and stories about doing things together (Kretzmann & McKnight, 1993). The purpose of progressive inquiry is to engage the same or similar community members in identifying issues that they would like to change. The issues are important for community members who would not normally have the opportunity or be willing to participate in the more formal assessment methods, such as questionnaires.

Progressive inquiry is similar to the meaning of Friere's (1972) dialogue: questioning and challenging the issues to identify a limiting situation that can be changed. The term *progressive inquiry* is used in postsecondary and computer-based learning in Scandinavian countries and is emerging in the same context in North America. In those situations, progressive inquiry is based on cognitive research in educational practices and the development of new knowledge based on the philosophy of science (Hakkarainen & Sintonen, 1999). Emphasis is on a systematic effort to advance shared knowledge (Muukkonen, Hakkarainen, & Lakkala, 1999). Although the application here is with people who are often unable or unwilling to participate in the usual assessment methods, the purpose of advancing shared knowledge is the same.

Progressive inquiry is "gentle" and sufficiently flexible to accommodate people's ability to respond to questions while using a systematic way of collecting and validating their information. Features of progressive inquiry:

- Is conducted individually or with people in small groups
- Can be quickly arranged
- Can begin as soon as questions and the approach are determined
- Is informal
- Is conducted face-to-face
- Promotes relationship building
- Accommodates people who have communication difficulties or would not speak in public
- Has a built-in validation feature that encourages the emergence of strongly felt concerns

Process

Before meeting with community members, team members decide on 1) one to three fairly simple questions that would help them to get to know the people and 2) how, when, and where people will be approached. Initially, start with questions that allow people to tell you their story about their experiences and the experiences of members of the community. You want to identify their own and the community group's assets, strengths, and stories about doing things together (Kretzmann & McKnight, 1993). As they learn to trust you, you can move into other areas such as their barriers to health and desired health.

Once decisions about the questions and approach are made, each team member individually follows the directions and asks the questions in a nonthreatening manner. A team member could approach people and ask the questions during normal conversation with one or more people in a place where they have already gathered. Team members record the responses they receive and the usefulness of the approach in field notes after the encounter has occurred. Other issues or items of interest may also be revealed during the discussion and are to be recorded as well.

After the cycle of questions is complete, the team meets to review and compare findings and determine the second cycle of questions and approach. At this point, the procedure for asking the questions may need to be changed. For example, if the community group has a very limited understanding of the language spoken by the team, the team may need to pretest the questions to be sure that the community members will be able to understand them. The cycles are repeated until the pertinent questions have been asked and most of the community members have been reached more than once, or people in a variety of settings are responding in the same way.

Progressive inquiry is a naturalistic approach that would develop from key informant interviews and participant observation. The approach promotes the development and maintenance of relationships. The method is particularly useful when communication is difficult, such as with people who are learning the language spoken by team members or those visually impaired, somewhat confused, or uncomfortable with formal procedures. Those people would be unlikely to participate in community meetings or surveys. The method has a distinct advantage over all other methods because the questions are not asked at just one point. When teams work with the same group of people, the questions become more specific and people have a chance to consider their responses between encounters. When teams work with different people in various settings, consistent topics can be identified.

Time considerations

When time is short, concentrate on asking different people the questions during each cycle of the inquiry and reduce the number of people or groups who are approached. Do not try to shorten the time taken to ask the questions and listen to the response. If you rush, community members will reduce the quality of their response and you may damage the relationship that you have built with them.

PRENATAL AND POSTNATAL HEALTH SCENARIO *(continued)*

CHINESE PROJECT: *During their interviews with Cantonese key informants and from their community observation, the students working with the Chinese community decided that their best opportunities for meeting with the community so far were the ESL class in the church and the contacts at the high-tech firm.*

They were not certain which methods they would eventually use, but felt that now they could eliminate a few. From their observations at the church event, they realized that most of the women would have difficulty speaking English and that fact ruled out focused discussions and phone interviews using a questionnaire.

They had obtained permission for two team members to spend as much time as they wanted in the ESL class. They considered using individual, face-to-face interviews there, but felt that they would get to know the women better by using progressive inquiry.

After their first time in the ESL class, the two students realized that the Chinese students' understanding of English varied greatly. For their second time in the classroom, the nursing students decided on one question about food that the teacher felt most of the students could understand. Both of the nursing students asked as many people in the class of 16 as they could about the food they liked to eat. After the class they compared their responses and found that they had talked to a total of 10 women and that most of them were interested in talking about the food they ate in their original country and the food they liked here. For the next week, the nursing students used two questions, augmented by pictures, on the use of healthcare services. Again the Chinese students talked about healthcare in China and healthcare here. The nursing students realized the importance of giving the Chinese students the opportunity to tell the story of their experiences. After being in the class five times, they had talked to everyone at least twice. They had kept very detailed field notes of the questions that they asked each week and the responses that they received. They felt very connected to the women in the class, and the women greeted them with smiles and nods whenever they went into the class. The other two students hoped to reach some Mandarin-speaking Chinese women through a meeting arranged at the high-tech firm.

LOW-INCOME PROJECT: The students working with low-income women found out that they would be able to go on a home visit with a public health nurse and attend well baby clinics in Fairway. They felt encouraged that they would be able to meet some of the women in Fairway, but were not certain about the best method to determine the area's strengths and needs. They called a project team meeting for the fourth week. At the meeting with the project team, they proposed developing a two-page questionnaire to use with the women at home and attending the clinics. However, during the discussion, they quickly realized that they would not have sufficient time to prepare the questionnaire, have the questionnaire reviewed, and pilot test it before the end of the placement. They went back to review the options open to them.

They decided that progressive inquiry was more appropriate to use in the home visit and well-baby clinic because of the time involved not only in developing the questionnaire but also in getting women to answer the questions. After determining two questions and asking them in the different situations, they found that the willingness of the women to respond varied. When one student asked a woman a question, the response was "Why do you want to know?" Another student found that she had a better response if she took time to talk to the woman first, before asking the questions. The students reconsidered how to approach the women. After they had been attending the well-baby clinic for three weeks and had adopted a new approach, they found that the attitude toward them was starting to change. They were being introduced to other women by women who they had already talked to, and the women were becoming more open in their responses.

DISCUSSION QUESTIONS

1. Chinese project: Explain how the key informant interviews and community observation helped determine the specific assessment methods and will help with the collection of the specific information.

2. Low-income project: Estimate how long it would take the students to prepare a two-page questionnaire, and how likely the women would be to fill out the two pages.

3. Consider why the students in the ESL classroom had a better response from the women than the students going on the home visits and attending the well baby clinics.

4. Do you feel that the women who were coming to the well baby clinic were the ones most at risk for poor prenatal and postnatal health? Explain.

Community meetings

Community meetings can take different forms depending on the purpose. A community forum, or town hall meeting, is held to obtain the views of as many people as possible. A more usual meeting is to obtain views of a group of people designated as important to the issue. This could involve joining a group that is already meeting or organizing a meeting of people who are interested in the issue. These types of meetings are called group meetings. Each type of meeting can provide valuable information in certain circumstances. Participants at meetings need to feel that their views were heard, something was accomplished, and future action will occur.

Group meetings

For some projects, a group with an interest in the issue may already be formed. The group could be a voluntary organization, coalition, or advisory board. In that situation, the team would seek a contact and opportunity to meet with the group in hopes of collaborating in the assessment.

In other situations, there may be considerable interest expressed in the issue, but those interested have not yet come together. For that situation, project organizers may suggest that the team brings people together either to obtain their views, support, and involvement in the assessment project if an issue has already been identified, or to determine an issue or focus for a project. The meetings can be the beginning of community development or coalition building. The people may be those living in a neighborhood or interested in the issue, representatives of organizations, or a combination of both. Organizing a meeting is necessary if neighborhood or community organizations and agencies have recognized the need to coordinate efforts on the project issue but have not yet formed a group. Features of group meetings:

- Are conducted with 4 to 20 people.
- Require one to four weeks to arrange, depending on the size of the group.
- Are semistructured or structured, depending on the number of people present and the purpose of the meeting.
- Allow decisions and plans to be made.
- Build relationships with organizations in the community or people who are comfortable speaking in public.

Process

A group meeting often evolves from key informant interviews when the team learns about other people or groups who would be interested in the assessment. If the people are not already meeting as a group, they can be invited verbally, on the phone, by email, or by written invitation. Be aware that people from some cultures and with certain personalities are not comfortable speaking in a group, especially a large group.

Meeting participants need to be included in planning the time, location, and points to be covered. The format for the meetings could vary but must include a listing of points and purpose and an opportunity for people to express their views. For a meeting with representatives from agencies and associations, an agenda can be developed from the outline in Appendix C.

At initial meetings, an open session to brainstorm the issues, approaches, and past experiences would be useful. In brainstorming, people are encouraged to contribute ideas that are listed on a flip chart without any discussion until everyone is finished or the time limit has been reached. Then a facilitator leads a discussion of the ideas and puts similar ideas together with the help of the participants. If more than eight people are present, they should work first in small groups to identify ideas. When the larger group is reconvened, the ideas can be discussed and grouped.

The initial meeting may be held simply to collect views and determine interest. If sufficient interest is not seen, further meetings will not be planned or attended. On the other hand, meetings can be the beginning of an ongoing relationship with the community. When a group is already meeting on a regular basis, the team needs to adapt to their schedule. If team members are not available when the group meets, possibly a few people from the group can be invited to join the team.

Comparison. In comparison to a community forum, the group meetings would involve fewer people and can move beyond a collection of viewpoints. In comparison to focused discussions, group meetings would probably occur more than once with the same people, and the format would involve determining views and making decisions.

Community forum

A community forum brings a large number of people together to exchange views. A forum is usually required when the community is concerned about an issue such as increased vandalism or an outbreak of head lice. Another use of a forum is to provide the community an opportunity to express their views on a proposed change in policy, such as a no-smoking bylaw. The purpose of a community forum is to provide the community with an opportunity to hear about an issue, express their views about an issue, or both. Community forums can indicate the number of people in a community who are willing to speak out on an issue and express their views. A community forum may have been the basis for developing an assessment project or could be a part of initiating action on specific issues. Forums involving a large community are unlikely to be part of small-scale projects unless they have already been organized by other groups. Features of community forums:

- Require a month of preplanning if there is no crisis.
- Are formal.
- Are held at a location able to accommodate many people.
- Are important when people are upset or want some action taken or when health professionals want the community's views on a particular issue.
- Contribute little to building relationships.
- Are likely to intimidate people with reduced communication abilities or difficulties speaking in public.
- Identify the number of people willing to voice concerns.

 Process. Community members are encouraged to attend the forum through notices, flyers, announcements, and word of mouth. A forum allows people to express their views, but the views will be of those people who are able to attend and are comfortable speaking in public. The purpose of the forum, which is to determine the community's views rather than determine action based on views, must be made clear when the team recruits for the forum and during the meeting. A forum that brings together people with differing views requires management and experienced leadership. When community members are frightened or angry, security measures need to be considered. Another consideration is to have someone prepared to deal with the media. This would include preparation of a fact sheet to ensure that accurate representation of the issue is reported.

An effective way of controlling the pace of the forum and ensuring that people are heard is to record key points in large type on flip charts or an overhead projector. People can see that their views are being acknowledged and note similarities and differences. More detailed notes should also be taken.

Comparison. A community forum can obtain the views of and provide information to a large number of people. In comparison to other community meetings, forums are much larger and are restricted to obtaining views and possibly identifying smaller working groups.

Time considerations

When time is short, each type of community meeting needs to be considered in terms of what it can provide in a limited time period. A group meeting is an effective and efficient use of time. Usually a minimum of two weeks is needed to organize a small meeting for people known to you, and a month is needed for a large meeting for comparative strangers. One way to reduce the amount of time needed is to organize the meeting to precede or follow an event that the people are already attending.

A community forum can be arranged quickly in response to a crisis situation. When there is no crisis, a community forum would probably take a month to organize.

PRENATAL AND POSTNATAL HEALTH SCENARIO (continued)

CHINESE PROJECT: *The two students working with the Chinese ESL students also maintained contact with the key informants that they had originally met at the church. The two English-speaking Chinese women had a sewing class in the church at the same time as the morning ESL class. The students met with the women at noon and discussed the issue of pre- and postnatal health. Soon others started joining them. They planned a community meeting to discuss the results at the end of the project.*

The two students working with the high-tech firm met with the manager of the personnel department, the occupational health nurse (OHN), and a Chinese woman who was on the firm's health and safety committee. At the start of the meeting, the students proposed that they would first describe their project and then open the meeting for discussion. The people from the firm agreed. After they explained their project and interest in finding out about factors related to pre- and postnatal health of Mandarin women, the OHN became very enthusiastic. She said that she had planned a women's health fair for employees and wives in two weeks, and the students could talk to the women then. They planned a meeting for the following week and exchanged email addresses so they could continue to plan during the week.

LOW-INCOME PROJECT: *The team working with the low-income women learned that a community forum had just been held because of vandalism in the area. A follow-up forum was being planned by the tenant association. They got the impression that few women would be interested in prenatal and postnatal meeting at that time.*

DISCUSSION QUESTIONS

1. How important is it to incorporate your issues into events or places where people naturally congregate?
2. When is a written agenda particularly important?

Focused discussions

Focused discussions use pretested questions to obtain people's views on a limited number of related issues. Focused discussions are most useful when you want to obtain extensive information on a particular topic from people who are knowledgeable and comfortable in expressing their views in a group. Focused discussions also provide an opportunity to recruit people interested in the project.

The term *focused discussion,* rather than focus group, is used because the format is less formal, it allows some flexibility in the questions that are asked, and people may come late or leave early. An example of a focus group is given in Application 4-2. The format in the example can be adapted to be used in situations where there is sufficient time to prepare and conduct a formal focus group.

The purpose of focused discussions is to obtain in-depth information about an issue from three to ten people who are knowledgeable about the issue. The participants need to be able to speak fairly well in the language of the team and to comfortably express their views in a group. Knowledgeable people can include program managers if you want discussion on motivating employees or teenagers if you want information about risk behaviors during adolescence. Features of focused discussions:

- Consist of meeting with groups of three to ten people for 30 to a maximum of 90 minutes. The more people, the more time is needed.
- Are structured by four to six open-ended, pretested questions.
- Can take two to four weeks to arrange and pretest questions.
- Are formal, with a moderator, recorder, and prepared material.
- Allow limited development of relationships.
- Are unable to accommodate reduced communication ability or difficulty speaking in public.

Process

The use of focused discussions necessitates advance planning to ensure that agency requirements are met and that the appropriate questions are asked of the correct people. First, the purpose of the discussions and the most appropriate participants need to be identified. Questions are then drafted from secondary data, key informant interviews, and participant observation and are reviewed by the project team. Revised questions are pilot tested by people who have characteristics similar to those of the expected participants. The organization may require that designated people, other than the contact person, review the questions. This extra review must be considered in the timelines. Once the questions are approved, a moderator's and recorder's guide must be prepared (see example in

Application 4-2) and the moderator/facilitator and recorder selected. A letter explaining the purpose of the focused discussion and the types of questions that will be asked needs to be prepared and reviewed. These measures are part of an ethical practice.

Comparison

The difference between a focused discussion and a focus group is that the former is more flexible and informal than the latter. In focused discussions, new questions or ideas can be explored as they arise. A disadvantage of shorter focused discussions can be that issues may not be discussed in great detail as they would be in a longer, more formal focus group.

In comparison to group meetings, focused discussions do not produce a conclusion or decision. However, the broader insight provided by focused discussions may help to raise the consciousness level of the community about the issue. Focused discussions should be avoided if participants have difficulty talking in a group or if the group includes a number of people who consistently dominate a conversation. If time permits, focused discussions can be used to develop the questions for a questionnaire and to assist with the analysis of the results.

Time considerations

When time is short (less than a month), some preparation work can be done by project organizers. They could draft questions and plan a focused discussion to follow another meeting that is already scheduled. The team members would then concentrate on rehearsing for the discussion.

When a committed time of at least 30 minutes is not available, the format can be changed to a meeting or one or two questions can be added to the agenda of other meetings. In these situations, more than 12 people may be present, and people could be coming in and leaving throughout the discussion. A meeting will not usually provide the time for an in-depth discussion, but a few specific questions can be answered efficiently. Otherwise, if sufficient time to prepare for focused discussions is not available, the discussions may be poorly attended or produce insufficient information.

PRENATAL AND POSTNATAL HEALTH SCENARIO (continued)

CHINESE PROJECT: *The students working with the two Chinese communities realized fairly early that focused discussions would not be appropriate. Many of the people in the community did not feel comfortable speaking English or speaking in a group.*

LOW-INCOME PROJECT: *The four students working with the low-income women organized two focused discussions with the PHNs working with mothers from the area. The PHN they had met during their third week of clinical placement suggested that nurses working in the Fairway area would probably be willing to meet with the students in three weeks (week six) because they all had a morning meeting. The discussions would be conducted by two students, each in separate rooms. The students checked with their project leader, who agreed that it was a good opportunity. Two rooms were booked and a list of 12 questions was prepared. The students felt ready when they went to their project meeting two weeks before the discussions.*

At the meeting the students learned that they had a lot more to do: The instructor pointed out that they had too many questions; they needed to pilot test the questions with at least a few PHNs before the discussions; and they needed to develop a moderator's and recorder's guide so a similar process would be used with each group. As part of the Public Health Department's procedures, they needed to prepare an information letter for the participants and have the questions approved by the project leader. They had hoped that the discussions could extend a half hour past the lunch time, but found that this extra time needed to have been approved by the manager at least a month before the event. They had to rush to prepare the needed information and to obtain approval from the project leader in time for the discussions. The following questions were approved:

1. How long have you been working with low-income mothers?
2. What factors limit low-income women from seeking or following pre- and postnatal health care?
3. What experience have you had or know about that could improve pre- and postnatal health?
4. What opportunities exist in the community or region that could benefit the health of pre- and postnatal women?
5. What ideas do you have about improving the pre- and postnatal health of mothers living in Fairway?

At the focused discussions, the students realized that the preparation time had been worthwhile. The participating nurses commented that the questions were very relevant, and they enjoyed discussing how things could be improved. The discussions also provided more ideas and opportunities to talk to women in Fairway.

DISCUSSION QUESTIONS

1. Why would the students want to have focused discussions rather than a meeting?
2. Why is the preparation and pilot testing of questions important for focused discussions?

Questionnaires

Questionnaires are a way to collect consistent information from individuals at different times and locations. In an assessment for a short-term project, the questions in a questionnaire need to be kept to a minimum, be clearly written, and be directly relevant to the development or evaluation of health programs. A review of draft questionnaires by the project team and a pilot test contributes to the clarity and relevance of the questions for the organization and community group.

Questionnaires developed to assess the present and preferred health situation of a specified group of community members are not the same as questionnaires used in research. Questionnaires used for health situations do not ask invasive questions but focus on determining people's interests and concerns related to the provision of services or resources. The KU Work Group (2002) uses the term 'concern survey' for this type of questionnaire. Features of questionnaires:

■ Are completed by interview or self-administered.
■ Are restricted to two pages or 15 minutes to complete.
■ Vary in preparation time according to the availability of previous questionnaires, number of questions, pilot test, and review process.
■ Can be structured or unstructured.
■ Distribution can be by email, mail, phone, or in person.
■ May be the only choice because of the need for quantitative data.
■ Able to accommodate people who have difficulty speaking in public.

Process

The first decision is to determine if questionnaires would have an advantage over other methods. Often the greatest advantage is that numbers derived from questionnaires are more readily accepted by decision-makers. You must first determine the purpose of the questionnaires and then consider the content. The purpose of using questionnaires in the community health nursing process is to identify assets and strengths along with needs. One of the disadvantages of questionnaires is that most types of questionnaires take time to prepare. Therefore, the decision about using questionnaires must be made quite early in the assessment process.

Type of questionnaire. Before questions are developed, a decision must be made about using an open-ended interview format or mainly structured, closed-ended questions. The interview format can only be used by one person at a time, face-to-face or on the telephone. The development and use of an interview would be similar to that of key informant interviews, which were described previously. These interviews differ from key informant interviews mainly in terms of the type of questions being asked. Key informant interviews focus on questions to orient the team generally; specific interviews focus on the details of the health situation. The remainder of this section will deal with structured questionnaires.

Structured, self-administered questionnaires can be delivered in a variety of ways. At the same time as the questions are being developed, the type of questionnaire needs to be determined so that specific people in the community can be reached.

Self-administered questionnaires are especially useful for large numbers of people who are comfortable reading, writing, and responding to questionnaires. Since questionnaires are impersonal, they may be most useful for programs dealing with sensitive issues such as sexual health programs and programs to reduce drinking and driving. The distribution of self-administered questionnaires needs to be considered to encourage a maximum return rate. In a community, questionnaires can be distributed and collected at a popular shopping mall or community event; or at work they can be distributed with pay checks. When there are few questions, encourage people to complete them immediately by providing tables, chairs and pencils. Otherwise, prizes, draws, and posters can be used to prompt people to return their questionnaires. Email is an inexpensive way to reach people if you have their email addresses. Within time and resources constraints, the criteria for the selection of the method is that it is the most convenient for the people you want to reach in the community.

Interviews in person or telephone interviews using a structured questionnaire provide an opportunity to include people who have difficulty reading and writing and need some explanation for the questions. Although fewer people will be reached with individual interviews than self-administered questionnaires, those people will likely have special needs that could not be determined any other way. However, because of past experiences in repressive countries or dealing with bureaucracy, some people are reluctant to respond to any structured questionnaires. In those cases, progressive inquiry would be more appropriate.

Cost is also a factor to consider in preparing the questionnaire. The unit cost and response rate are the lowest with self-administered questionnaires, increases with telephone surveys, and is the highest with face-to-face survey interviews (KU Work Group, 2002; The Health Communication Unit, 2000; Wass, 1999). Face-to-face interviews provide the opportunity to explore complex issues and accommodate difficulties with literacy.

Questionnaires can provide data that support a change in practice, but can be costly in terms of time and resources. To ensure a good return for the investment, sufficient time must be spent in developing and testing the questionnaires. The major part of your assessment project may be to pilot test questionnaires that you have developed. On the other hand, part of your assessment project may be to conduct a limited number of telephone or face-to-face interviews using a questionnaire developed by others. In both situations, you will gain valuable experience in learning how people think and respond to certain questions.

Developing questions. Questions in a collaborative assessment need to be developed with some community involvement. Preferably some people from the community group, or at least people who work closely with them, will be involved. Ideas for questions can come from issues identified in the secondary data, especially previous questionnaires, and from key informant interviews, progressive inquiry, meetings, or focused discussions. The development of appropriate questions to meet the purpose of the assessment takes considerable knowledge and experience. To shorten the preparation time, model the questionnaire on others that have been used with a similar community group or on the same issue. The KU Work Group (2000) provides indices on their site for developing properly worded items and examples of demographic questions. If there are no appropriate questionnaires available, a Web search can provide some useful prototypes.

The two main types of questions on a questionnaire are content questions and sociodemographic questions. Sociodemographic questions aid in the development of services. For example, questions on age, gender, family size, language, and transportation methods help define the community of interest. For the content questions, specific issues and strengths that were identified during preliminary assessment work need to be explored.

For the assessment project, restrict the length of questionnaires to two pages or a time limit of 15 minutes (KU Work Group, 2000). This will improve the response rate and reduce the amount of time needed to analyze the results. To achieve that length, each question must be weighed in terms of the information it will provide. For each question, ask "What will we do with this information?" If your response does not relate directly to the goal of the assessment, remove the question.

Another consideration related to response rate is the type of questions—open or closed ended or a mixture of both. Open-ended questions allow a variety of answers; closed-ended, multiple-choice questions restrict the number of responses. Not everyone will respond to the open-ended questions, but they are useful in identifying issues unknown to the team. People usually find it easier to respond verbally. After people have given their written responses, you might ask participants one or two open-ended questions that you record for them.

Questionnaires need to be pilot tested by people with similar characteristics. The pilot testing helps ensure that people understand the questions that are being asked. Most people have had experience with ambiguous multiple-choice questions on an examination. If ambiguous questions occur on a questionnaire, the responses to these questions will be of no use.

Organizations may require that questionnaires be reviewed by someone other than the contact person. Determine the procedure for the organization and the timeline. When preparing questionnaires, also prepare an information letter for the questionnaires.

Everyone asked to complete the questionnaires must be given an explanation and has the right to refuse to participate. These measures are part of an ethical practice.

Comparison

In comparison to focused discussions, self-administered questionnaires offer the possibility of obtaining information from a great number of people privately, as long as they can read and write and are motivated to respond. Face-to-face interviews are more comfortable for people who avoid groups or have difficulty with language. More formal assessment methods, such as focused discussions and questionnaires, tend to be avoided by people who feel disenfranchised.

In comparison to a questionnaire used in research the questions used in a health situation assessment are focused on identifying interests and services rather than on describing what people do or think. This means asking questions about interest in smoking cessation information or in a sports or activity program rather than asking about the number of cigarettes smoked or how much people watch TV.

Time considerations

In planning the use of questionnaires, consider their development, approval, distribution, and analysis. To reduce development time, work from questionnaires that have already been developed and tested. The use of revisions of previous questionnaires will also reduce approval time. Consider distributing the questionnaire in a location that allows for immediate completion and collection. Analysis is more straightforward with quantitative data (closed-ended, multiple-choice questionnaires) rather than qualitative data (open-ended interviews), although the latter are quicker to prepare.

PRENATAL AND POSTNATAL HEALTH SCENARIO (continued)

CHINESE PROJECT: *At first, the students working with the high-tech firm were quite excited about the opportunity to talk to the Mandarin women at the healthy women's fair—then they realized the amount of work that they would have to do in two weeks. They talked with the other team members who were working with the ESL students and came up with the following list of questions that they sent to the OHN:*

1. *Should we prepare close-ended written questionnaires or open-ended interview questions? We feel that closed would be better because our classmates find that many of the Mandarin women can understand written English better than spoken English.*
2. *Can we have the women complete the questionnaires while they are at the fair?*
3. *Do you have any questionnaires that you have used with this group in the past?*

The OHN agreed that written questionnaires would be the best choice. She wasn't certain about the women having enough time at the event to complete them there. She also had been revising a pre- and postnatal questionnaire that had been used at another firm. The project leader gave the students a questionnaire on pre- and postnatal care that had been used with multicultural groups the previous year.

At the meeting with the OHN and safety committee member, everyone went over the two short questionnaires and found a lot of similarities. The two students added two items that their teammates had found in their work with the ESL class. Otherwise, just minor changes were made to the multicultural questionnaire. The OHN took responsibility for typing up the revised questionnaire. The safety committee representative was responsible for conducting the pilot test with two women during the week. Revisions after the pilot testing would be by email. The two students were to prepare the information about the purpose of the questionnaire.

On the day of the health fair, the OHN, the project leader, and the student team were pleased with the final questionnaire. More than 20 Mandarin Chinese women attended the health fair and willingly took the questionnaires. However, only five questionnaires were completed by the end of the fair. The women said that they needed time to carefully read and answer the questionnaires. Everyone felt discouraged at first until the safety representative said that the women would return them by next week when they or their husbands came to work. The OHN and project leader announced that these questionnaires would be a pilot test for a large survey involving the high-tech firm and the Chinese Mandarin community.

DISCUSSION QUESTIONS

1. Would questionnaires have been possible within the timeframe without the two previous questionnaires? Support your answer.
2. What aspects of distributing questionnaires would need to be pilot tested if they were going out to more than a few people?

Summary of methods used in assessment

Throughout the presentation of various assessment methods, five criteria were used to match a method with a specific community group. The methods needed to

1. Build relationships
2. Accommodate difficulty with communication
3. Accommodate discomfort speaking in public (or a group)
4. Consider the amount of advance planning needed
5. Provide for recording required numbers and statistics

Table 4-4 provides a comparison of the various methods according to the five criteria.

Teamwork during the assessment

As teams work through the assessment steps using the community health nursing process, they are faced with certain challenges. Some are a result of the stage of group development; others result from the different tasks that are required during assessment. The aspects of the assessment that are relevant to team building are indicated during the orientation period and during the planning and conducting of the specific assessment.

Teamwork during orientation

All projects will include some time spent on orientation to the assessment project and to the project team. The team tasks at this stage are the same as those in the forming stage identified in Chapter 2:

1. Select an initial group leader.
2. Make decisions together.
3. Document and communicate the decisions.
4. Conduct initial individual and group reflection and evaluation.
5. Involve community members.

TABLE 4-4	Summary of Assessment Tools				
TOOL	**BUILD RELATIONSHIP**	**ACCOMMODATE DIFFICULTY IN COMMUNICATION**	**ACCOMMODATE DISCOMFORT SPEAKING IN PUBLIC**	**AMOUNT OF ADVANCE PLANNING**	**PROVIDES NUMBERS**
Area/setting/ resource observation and mapping	Contributes	N/A	N/A	0–2 weeks	N/A
Key informant interviews	Yes	Yes	Yes	1–2 weeks*	No
Progressive inquiry	Yes	Yes	Yes	1–2 weeks	Limited
Community meeting—group	Yes	No	No	2–4 weeks*	No
Questionnaire, individual, open-ended	Yes	Yes	Yes	2–4 weeks*	Limited
Focused discussion	Contributes	No	No	2–4 weeks*	No
Questionnaire— telephone	No	No	Yes	2–4 weeks*	Yes
Questionnaire— written Self-administered	No	No	Yes	2–4 weeks*	Yes
Community meeting—forum	Contribute	No	No	1 month unless a crisis*	Limited

*Time can be reduced by prior organizing and development.

Successful completion of several of the tasks is apparent in the work of the Chinese project team. That team seemed to be clearly working together because they scheduled weekly meetings and expressed a common concern about working with people from a different culture. Those actions indicate that they had a leader, made decisions together, could communicate concerns at the scheduled meetings, and had defined tasks such as collecting the names and contact information for key informants. They followed through with the contacts they had and involved people in the community. They need to evaluate and document their ability to collaborate with others in step 6 of the workplan.

In contrast, the low-income project team did not show any team direction because they did not schedule meetings, asked different questions of different people, and only showed an interested in conducting focused discussions. Even when they made a trip to Fairway, they lost an opportunity to talk to the women at the playground. Their team's initial lack of direction was costly for them, the project organizers, and the women in the community. At the beginning of projects, people who have been doing the preplanning are usually ready to put extra effort into orienting new people and offering assistance. If the assistance is not accepted, it is not offered again or as readily. The same is true in following up on subsequent offers of help. The team's lack of direction for three weeks indicated a need to review the team's functioning with the project leader. Their difficulties with collaborating need to be identified in step 6 of the workplan.

Although not apparent in the scenario, documentation and communication can be a problem initially. One thing that a team needs to work out is the relationship between the weekly summary and the assessment workplan. Think of the weekly summary as the minutes of your meeting or the charting you would do on a patient in an institution. You need to include the decisions that you made and why you made them. You then summarize that information and put it in your workplan. Anyone should be able to pick up your assessment workplan at any time and be able to tell what you have done and what you are planning to do. Your workplan is also invaluable to people who want to carry on with your work without repeating the problems you encountered.

Teamwork while planning and conducting specific assessments

Once the team has completed the orientation to the project, issue, population, and community, they have been together long enough to have faced some differences of opinion and hopefully have found ways to resolve their differences and move into performing (see Chapter 2 for a discussion of storming, norming, and performing) in relation to leadership, group decision making, and documentation and communication. They also need to maintain or expand community involvement and conduct a team evaluation of roles and functions.

At the midpoint of the time available for the assessment, the team is encouraged to take time to review and evaluate their team and the team agreement (Appendix C). The review must also include each person's feelings about the team's support for each member and each member's support of the team. Often items such as leadership, communication, and task allocation have become issues and need to be resolved through a conflict resolution process described in Chapter 2.

Often during specific assessment, team members work separately to complete all the tasks. This requires that greater attention be paid to documentation and communication by all members. At meetings when tasks are allocated, names and deadlines are given in the weekly summary. The responsible members are expected to complete the task by the due date or propose an alternative if they are having difficulty completing the task. Members' difficulties in fulfilling obligations must be dealt with first at the team level. This discussion could help the team deal with their differences. If issues cannot be resolved within the team, the team must decide how to seek a resolution. The rule is that issues do not go away if ignored; they ferment and explode when there is little time to deal with them. Difficulties occur in every team. What distinguishes successful teams from unsuccessful ones is the ability of team members to quickly use a fair and considerate approach to deal with difficulties.

Another challenge when members work separately is that they may be led in other directions because of the interests of the community people who they are encountering. For example, a community member may see the project as a means to promote his or her own issue, such as reducing violence against women or getting a traffic light on a busy street. These issues are difficult to ignore, especially when you want the person to work with you. You may find it helpful to include a statement in your team agreement that requests from the community will be dealt with by 1) listening carefully and recording the request, 2) stating that the request will be taken back to the team and the person will be informed of the result, and 3) cautioning the community member that you have a limited time to accomplish your assessment project and need to consider each activity carefully. Although the request may not directly relate to your project, it may provide a way to meet with the community that may not otherwise have been available. Weigh the request in terms of time and possible contribution to the project.

The teams in the scenario began working differently once planning was completed. The Chinese project team obviously went through a change in leadership because two subteams were formed. One worked mainly with the Chinese women at the church, while the other worked with the high-tech firm. This could have resulted in two separate projects, but that did not happen because the students with the high-tech firm used information from their teammates in their questionnaire.

The Chinese project team members expanded their group to include more women from the community at the church location and one woman from the Chinese community at the high-tech firm. Because of the direct involvement of the community members, these students had an opportunity to appreciate the lives of these women and adapt their approach accordingly. The community women learned to work with others on identifying issues and organizing an assessment.

The low-income project members turned things around quickly after the fourth week. Presumably they evaluated and made changes in their leadership, decision making, and task allocation after going through a conflict resolution process or evaluating the team. Their ability to organize the focused discussions in a short period of time and change their approach to the women in the well baby clinic indicated that they could now work together and adapt. Although low-income women did not become involved in the direction of the project, the students did learn the value of "listening to learn."

Summary

Collaborative assessment involves working directly with the people in the community group to determine their issues, strengths, assets, barriers to health, and desired health. Collaborative assessment also relies on planning of the assessment by selecting assessment methods that foster a good exchange of ideas between the project team members and the community group. These methods should be useful for building relationships, accommodating difficulty with communication (e.g., language and public speaking), providing enough preparation time to process the assessment for the most useful results, and recording supportive statistical data.

Among effective assessment methods are community mapping, key informant interviews, progressive inquiry, community meetings and forums to exchange viewpoints and discuss issues, focused discussion, and questionnaires. Of course, a useful and effective community health nursing assessment requires a high a degree of teamwork. Team members need to be able to deal with challenges that arise as groups develop and tasks accumulate. Among team challenges are selection of group leaders; decision making as a team; documentation, communication and evaluation of decisions; and continuous involvement of the community.

PRACTICE AND APPLICATION

1. In the prenatal scenario, use the information provided on the team working with women speaking Chinese to create what you would imagine would be in
   a) The weekly summary (Appendix C) at week five
   b) Items 3 and 4 in the Assessment workplan (Appendix C)

2. Using information from the scenario, prepare a table to compare the assessment methods and results in terms of numbers of participants and relationship for each team. Present and compare your findings to those of others.

3. Imagine that the team working with low-income women in the scenario decides to review their team roles and process after the assessment project meeting in week four. Using methods in Chapter 2, identify actions that they could have done differently and actions that they could do in the remaining weeks to improve their progress.

4. Use the focused discussion example in Application 4-2 to
   a) Conduct a focused discussion with 4 to 12 people including a moderator and recorder
   b) Discuss the preparation and skills that are needed by the moderator and recorder
   c) Compare the use of focused discussions to other specific methods

5. Determine which assessment methods would be most appropriate to engage the highest number of participants and promote a relationship for the following community groups or issues:
   a) Workers in a small manufacturing plant
   b) Reducing smoking initiation in teens
   c) Seniors' drop-in center

REFERENCES

Anderson, E., & McFarlane, J. (2000). *Community as partner* (3rd ed.). Philadelphia: Lippincott.

Canada Perinatal Surveillance System. (2003). *Maternity experiences survey*. Retrieved July 21, 2003, from http://www.hc-sc.gc.ca/pphb-dgspsp/rhs-ssg/mes-eem_e.html.

Freire, P. (1972). *Pedagogy of the oppressed*. New York: Herder and Herder.

Hakkarainen, J., & Sintonen, M. (1999, September). Interrogative model of inquiry and computer-supported collaborative learning. Paper presented at the Fifth International History, Philosophy, and Science Teaching Conference, Como-Pavia, Italy.

The Health Communication Unit. (2000). *Conducting surveys: workshop material*. Toronto, ON: University of Toronto, Centre for Health Promotion.

Janesick, V. (1997). The dance of qualitative research design. In N. Denzin & Y. Lincoln (Eds.), *Handbook of qualitative research* (pp. 209–219). Thousand Oaks, CA: Sage.

Kretzmann, J., & McKnight, J. (1993). *Building communities from the inside out*. Chicago: ACTA Publications.

KU Work Group on Health Promotion and Community Development. (2000). *Conducting concerns surveys*. Lawrence, KS: University of Kansas. Retrieved July 21, 2003, from http://ctb.lsi.ukans.edu/tools/EN/sub_section_main_1045.htm.

Minkler, M., & Wallerstein, N. (1997). Improving health through community organizing and building. In M. Minkler (Ed.), *Community organizing and community building for health*. New Brunswick, NJ: Rutgers University Press.

Muukkonen, H., Hakkarainen, K., & Lakkala, M. (1999). Collaborative technology for facilitating progressive inquiry: Future learning environment tools. In C. Hoadley & J. Roschelle (Eds.), *Proceedings of the Computer Support for Collaborative Learning (CSCL) 1999 Conference, Dec. 12–15*, Stanford University, Palo Alto, CA.

Nyswander, D. (1956). Education for health: Some principles and their application. *California's Health, 14*, 69–70.

Wass, A. (1999). Assessing the community. In J. Hitchcock, P. Schubert, & S. Thomas (Eds.), *Community health nursing*. Albany, NY: Delmar.

WEB SITE RESOURCES

General assessment methods

The Health Communication Unit. (2002). *Information and resources*. University of Toronto, Centre for Health Promotion. Retrieved July 21, 2003, from http://www.thcu.ca/infoandresources.htm.

KU Work Group on Health Promotion and Community Development. (2000). *Community tool box*. Lawrence, KS: University of Kansas. Retrieved July 21, 2003, from http://ctb.lsi.ukans.edu.

Focus groups

KU Work Group on Health Promotion and Community Development. (2002). *Conducting focus groups*. Lawrence, KS: University of Kansas. Retrieved July 21, 2003, from http://ctb.ku.edu/tools/en/section_1018.htm.

National Center for Chronic Disease Prevention and Health Promotion. *Using focus groups to gain an understanding of living with diabetes in various communities*. Retrieved July 21, 2003, from http://www.cdc.gov/diabetes/pubs/focus/step1.htm. (This site is applicable to other situations, and provides cultural perspective.)

Questionnaires and surveys

Centers for Disease Control and Prevention: http://www.cdc.gov. On the site, search for "questionnaire," "survey," or a particular issue or population group.

The Health Communication Unit. (2002). *Information and resources*. University of Toronto, Centre for Health Promotion. Retrieved July 21, 2003, from http://www.thcu.ca/infoandresources.htm.

KU Work Group on Health Promotion and Community Development. (2000). *Conducting concerns surveys*. Lawrence, KS: University of Kansas. Retrieved July 21, 2003, from http://ctb.lsi.ukans.edu/tools/EN/sub_section_main_1045.htm.

Search strategy

To obtain information on the Internet about questionnaires or assessment methods, type the following into your search engine: "community questionnaire" or "community assessment." Other terms such as "community needs assessment," "community asset assessment," or "survey" can also be used, as well as terms such as "health promotion," "food," "exercise," "immunizations," and "childcare" along with "questionnaire" or "survey." See Chapter 1 on Web site resources to limit your search to reputable sites.

APPLICATION 4-1

ASSESS SECONDARY DATA (STEP 2) ON PRENATAL AND POSTNATAL HEALTH

2a. National Policy Documents

Investing in prenatal health and the first five years is good for children and the economy and must become a priority in order to reduce inequities between children living in different socioeconomic situations and support parents and families (Federal, Territorial, and Provincial Advisory Committee, FTPAC, 1999). Two groups were identified as at risk for poor perinatal outcomes: recent (within 5 years) immigrants and teenage mothers (Health Canada, 2003b).

Local policy documents: Health Department presently working on a document

2b. Sociodemographic Data

Poverty: The average birth weight of infants from the poorest urban areas is 120 grams or a quarter pound less than those born in the richest neighborhoods (Statistics Canada, 1999).

Low maternal educational level: Consistently related to poor perinatal health outcomes including preterm birth, small-for-gestational age, stillbirth, and infant mortality rates (Health Canada, 2003a). The outcomes are likely a result of intermediate variables such as maternal age, health care utilization, and the prevalence of risk behaviors such as maternal smoking (Health Canada, 2003a).

Immigration: Since 2000, the highest percentage of immigrants to the city is Asian, and highest percentage of Asians are those from China (reference, 2003)

Census tract data: The areas with the highest percentage of lone-parent families also had the highest percentage of low-income families.

TABLE 4-1A	Census Tract Data: Total Lone-Parent Families by Incidence for Selected Municipalities, 1986–1996*		
SPECIFICS	**% LONE PARENT FAMILIES**		
	1986	*1991*	*1996*
Region	13.1	13.7	15.6
City	16.5	17.6	19.7
Subdivision: Fairway	20.7	25.0	28.1
Lowertown (includes Chinatown)	16.0	18.0	22.4

*Fictional figures used to demonstrate type of information available.

2c. Epidemiology

Low birth weight: Associated with premature birth, or birth before 37 weeks, and growth retardation due to lack of nourishment in utero, pregnancy-induced hypertension and/or heavy smoking by the mother during pregnancy (Federal, Territorial, and Provincial Advisory Committee, FTPAC, 1999). Smoking a pack of cigarettes a day can lower birth weight by 150 to 200 grams or ⅓ pound (Statistics Canada, 1999).

Causes of growth retardation: Poor nutrition, pregnancy induced hypertension, and excessive smoking (Federal, Territorial, and Provincial Advisory Committee, FTPAC, 1999).

Poverty: The average birth weight of infants from the poorest urban areas is 120 grams or ¼ pound less than those born in the richest neighborhoods (Statistics Canada, 1999).

2d. Local Survey: No previous surveys completed

Program utilization figures

TABLE 4-1B — Attendance at Prenatal Classes by % of Total Births		
AREA OF CITY	**2002**	**2003**
North End	40%	35%
Middle Town	50%	50%
Lower East End	35%	40%
Fairview	20%	15%
Chinatown	10%	10%

2e. Literature Review: Factors associated with poor perinatal outcomes identified in government reports

Relevant best practice guidelines:
Registered Nurses of Ontario (2004):
Integrating smoking cessation into daily nursing practice
Breastfeeding best practice guidelines for nurses
Supporting and strengthening families through expected and unexpected life events

2f. Summary

Poor perinatal outcomes are associated with recent immigration, teenage pregnancy (Health Canada, 2003b), and poverty (Statistics Canada, 1999). Families living in Fairway have a higher percent (9%) of lone-parent and low-income families than the city and a low percent of attendance at prenatal classes. Newcomers from China living in Chinatown have a very low attendance at prenatal classes. Factors that need to be considered in the assessment are use of health services, smoking, nutrition, and educational level. Three best practice guidelines related to pre- and postnatal health are available.

REFERENCES

Registered Nurses of Ontario. (2004). Completed guidelines. Retrieved June 2, 2004, from http://www.rnao.org/bestpractices/completed_guidelines/bestPractice_firstCycle.asp.

Federal, Territorial, Provincial Advisory Committee, FTPAC. (1999). *Toward a healthy future: Second report on the health of Canadians.* Ottawa: Minister of Public Works and Government Services of Canada. Retrieved June 2, 2004, from: http://www.hc-sc.gc.ca/hppb/phdd/report/toward/index.html.

Health Canada (2003a). Canadian perinatal health report 2003. Retrieved June 2, 2004 from http://www.hc-sc.gc.ca/pphb-dgspsp/publicat/cphr-rspc03/index.html.

Health Canada (2003b). Maternity experiences survey-background. Retrieved June 2, 2004 from http://www.hc-sc.gc.ca/pphb-dgspsp/rhs-ssg/mes-eem_e.html.

Statistcis Canada (1999, winter). Health status of children. Health reports, 11, 25-34.
Retrieved June 1, 2004 from
http://www/statcan.ca/english/indepth/82-003/archive/1999/hrar1999011003s0a02.pdf.

APPLICATION 4-2

DEMONSTRATION OF A FOCUSED DISCUSSION

Focused Discussion on Factors to Reduce Smoking by Youth
Moderator's Guide

Thank you for agreeing to participate in this discussion. I would like you to introduce yourselves.

Statement of Purpose and Confidentiality (moderator reads this)

In community health nursing, focused discussions are one of the methods used to assess the community group's needs and interests. This experience will give us some idea of what it is like to be in and conduct a focused discussion. Focused discussions are less formal than focus groups, which are used in research and are often recorded. The topic of discussion for today is about smoking and what we could do to reduce smoking by youth.

We only have 40 minutes for our discussion, so it will be a much shorter version than most discussions, which can take an hour to an hour and a half for a group of 10 to 12. However, we already know each other and have been working together before so we can probably accomplish a lot in 40 minutes.

In the first part of this discussion, I will be asking for your experiences as smokers or nonsmokers and the different factors affecting this behavior. In the second half, we will be looking at the ways we can approach this problem, individually or as a group. In particular, I would like to know how you feel about:

1. The factors contributing to smoking and nonsmoking.
2. The influence of the media and tobacco industry.
3. The influence health professionals could have to decrease smoking rates.

Your comments are completely confidential. Your name will not be associated with any comments you make during this discussion. This is an opportunity to be heard, and I encourage you to speak up. I also encourage you to speak about yourself and your experiences. There are no right or wrong answers. Please feel free to be totally honest.

_____ (recorder's name) will be taking notes using a number to represent each person.

I want everyone to have an opportunity to speak, so as moderator, I will sometimes call upon you to share your ideas, or, if you are speaking more than others, I may have to interrupt you to give other people an opportunity to comment. Please don't be offended. It is not that I do not want to hear what you have to say, it is just that we have only 40 minutes and I want everyone to have equal opportunity to comment. Are there any questions or concerns?

End of discussion. Moderator thanks participants.

Recorder's Guide

Notes on recording for focused discussions include the following:

1. Write each of the questions from the focused discussion on the top of a separate sheet of paper. Try to capture the essence of the conversation and important quotes. Write some observations about the nonverbal communication from group members.

TABLE 4-2A	**Focused Discussion Questions**
QUESTIONS: FACTORS AFFECTING SMOKING STATUS OF YOUTH	**PROBES**
1. Thinking back as far as possible, what was your first experience with cigarettes?	As a child were you exposed to advertisements, parents or siblings who smoked, ads on TV, or tobacco paraphernalia?
2. Thinking of yourself and/or other people, what factors do you think encourage youth to start smoking and why do they continue?	Partying and smoking with friends, occasional or social smoker, smoking in family, wanting to belong, wanting to make choices independent of parents, stress, weight concerns, being "cool," fashion, addiction
3. Consider mass media and advertising. a. What messages encourage smoking? b. What messages encourage nonsmoking?	Movies, TV, magazines, ads
4. How does the tobacco industry influence smoking by youth?	Lawsuits, labeling, young models, smoking in movies, sponsorship or sports/cultural events—Are particular methods used to get youth to start smoking?
5. As a group of future healthcare professionals, what could we do to a. Help youth refrain from smoking? b. Help youth quit smoking?	Increase awareness of the influence from media and the tobacco industry, cost of cigarettes, be supportive for those who are in the process of quitting, help people deal with stress and/or body image issues, be aware of the addictive nature of nicotine, refer to a nicotine addiction clinic, advocate for smoke-free indoor air, "take it outside," offer "munchies" to quitters (celery, carrots)

TABLE 4-2B	Information about the Focused Discussion
Date	
Location	
Number of participants	
Name of moderator	
Name of recorder	
Name of facilitator to assist and lead debriefing (optional)	
Other comments	

2. Usually a recorder does not speak until the end. However, if you want to clarify a point or contribute to the conversation, do so. You need to remember to return to your note taking.
3. At the end of the discussion, clarify any questions you have on what a person said.

Debriefing Session after Demonstration

This debriefing can be led by the facilitator or another person in the group. Questions to ask include the following:

1. Did you feel that there was good discussion of the questions? Why or why not?
2. The advantages of focus groups are in depth discussion and probing, provision of more information at less cost than interviews or quantitative measures, and provision of more information in less time than individual interviews (The Health Communication Unit, 2000). Do you feel that these advantages were realized in this discussion? Why or why not?
3. The disadvantages of focus groups are that the participants may influence each other's opinions, data are not quantifiable, a limited number of questions can be asked, the discussion is more difficult to analyze than answers to quantitative questions, the quality depends on the skill of moderator, they are not effective in some social contexts, and they are difficult to conduct with populations with hearing, cognitive, or communication impairments (The Health Communication Unit, 2000). Did these disadvantages affect this discussion? Why or why not?
4. How did the size and location of the group affect the results?
5. Consider how easy or difficult it was for the moderator to meet the following characteristics of a good moderator: establish rapport, probe for deeper meanings, lead discussion without domination, control opinionated participants, draw out quiet participants, focus (return to questions), encourage discussion among all (The Health Communication Unit, 2000).
6. How easy or difficult was it to record the responses?
7. Is anyone planning to use focused discussions in their projects? Was this demonstration useful to prepare you about what to expect?
8. What main points on smoking among youth were identified during the discussion?

CHAPTER 5

Determining Action Statements from Collaborative Assessment

ELIZABETH DIEM

PRENATAL AND POSTNATAL HEALTH (continued from Chapter 4)

The two teams were working on prenatal and postnatal health projects in the city of Old York. The low-income team was working with women living in an area of the city called Fairway. The other team was working with Chinese-speaking women in two locations: in Chinatown at a church and in an English as a second language (ESL) class at a high-tech firm called Computer Age with many Mandarin-speaking employees. The information from secondary sources is given in the previous chapter in Application 4-1.

LOW-INCOME PROJECT: With four weeks to go on the project, the team working with the low-income women in Fairway had primary data from two key informant interviews, a limited mapping of the Fairway area, and two focused discussions with 16 public health nurses. They were continuing with progressive inquiry with low-income women seen on home visits and at a well baby clinic for another two weeks. On the last week of the project, they were to give a presentation to the public health nurses working with mothers in the Fairway area.

CHINESE PROJECT: The four students working on the prenatal and postnatal health project for women from China had primary data from three weeks of progressive inquiry with women in the ESL class and women meeting at the church and had two weeks to go. At Computer Age, they had obtained the firm's policy statements on health services to employees and their families and had five questionnaires completed by Mandarin-speaking mothers. They expected another 15 in the next week. They were planning to sit down as a team this week and brainstorm about all the things that they needed to do by the end of the project. They were excited about the opportunity to present their information to the women at the church and prepare a short article on their preliminary data for the newsletter of Computer Age.

OBJECTIVES   After reading this chapter and answering the questions throughout the chapter, you should be able to

1. Identify different types of groups in the community.
2. Analyze primary and secondary data.
3. Prepare and conduct a presentation to validate the collaborative assessment and analysis, and define the issues for action.
4. Develop action statements to address the issues for action.
5. Document and communicate decisions.
6. Complete a collaborative assessment report.

KEYWORDS   action statement ▪ collaborators ▪ community of interest ▪ gap analysis ▪ issues for action ▪ preferred situation ▪ present situation ▪ qualitative data ▪ quantitative data ▪ stakeholders

People involved in collaborative assessment

The purpose of collaborative assessment is to identify ways to improve the health of certain people in the population. These people are called the **community of interest** for the project. **Stakeholders** are people or organizations who have a "stake" in improving the health of the people in the community of interest. **Collaborators** are the people from the community of interest and the stakeholders who are involved in the project. Table 5-1 provides an explanation and description of the terms.

When the collaborative assessment is initiated, the community of interest and the stakeholders may not be defined. After interacting with people for a few weeks, the people and their relationship to the project become more apparent. During the analysis and

TABLE 5-1	Definitions of Groups in the Community	
CATEGORY	**CHARACTERISTICS**	**EXAMPLES**
Community of interest	Defined group of people expected to receive health benefits from project	Seniors attending the mall walking program Breast-feeding mothers in the city Children in grades 5 and 6 living downtown Women living on farms in County X
Stakeholders	People and organizations who can contribute to the health benefits of the community of interest	People who are associated with the community of interest, such as parents of children, adult children of elderly persons, or nonsmoking friends of smokers Health professionals including nurses, doctors, and social workers Service providers that are healthcare organizations such as public health departments, community health centers, clinics, and hospitals Other professionals such as teachers or police Voluntary health associations for conditions such as heart disease and stroke, diabetes, or lung cancer Public service organizations such as Mothers Against Drunk Driving (MADD), Shriners, or seniors' associations Managers of businesses or organizations Regional and municipal governments
Collaborators	People from the community of interest and stakeholders who work closely with the team	A small number of individuals from the community of interest who become part of the team People from different agencies or organizations who are ready to provide assistance as needed

definition of issues, the community of interest and stakeholders must be clearly identified. Both are crucial in determining the direction and sustainability of the project.

Collaboration during assessment and analysis

The team and collaborators develop a responsive relationship while completing the steps in the collaborative assessment. The development depends on the different parties making complementary contributions throughout the assessment and project. The main contribution of the team is to provide information and a process that supports collaborative decision making. The contribution of the collaborators is to provide advice and information and engage in the decision making to identify an issue for action that would be

TABLE 5-2	Team and Collaborator Contribution Leading up to Analysis	
STEP	**TEAM CONTRIBUTION**	**COLLABORATOR CONTRIBUTION***
Step 1: Establish relationships with community contacts.	Ask questions to begin to clarify the characteristics of the community and the issues that concern them.	Provide information/advice on community and issues to begin orientation of team.
Step 2: Assess secondary data.	Identify issues from the secondary data that pertain to the community group and issues.	Indicate whether the information found in the secondary data is consistent with that found in the community.
Step 3: Initiate assessment.	a. Observe and map area, situation, and resources and report findings to community contacts. b. Meet, talk to, and interact with key informants to define community and issues, and identify possible approaches to systematically collect assessment information from community group.	a. Respond to the usefulness of the observations and mapping. b. Discuss various approaches and questions that would be relevant to the community group.
Step 4: Conduct specific assessment.	a. Collaboratively determine specific assessment tools and timing after presenting and discussing: 1) Options for collecting information 2) Content to be included in assessment 3) Means and timing to collect information b. Conduct specific assessment.	Provide information/advice/assistance on what is likely to work the best, how to deal with difficulties, and how to increase the involvement of people who do not readily attend meetings.

*This is the minimum contribution that is expected. Any additional help would be welcomed.

relevant to the population group. Preferably the collaborators will become or have been part of the team and engage in all activities. However, they may not be available to attend all the meetings. Table 5-2 summarizes the contribution from the team and collaborators leading up to analysis.

Step 5: Develop action statements

The relationship of the team members and collaborators is particularly important during the analysis of assessment data and development of action statements (step 5 of the workplan, see Appendix C). During the analysis, the team draws inferences regarding the rationale for the project, the issues, and the strengths and presents preliminary conclusions to the collaborators. The collaborators are involved in validating the accuracy of the present situation, determining the vision for the future, and participating in a gap analysis between the present situation and the vision to determine the issues for action.

The project team uses the issues for action to generate **action statements** to indicate where the team and community could take collaborative action on the issue. The activities associated with the substeps and the results are documented in the workplan (Appendix C). The substeps for step 5 follow:

- Analyze data and prepare presentation.
- Validate findings and devise three action statements.
- Prepare collaborative assessment report.

Analyze data

Data analysis involves condensing and converting the data into pieces or "chunks" of information that people can comprehend fairly quickly. Analysis involves either four phases ("categorize, summarize, compare, draw inferences" [Anderson & McFarlane, 2000, pp. 219–221]) or five phases: the previous four plus "validate" (Helvie, 1998, p. 210). Analysis entails finding answers to questions about the data for each phase. The questions are formed from the items given for each phase in Box 5-1.

Categorize

In the initial categorizing phase, the data is simply grouped into one of three categories: background, issue, or strength. To determine whether the data is background data ask: "What is background information that provides a reason for doing the project?" The remaining information is sorted into issues and strengths.

Summarize

The data within each category is then summarized. Questions are particularly important in identifying themes in **qualitative data** (information that can be described rather than

BOX 5-1	**Phases of analysis for collaborative assessment data**

Categorize into Areas Appropriate for the Project:
- Background or rationale for the project based on secondary data sources such as socio-demographic statistics, mortality and morbidity statistics, utilization data, and government and organizational policy statements
- Issues that are strongly felt by assessment participants such as barriers to health and preferred health
- Strengths of community members and stakeholders including individual and group assets, previous initiatives, amount of interest, and available resources

Summarize:
- If the primary data is quantitative, determine statistics; if the data is qualitative, use themes for the three categorized areas.
- Identify main points.

Compare:
- Identify data gaps, inconsistencies, and omissions with collaborators.
- Compare with similar data, if available.
- Compare with objectives identified by the community or agency and government reports.

Draw Inferences or Conclusions:
- Prepare conclusion statements that allow collaborators to make decisions, such as major points from the secondary data, or determine where they are now and where they would like to be from the primary data.

Validate and Define Issues for Action with Collaborators:
- Determine the accuracy of the collaborative assessment data.
- Determine the present health situation (barriers to health and strengths).
- Determine the vision of where the community would like to be (preferred health situation).
- Define the issues for action by conducting a gap analysis between the present situation and the preferred state.

measured). The first question could be: "What are some people saying that is similar to what others are saying?" The next question could be: "What are only one or a few people saying?"

The **quantitative data** (the information that can be measured definitively, usually numerically) is easier to analyze. Descriptive statistics are used to identify the items with the highest percentage of responses. Only items with five or more responses are reported to avoid revealing participants with particular interests. This usually means that for questionnaires with ten or fewer people responding only one or two items will be identified. The responses to all questions are documented as summary statements.

Compare

Once the information has been summarized, the next step is to identify missing or inconsistent data with collaborators. Either complete the missing data or identify it as a limitation in the collaborative assessment report. Comparisons are then made with other secondary data, such as comparing socioeconomic status and utilization patterns in one area to another. Data from two different groups, such as health professionals and community members, provides another means of comparison.

The mission statement or mandate of the agency or organization is an important source for comparison. Resources for most projects are provided by an agency or organization, so the projects must support or further the mandate or mission. This decision is made by management comparing the identified issues and community of interest to the mission or mandate of the agency or program within the agency. Usually the mission statements are quite broad and can cover a variety of projects, but they also provide some restrictions. For example, if the mission statement is to "Promote the health of families living in the Bayview Ward of the city," a project for single adults or for families living in a different area would not be consistent with the mission of the agency.

Draw inferences or conclusions

Before presenting the assessment information, the team and available collaborators need to draw some preliminary inferences or conclusions. At this point, the team members and collaborators have probably formed their own ideas about what conclusions can be drawn from the data. A brainstorming session is useful to elicit each person's views about the main findings. The first round would involve asking each person how they would describe 1) the **present health situation** (barriers to health and strengths) of the people who participated in the collaborative assessment and 2) the participants' **preferred health situation.** The responses are documented without discussion. This procedure of equitably giving everyone a chance to express his or her ideas and recording the ideas so everyone can see them, encourages a more objective view of the ideas. After everyone has contributed, the responses are compared with each other and with the data.

To determine whether consensus is possible on the two questions, team members need to keep comparing their responses to the data. This process is best done in at least two sessions to allow ideas to emerge after team members have had a chance to consider different perspectives. Without sufficient time to allow ideas to emerge, premature conclusions might result. Teams are encouraged to remain open to various conclusions, especially if collaborators from the community are not available to attend the analysis sessions. If the team offers a range of options in the presentation to the collaborators, the collaborators would probably feel more comfortable expressing their true feelings.

PRENATAL AND POSTNATAL HEALTH SCENARIO (continued)

LOW-INCOME PROJECT: Three weeks before the end of clinical placement, the team working with the low-income women met in a seminar with two other teams to discuss the analysis and presentation of assessment data. Because time was limited, each team was allowed to ask only two questions about their analysis.

The team had started to categorize the data. They realized that they would be using the secondary data to make two or three statements about the importance of working in a low-income area. This would be called background data. They felt that they had sufficient information to do that. Most of their concern *related to how to summarize the data they had collected from the focused discussions with two groups of public health nurses working in the Fairway area. They had put the responses from both discussions together in one document according to the discussion questions. They presented the data from one question to the seminar group and asked the group members to look for common themes. Just by presenting the data, the team members themselves started identifying themes. The members of the seminar group asked questions that helped to clarify the issues. The team quickly had two themes identified: one on transportation and the other on health information.*

CHINESE PROJECT: *At their brainstorming session a month before the end of their clinical placement, the Chinese project team members listed all the remaining work that they had to do on their workplan. They also decided that during data analysis they would work with a different person so that more team members would know about the two types of data collection and analysis. They were amazed by all the things that needed to be done to complete the project, but felt more relaxed now that they knew that they would have data to analyze.*

The two team members working with the Chinese women in the ESL class found that by using progressive inquiry they had really been analyzing the data as they were going along. With each of them asking the same few questions of a number of ESL students, they were able to determine the concerns and interests of most and could ask more specific questions the next time around. After a few weeks, they repeated a few of the questions and received the same type of response. By the end of the five weeks, they felt quite confident that the ESL students understood the questions and that the issues they found were important to most of the students. The three issues with the most support were 1) prenatal and postnatal information written in Cantonese and Mandarin or in simple English, 2) nutritious food, and 3) sleep.

DISCUSSION QUESTIONS

1. What data can the team working with the low-income women use for comparison with the themes from the focused discussions with the public health nurses?
2. Why did the team members working with the Chinese women in the ESL classes repeat some of the previous questions they had used?

Prepare and conduct presentation for validation

Once some conclusions from the data analysis have been prepared, the preliminary conclusions need to be presented in a meaningful way. The collaborators need to be involved in decisions about the accuracy of the collaborative assessment of the present health situation (where they are now) and the preferred health situation (where they would like to be).

Prepare for validation presentation

To prepare for the presentation to validate the assessment data, the team should consider the information that the collaborators need to make informed decisions. They first need a description of how the data were collected. Even if they have been working with the team, they are unlikely to know everything or to know it from the team's perspective. The analysis can be presented by following a simplified version of the process given previously in Box 5-1. The list that can be used for outlining the presentation follows:

1. What and how data were collected
2. Background: Why the issue is important
3. Summary of the major issues found in the qualitative and quantitative data

4. Summary of the strengths found in the qualitative and quantitative data
5. Comparison of the issues and strengths with different groups who participated, with background statistics, and with the agency mandate
6. Preliminary conclusions on the present and preferred health situation

When preparing for the presentation, the team members should draw on their experience with the collaborators to make the presentation interesting and interactive and also include the collaborators in the preparation and presentation. For example, the team could ask themselves or the collaborators which questions sparked the most interest, what approach made the collaborators more comfortable, and whether the collaborators like pictures or jokes. The responses to the questions will help the team tailor the presentation to suit the collaborators. Further suggestions and a process to prepare for the presentation are given in Appendix A.

Another consideration is the language that is used. Information on using plain or simple language is given in Appendix B.

People can be encouraged to respond in various ways. Often people find it easier to respond if they are given options to choose from. For example, in the area of barriers to health, the team could present the following: "In our questions, we found that most people mentioned a difficulty in getting nutritious food. We did not know if this was because of the cost of food, transportation to grocery stores, knowing what food was nutritious, or some other reason." Depending on the number of people present and the team's past experience with the collaborators, the team needs to structure the meeting so people will be comfortable responding to questions and will not be overwhelmed with the amount of information presented.

As mentioned earlier, the team is encouraged to present possible or preliminary conclusions that are open to change through discussion. This will not only reduce the pressure of the team feeling that they need to have all the answers but also encourage others to provide more comments or suggestions. This approach would identify whether the team has done the best it could in the situation to collect and analyze the data but is open to hearing from others. The approach also acknowledges that the people in the community and the stakeholders have a more intimate knowledge of the situation than the team does.

As an example, a survey was conducted with girls being asked various questions about health and social behaviors. The survey team learned that a high percentage of the girls brushed their teeth regularly. The team was impressed until two teachers reported that the girls brushed their teeth to remove the smell of smoking tobacco! In another example, a team of nurses working with native groups in Australia had difficulty understanding why a high rate of infants were born with anomalies. During conversations with the nurses, the mothers of the infants said they knew about the dangers of drinking alcohol when pregnant. After further discussions with the women, however, the nurses realized that the women did not consider themselves pregnant until the fetus first moved at approximately four months. With that information about the women's beliefs, the nurses needed to consider a different approach.

Conduct presentation

The purpose of the presentation is to obtain feedback on the six items in the presentation outline given above. As each item is presented, allow the participants time to discuss the information. If they have been involved in the assessment, they should already have a fairly clear idea of what you are going to say.

If concerns are expressed about how the data were collected or incompleteness of the data, that limitation needs to be recorded and included in the limitations section of the collaborative assessment report. Once the data and methods have been considered, the next items on background, issues and strengths, comparisons, and possible conclusions are presented for discussion and validation.

The final step is to define the present health situation and preferred health situation and conduct a **gap analysis,** which is the difference between the two situations. The gap analysis is best done in small groups of four to eight. Each group would be asked to identify the difference between the present and preferred situations. The common differences identified by the groups are the **issues for action.**

PRENATAL AND POSTNATAL HEALTH SCENARIO (continued)

LOW-INCOME PROJECT: *The team working with the low-income women felt well prepared for their presentation with the public health nurses. Because 14 to 20 nurses would be present, the team considered various ways to present the information so everyone could see it. They chose to do a computer slide presentation because a team member was familiar with the presentation program and the equipment was available. Box 5-2 is one of the slides they showed their project leader a week before the presentation.*

The project leader said that they would first need to provide an overview of progressive inquiry (Chapter 4), so that people would have an idea of what they did. They also had to reduce the amount of detailed information they had on the slide. Boxes 5-3 and 5-4 show the two slides that replaced the original slide.

During the presentation, the low-income team felt that it was important to provide some context to the situation of the low-income women. They presented the following story told to them by a woman in the second week of their progressive inquiry:

I moved into a low-cost apartment building just a month before I was due to deliver my second baby. Jenny was two. I hadn't seen Roger for about two weeks, and I sort of hoped that he had left for good. On the first night I was there, the pains started at two a.m. I was scared! I didn't know anyone! I knocked on the door of the apartment next door. I saw an older woman go in there earlier in the day. Well, Ruth called the president of the tenants association and they took right over. Someone called the doctor and got me to the

BOX 5-2	**Original slide on progressive inquiry**

Last Two Weeks of Progressive Inquiry During Clinic and Home Visits
Week 10 Questions (12 of 12 mothers):
What/who helped you keep yourself healthy when pregnant or had new baby?
What/who helped keep your baby healthy?
   Information provided by another woman they respected/trusted
   Pamphlets from PHN that they could understand.

Week 11 Questions (14 of 14 mothers):
What additional help would have been useful when pregnant? Now with a new baby?
   Help when pregnant and someone they could call or talk to about swelling legs and food.
   New baby: Sharing ideas on food and sleep and help with other nearby mothers.

BOX 5-3	**First slide on progressive inquiry**

Four Weeks of Progressive Inquiry with 30 Mothers at Home or Clinic Visits

Week	Approached	Participated	Repeats
1	10	6	
2	12	9	2
3	12	12	4
4	14	14	6

hospital, and Ruth stayed with Jenny. Now I have friends, and I find out about things like this clinic. Ruth is like the mother I never had!

Everyone was impressed with the information and how the team presented it. The team members documented the comments from the public health nurses and their project leader in their weekly summary.

CHINESE PROJECT: A week before the presentation with the Chinese women at the church, the team was puzzling over how to explain progressive inquiry. Each week for five weeks, the two students prepared two questions. Each of them asked as many people as possible the questions in the course of normal conversation, and at the end of the class they compared the responses.

The team took a while to come up with possible ideas on how to present their information to the ESL students. They first remembered that the teacher had used a calendar and knew that the students liked the use of pictures and understood that stick figures could represent the number of people. They asked the ESL teacher and their collaborators at the church if they had any ideas. The teacher agreed that the use of the calendar and pictures would be appropriate. She checked the words they would be showing and helped them change a few to words with fewer syllables.

When they asked the collaborators at the church how they could present the information, one of the women started talking about the puppet plays she saw in her village while growing up. Another mentioned that when actors came to perform, everyone came to watch. The students looked at each other and almost said together "role play!" They talked more to the women to develop ideas for the script. A few sat in on their rehearsal and, after applauding enthusiastically, very politely reminded them to speak slower.

At the presentation with the ESL students and the other Chinese women, the team first performed the role play to demonstrate how they got their information. They showed through pictures and the number of stick people how many women were interested in different topics related to prenatal and postnatal health. The women kept nodding and pointing to the pictures to indicate the ones they supported.

BOX 5-4	**Second slide on progressive inquiry**

What Keeps or Would Keep Them and Their Babies Healthy? (Questions from Weeks 3 and 4, Respectively)

Present Situation (12 mothers)	Preferred Situation (14 mothers)
■ Information from other trusted women—all ■ Pamphlets—2	■ Other mothers who are nearby who they could talk to and share ideas with ■ Relevant information on nutrition and baby food that they could discuss with other mothers

The team checked out these topics by having each of the four team members hold up a card. The first card was on information they could understand, the second was on food, and the third was about sleep. The fourth had a question mark and other items that were mentioned by a few people. The audience was asked to go and stand by the picture that they felt was the most important. Eight of the 22 women present quickly moved to stand by the information card. The cards for food and sleep had six women each. Two, who felt that exercise was important, stood by the card with the question mark. These four items became the issues for action.

When the team evaluated their ability to collaborate, they included comments from the teacher and students on how clearly they provided information so everyone could take part.

DISCUSSION QUESTIONS

1. Low-income project:
   a. Why did the team show a table with the number of women participating in progressive inquiry?
   b. Explain how the second slide (Box 5-4) would help with the gap analysis.
2. Chinese project:
   a. Why would the team working with the Chinese women bother with doing the role play?
   b. What aspects in the presentation made it easy for the Chinese women to provide their responses?
   c. Can you think of other ways in which the information could be presented?

Develop draft action statements

After the team has determined the issues for action with the collaborators, members are ready to develop draft action statements that are expected to address the issue. Action statements are developed by nurses from the issues for action determined with community members and stakeholders to provide alternative means for achieving the community's preferred status.

The development of draft action statements is an intermediary phase in the decision-making process with the community. The action statements provide options to address the different issues and indicate what the team or nursing could contribute to collaboration action with the community members or stakeholders. Action statements provide options that community health nurses believe are feasible. The three parts of the action statements are defined in Table 5-3.

TABLE 5-3	*Three-Part Action Statements*		
COMPONENTS	**PART 1: COMMUNITY OF INTEREST**	**PART 2: ISSUE FOR ACTION OR STRENGTH**	**PART 3: "RELATED-TO"**
Description of part	Specific description of community of interest	State in terms of risk or strength from analysis and validation of assessment data	Factors related to preferred state that nursing in collaboration with others can change

The term *action statement* is used instead of nursing diagnosis or community diagnosis for several reasons. The terms *diagnosis* and *community diagnosis* are associated with a medical, prescriptive approach to healthcare. The term *nursing diagnosis* is more closely associated with nursing care for individuals and individual families, rather than communities. The term *action statement* is also more understandable to people in the community. (*Note:* The term *action statement* was defined from discussions on the electronic mailing list of the Community Health Nurses Initiatives Group of the Registered Nurses of Ontario, www.chnig.org, November 2002 to February 2003.)

Formats for community or nursing diagnosis relevant to community health nursing practice use a four-part statement that identifies the following (Anderson & McFarlane, 2000; Ervin, 2002; Helvie, 1998; Neufeld & Harrison, 2000):

- Name or description of group
- Situation or response
- Related to factors
- Evidence

Action statements use the first three parts, similar to the three-part community-oriented nursing diagnosis (Shuster & Goeppinger, 2003). The evidence is not repeated in the action statement because it has been validated previously by the collaborators and has already been documented in relation to the findings. When action statements are presented without the validated findings and evidence, the evidence can be added at the end the statement.

The two parts of the action statement that have definitions different from that of community or nursing diagnosis are the situation or response and the "related-to" clause. For the situation or response, only three references (Ervin, 2002; Neufeld & Harrison, 2000; Stolte, 1996) mention the possibility of using strengths or a healthy response along with adverse situations or unhealthy responses. For example, community-oriented nursing diagnosis describes only risk statements (Shuster & Goeppinger, 2003). In this text, both risk and strength action statements are included.

In statements or examples from most references (Anderson & McFarland, 2000; Helvie, 1998; Neufeld & Harrison, 2000), the related-to factors must be those that nursing (or nursing in collaboration with others [Neufeld & Harrison, 2000]) can change or use for planning. In this text, the related-to must be within the realm of nursing in collaboration with others.

Community of interest

The community of interest is the people in the community who are expected to receive health benefits from collaborative action. The community of interest can change, depending on the availability of resources. For example, the community of interest for the Chinese project could be the prenatal and postnatal Cantonese- and Mandarin-speaking women living in the city, the prenatal and postnatal Cantonese-speaking women living in Chinatown, the postnatal Mandarin women associated with the high-tech firm, and so on.

Issue for action or strength

The issues and strengths are determined during the analysis and validation of the data with collaborators. At least one strength should be included. The strengths are incorporated into the collaborative action.

Most issues will become risk statements by including the words "are at risk for" because the team would not have sufficient information on most of the population. For example, poor nutrition in Fairway is presumed, based on the poverty in the area and the accounts of some of the public health nurses and 30 women. The team does not have information on their daily intake of food or information from a high percentage of the women in the area.

A properly constructed risk action statement includes a specific community group with a defined risk or issue that is related to the lack of something. For example, the following is a properly constructed risk action statement: "Prenatal and postnatal Cantonese women in Chinatown are at risk for fatigue, poor nutrition, and poor fitness related to lack of understandable and available information on healthy pregnancy." In this example, note that both the status and related-to clause are negative.

The strength action statements will often use the words "have potential for" followed by an improved health status. A properly constructed strength action statement includes a specific community group with a strength or potential strength that is drawn from a particular characteristic of the group. For example, the following is a properly constructed strength action statement: "Prenatal and postnatal Cantonese women in Chinatown have potential for increased prenatal and postnatal health related to interest in learning about better nutrition, promoting sleep, and exercise." In the example, note that both the status and the related-to clause are positive. A low knowledge score on a topic should not be interpreted as showing an interest in the topic. The women's interest could be determined only if they were asked a question about their interests or demonstrate interest through their actions.

The issues, strengths, and preferred health situation state are usually determined by first collecting primary data from community members and stakeholders. When secondary data alone is used, these three elements can be inferred from the data and need to be confirmed by stakeholders.

"Related-to" clause

This clause identifies the factors that contribute to the issue or strength that nursing in collaboration with others can address. Four types of characteristics of related-to clauses are important to take into consideration when action statements are developed. The four characteristics are the following:

1. Factors that promote collaboration
2. Factors that can be changed
3. Factors that define a nursing role
4. Factors that are manageable within a short-term project

The factors are described in Box 5-5.

PRENATAL AND POSTNATAL HEALTH SCENARIO (continued)

LOW-INCOME PROJECT: *The team working with the low-income women was concerned about writing action statements. Team members spent a considerable amount of time developing nursing diagnoses for individuals and families in their institutional practice and did not know whether it would be easier or more difficult in the community.*

They found that the validation of the information from the focused discussions with the public health nurses and the progressive inquiry with the women living on a low income provided several possible action statements. They felt that there were three possible communities of interest and three related-to clauses.

| BOX 5-5 | **Four important characteristics of the "related-to" clause in a short-term project** |

1. Factors That Promote Collaboration

To promote collaboration and engage the interest and support of community members, the terms in the related-to clause need to be understandable, nonjudgmental, and relevant.

Tips:

- Use terms familiar to the community rather than medical terms such as 'maternal attachment'
- Select actions that would be strongly supported
- Define reasons why an action is not being taken rather than passing judgment on people. For example, terms such as 'lack of knowledge' or 'knowledge deficit' can convey a total lack of knowledge or understanding by everyone, which is rarely the case. The reasons for the lack can be beyond the control of the group or, specifically in terms of information, could be that the information is inaccessible or unavailable in plain language or in the language spoken by the community group. Also avoid more obvious negative terms such as 'neglect' and 'do not control.'

2. Factors That Can Be Changed

During the collaborative assessment, issues and strengths that can be changed or supported need to be identified. Those that cannot be changed, such as survey results, age, or developmental stage, need further explanation or expansion. For example, rather than simply stating "survey results," explain how respondents have indicated that they were very interested in obtaining certain information or a program to deal with a problem such as discipline or nutrition for children that is specific to a particular age.

3. Factors That Define a Nursing Role

Although community health nurses consider all the social determinants of health such as socioenvironmental conditions, psychosocial relationships, and behaviors (The Health Communication Unit, 2001), they do not necessarily have the expertise to directly provide all needed services. Often nurses will need to work in collaboration with others, and within that collaboration, their role needs some definition. For example, the term "language barrier" can be interpreted to mean that nurses are to teach language skills, and the term "unemployment" could indicate that nurses are expected to provide job search strategies. In contrast, nurses working with people who do not communicate in the dominant language can collaborate with language teachers to provide meaningful information that is illustrated and written in plain language. Nurses working with people who are unemployed might refer people to employment counselors or arrange information sessions with them.

4. Factors That Are Manageable within a Short-Term Project

Broad determinants of health, such as poverty, need to broken down into manageable steps for short-term projects. Some suggestions to deal with poverty are increased communication among community members or service providers, a location or structure to bring people together, or provision of accessible information on community resources. Those directions are feasible for nurses to initiate alone or in collaboration with others.

Their work is displayed in Table 5-4 to indicate how they followed the three-part format. By using each of the communities of interest and each of the related-to clauses, they would have nine possible action statements on nutrition. Action statements on poor prenatal and postnatal medical care and social isolation could also be considered. Usually the team would narrow down the action statements to three to five, with at least one indicating a strength.

TABLE 5-4	**Draft of Action Statement Showing Three-Part Format**	
PART 1: COMMUNITY OF INTEREST	**PART 2: ISSUE FOR ACTION OR STRENGTH**	**PART 3: "RELATED-TO"**
1. Prenatal and postnatal women living in Fairway 2. Women and infants in Fairway visited by public health nurses 3. Women and infants attending the Fairway Well Baby Clinic	Are at risk for poor nutrition	Related-to: 1. No access to a program for cooperative food buying, food preparation, or gardening 2. No access to appropriate information on nutritional, economical food 3. No access to local support groups on prenatal and postnatal health

The team found that the most challenging parts of creating the action statement were identifying the different communities of interest and all the different data sources that they used during their assessment. They found that those two parts were quite different from a nursing diagnosis with an individual or family.

CHINESE PROJECT: The students working with the Chinese women also struggled with defining the various communities of interest that could be involved. They had difficulty trying to bring together the information on the Cantonese and Mandarin women. Although both groups were fairly recent immigrants and were learning to converse in English, they differed in many factors related to education, ability to read English, and availability of social support. They finally decided on three action statements. The action statements are provided in their assessment report in Application 5-1 at the end of the chapter.

DISCUSSION QUESTIONS

1. For each of the projects, identify another community of interest or "related-to" clause and the type of evidence that would be expected.
2. What do you see as the difference between action statements and nursing diagnoses used with individuals and families?
3. How do you feel that the community members would respond if they were told that they had a "lack of knowledge," as opposed to needing appropriate resources?

Prepare collaborative assessment report

The final task for the team to complete is the assessment report. The collaborative assessment report is prepared for the project organizers and is a very condensed summary of what the team has done and found. Attached to the assessment report are the questionnaires, focused discussion questions, tables of data, excerpts of comments (with revealing information removed), reference list, and so on. The assessment report is expected to assist the organization and others to carry on with the work that the team has started during this assessment.

The report should be no more than two pages long. The format is given in Appendix C. At the halfway point in the clinical placement, the team is encouraged to start filling in the information for each section so everything is not left to the end. If the workplan is fully

TABLE 5-5	Source of Information for Sections of the Collaborative Assessment Report

SECTION OF ASSESSMENT REPORT	SOURCE OF INFORMATION
Importance of issue/problem	Summarize national, provincial, local statistics, and literature review (step 2 in workplan with references)
Agency mandate	Mandate/mission from agency policy documents
Agency priority or issue	Priority from original purpose of project
Community of interest	Defined initially, may be changed
Assessment goal	Defined initially, may be changed during planning for specific assessment
Assessment methods, timelines, number, and description of participants for primary data	Summarize from workplan For participants, indicate number and particulars if there are more than 5 in a category such as age, sex, SES, residence
Validated key results/findings: —Present health situation including barriers to health and strengths (assets, previous initiatives, amount of interest, resources) with evidence —Preferred health situation with evidence	Summarize from analysis
Issues for action	Summarize from consultation
Limitations	Identified during analysis and consultation
Possible action statements to address issue for action including one strength (3)	Developed after consultation with collaborators

completed, the team will have all the appropriate information to condense into the assessment report.

Table 5-5 provides the sections of the report and the sources for the information.

PRENATAL AND POSTNATAL HEALTH SCENARIO (continued)

LOW-INCOME PROJECT: The students working with the low-income women started to fill in the sections on the collaborative assessment report when they began their analysis. They were progressing well but had some questions that they brought to their project leader. The first one was "What is a good title for the project?" The project leader responded by asking them what they had been calling the project. They responded with "The Low-Income Project." She asked them if they felt that this title would explain the project to other people. They said "No" because the name could represent many different things such as housing, employment, or child care. After they discussed it for a while, they came up with the title: "Assessment of Prenatal and Postnatal Health of Women in Fairway."

Their second question was: "How much information should we put in the assessment methods? We have documented considerable information in weekly summaries and condensed it in our workplan." The project leader explained that they needed to provide the reader with sufficient information to indicate clearly how they obtained their information, how long they took, and how many people were involved. That information

TABLE 5-6	Use of a Table to Display Method, Timelines, and Participants		
METHOD	**TIMELINES**	**NUMBER OF PARTICIPANTS**	**DESCRIPTION OF PARTICIPANTS**
Collection and review of secondary data	Sept. 10–Oct 1	Not applicable	
Key informant interviews	Sept. 17–24	2	Both public health nurses
Two focused discussions	Oct. 15	16	Public health nurses with 2 to 12 years experience working with mothers
Progressive inquiry	Oct. 22–Nov 12	31	Women seen: Fairfield home visits: 12; well baby clinic: 19 Number of children involved: 1 year old–18; 2 years old–10; 3 to 5 years old–3

provides evidence for the efforts that were made to include a variety of resources and people. Table 5-6 shows how the team decided to display their information on methods. Different formats can be tried to find one that uses the least space.

While the team was completing their assessment report together, members started to reflect on their experience. One student said: "It really hit me that I had some prejudice against single mothers. I guess that I somehow felt that they were different from me. When that mother told her story about being in labor in a new apartment where she didn't know anyone, that really got me!"

Another student added, "The whole effect of poverty never really meant a lot to me until I saw how these mothers struggle each day to provide food and clothing. Something like going to a movie is a big deal to them."

"Well, I am a single mom, so I know how difficult it is," declared a third member. "I was upset by statements made by one or two of the nurses in the discussions. I felt that our presentation showed that the moms without much money want to keep healthy and keep their babies healthy. The system needs to be changed to make it easier for them to do that!"

The team leader had the final word: "I know that we didn't start off too well, but we have our act together now! I think what made the difference is that we started to really listen to what people were saying to us rather than just thinking about getting things done. I learned that a team can learn to work together. I am proud of the work we did. We provided a different perspective on the lives of single mothers!"

CHINESE PROJECT: The team working with the women from China also had two questions on completing the assessment report. The first was: "What is the difference between the community of interest and the agency priority?" They added that they knew the definition for the community of interest, but this section was right after the agency mandate and priority. The project leader asked them to describe the women who had been originally identified for the project. They remembered that initially the project identified the fact that Chinese women were underserved and that later the team further specified two groups, Cantonese- and Mandarin-speaking women. The first description would be the agency priority, and the specified description would be the community of interest. They knew for some projects that the priority and community of interest might remain the same or that the priority might be an issue such as smoking reduction, without a designated population.

For their second question, they said they did not know what to include in the section on limitations. The project leader responded by asking them how confident they were with the data and validation of data collected from discussions and progressive inquiry with the Cantonese women. In other words, if someone else repeated what they had done, would they get the same results? After thinking for awhile, the team members said that they were very confident about the results from their progressive inquiry because they had the time to explore different questions with all the women. In contrast, they did not feel the same way at all about the questionnaires that were completed by the Mandarin women at the high-tech firm. They felt that they needed more time to pilot test the questions and the method of distribution and to reach more of the women. Those would be the limitations of their collaborative assessment. The team's assessment report is given in Application 5-1.

As the team reflected on their experience, they all felt good about how they had stayed focused on forming relationships with people in the community. The women that they had met with each week at the church in Chinatown helped them connect to other people and keep on track with what would be relevant. Their suggestion of putting on a play for the ESL students worked well for everyone. After their presentation, all of the students were given a small scroll that the women translated as being a good luck message based on their birth date and year. The collaborators agreed to keep working with the public health agency to increase Cantonese language prenatal and postnatal services in Chinatown.

DISCUSSION QUESTIONS

1. What is the benefit of having a two-page collaborative assessment report?
2. Why would readers want to know about the methods and number and type of participants before they consider the findings?
3. What are the benefits of reflecting on experiences with teammates?

Teamwork during analysis

The two challenges during analysis are dealing with time and coordinating tasks. You will probably feel that you are doing a juggling act to complete the assessment on time and deciding when to finish data collection and start analysis. Coordination involves monitoring all the tasks and keeping everyone informed.

Time

The decision related to time involves determining when to complete the collection of primary data so you will have time to analyze what you have collected. You might be tempted to keep collecting data because you do not feel that you have a sufficient number of participants. The approximate numbers expected for the projects are indicated in the scenarios. For example, the four team members on the low-income project team held two focused discussions and involved 31 women in progressive inquiry over four weeks. The four team members on the Chinese project involved 22 women over five weeks in progressive inquiry and received 20 responses to a questionnaire.

As an approximation of expected numbers, based on four team members, at least 30 participants would be appropriate for a survey of people who read and write English and are fairly easy to access. However, when the community of interest is composed of people who are difficult to reach or have some difficulty with English or making their views known, the quality of the data you are collecting becomes more important than simply the quantity. Conducting a face-to-face interview with 8 to 12 people who barely speak English would be equivalent in effort and time to conducting a survey with more than 30 people who read and write English.

Another aspect of timing is to allow sufficient time for the team to study and analyze the data so that they can make careful and accurate inferences. Often you can complete parts of your analysis earlier than other parts. For example, you can summarize your background data into two or three sentences as soon as it has been collected and reviewed. You will use the summary in your presentation and assessment report.

Be aware that the analysis of data from focus groups and complex questionnaires is particularly time consuming. Allow a few weeks for the analysis so that all the team members will become familiar with the data. One way to facilitate team members learning new skills is to have different people work on the preliminary analysis than those who collected the data. Once everyone knows the data, you can choose the questions to direct the analysis and everyone can contribute. When you present the findings, you want to feel confident that you have done a thorough analysis.

Coordination

Coordinating activities as the assessment is ending is particularly important. Because of the many tasks associated with completing data collection, starting data analysis, preparing presentations, and completing the assessment report and team evaluation, important details can be missed unless a person is responsible for coordination and communication. By this period in the project, the chairing function may have become shared among the team members. Although that shows maturity in the development of the team, a person who will be responsible for the overall completion of tasks for the project needs to be designated at this stage. Also, communication of the team decisions, especially those concerning the analysis and preparation for the presentation, needs to be maintained. The distribution list may need to be expanded as more people become involved or want to know about the findings from the assessment.

As an assessment project is nearing completion, there is a tendency to focus on tasks and neglect personal and team morale. Teams are encouraged to look back to what they felt when they started the project and ask themselves some questions: Did we learn what we wanted to learn? Did we learn what we expected to learn? Did we learn more than we expected to learn? What individual and group skills can I now add to my resume?

During the final stages the team members will be spending considerable time working together. This is when you are likely to see that the team has reached the performing stage and to see the benefits of your hard work. If your team will be taking action based on your assessment, your team is ready for the next stage.

If this is the end of your project, take some time to enjoy yourselves. In the future you will probably have fond memories of feeling part of a team that was doing something worthwhile. Also take some time to show appreciation for the people who have worked with you. In your presentation, mention people who have been especially helpful. You may also want to give people a thank-you card or a letter that they can put in their personal file. Plan a party or some form of celebration to commemorate the work you have done and the friends you have made. Chapter 8 has more ideas for ending well.

Summary

Analysis of the data, validation of the results, and preparation of action statements require both time and collaboration with community members. Data collection needs to be stopped so that the team has the time to focus on analysis and the preparations needed to involve the collaborators in determining the issues for action. Decision making with the collaborators at this stage is important to ensure that the direction of the project is relevant for the community. These decisions in the form of action statements are ready to be carried into the planning stage, either by the team or by the organization in the future.

PRACTICE AND APPLICATION

1. Identify the final community of interest and stakeholders for the low-income and Chinese projects.

2. Explain each phase of the data analysis for the low-income project.

3. Using the available information in Chapters 4 and 5, complete a collaborative assessment report for the low-income project.

4. Using at least two sources of data that you have available, describe the analysis process you would use to prepare for a presentation to community members and stakeholders.

5. Using the information from question 4, explain how you would structure the presentation to obtain feedback on 1) the assessment data, 2) the present health situation, 3) the preferred health situation, and 4) the issues for action.

REFERENCES

Anderson, E., & McFarlane, J. (2000). *Community as partner* (3rd ed.). Philadelphia: Lippincott.

Canada Perinatal Surveillance System. (2003). *Maternity experiences survey.* Retrieved July 21, 2003, from http://www.hc-sc.gc.ca/pphb-dgspsp/rhs-ssg/mes-eem_e.html.

Ervin, N. (2002). *Advanced community health nursing practice: Population-focused care.* Upper Saddle River, NJ: Prentice Hall.

The Health Communication Unit. (2001). *Introduction to health promotion planning.* Toronto, ON: University of Toronto, Centre for Health Promotion. Available online at http://www.thcu.ca/infoandresources/planning.htm.

Helvie, C. (1998). *Advanced practice nursing in the community.* Thousand Oaks, CA: Sage.

Neufeld, A., & Harrison, M. (2000). Nursing diagnosis for aggregates and groups. In M. Stewart (Ed.), *Community nursing: Promoting Canadians' health* (2nd ed., pp. 370–385). Toronto, ON: Saunders.

Shuster, G., & Goeppinger, J. (2003). Community as client: Assessment and analysis. In M. Stanhope & J. Lancaster (Eds.), *Community and public health nursing* (6th ed., pp. 342–373). St. Louis, MO: Mosby.

Stolte, K. (1996). *Wellness nursing diagnosis for health promotion.* Philadelphia: Lippincott.

WEB SITE RESOURCES

Nursing diagnosis: http://www.nanda.org

Search strategy: To obtain information on the Internet about community diagnosis, type the term "community diagnosis" into your search engine. Limit your search by adding "site:.edu" to limit the search to educational sites; use "site:.org" to restrict the search to organizational sites (commercial and noncommercial), and use "site:.gov" to limit it to government sites.

APPLICATION 5-1

EXAMPLE OF A COMPLETED COLLABORATIVE ASSESSMENT REPORT

Nursing University of North America, Division of Community Health Community Health Nursing Project in Collaboration with City of Old York, Department of Public Health, Child-Bearing Families Program

Assessment of Prenatal and Postnatal Health of Cantonese- and Mandarin-Speaking Women

Date: November 30, 2004

Students: Fiona Gilchrist, Hoa Nguyen, Doncia Garcia, Tracey West

Project leader: Lien Lee, RN, PHN

Manager: Maria Stellhorn

Clinical Instructor: Joanne Gilchrist

Importance of issue/problem: Immigrants from China outnumber all other immigrants to the city (reference, 2003), and recent immigrants are at higher risk for adverse prenatal outcomes (Health Canada, 2003b). Only 10% of pregnant Chinese-speaking women attend prenatal classes (reference, 2002).

Agency mandate and priority: Improve the prenatal and postnatal health of mothers and infants in the City of Old York. Priority in 2004 is for immigrants from China and women living on a low income.

Community of interest: Prenatal and postnatal women speaking Mandarin or Cantonese and living in Chinatown or associated with the Computer Age firm.

Assessment purpose: Determine the factors influencing the prenatal and postnatal health of the community of interest.

Assessment methods and participants:

■ Collect and review secondary data, Sept. 10–24
■ Community mapping, Sept. 17–24
■ Interviews with key informants: Sept 24–Oct. 8; five people including multicultural worker and executive, Cantonese community leaders
■ Progressive inquiry: Oct. 15–Nov. 12; 22 women speaking Cantonese and Mandarin attending ESL class and church meeting
■ Questionnaire: Oct. 29–Nov. 12; 20 women speaking Mandarin associated with the Computer Age firm

Validated Key Results/Findings with Supporting Evidence

Present situation: No information available on prenatal and postnatal healthcare services in Cantonese, Mandarin, or simple English. No information on nutrition, exercise, and sleep.

Evidence: Progressive inquiry with 22 women over five weeks; 15 of 20 responses to question in questionnaire; no prenatal classes in Cantonese or Mandarin; most women unable to understand written information in English.

Strengths: Anxious to learn English and ways to keep themselves and their children healthy.

Evidence: Responses in progressive inquiry and 20 questionnaires. Cantonese women organized ESL classes held in church. Mandarin-speaking women experienced in using Internet and interested in support group.

Evidence: Responses in 18 of 20 questionnaires.

Support available: Meeting rooms available at church in Chinatown; Public Health Department has mandate to support child-bearing families and is willing to tailor information; Computer Age firm has mission statement that includes promoting the health of employees and their families, and management is willing to organize a support group for pregnant women and new mothers.

Evidence: From key informant interviews, meetings, and policy documents.

Preferred health: Have energy from good food, exercise, and sufficient sleep.

Evidence: Progressive inquiry.

Issues for Action

Prenatal and postnatal information in Cantonese and Chinese or simple English, especially on nutrition, sleep, and exercise is unavailable.

Limitations

Insufficient time to sufficiently pretest questionnaires, distribute broadly, or validate with Mandarin-speaking women, although most items were similar to results from progressive inquiry.

Possible Action Statements to Address Issue for Action

1. Cantonese and Mandarin prenatal and postnatal women living in the city are at risk for fatigue, poor nutrition, and fitness related to lack of understandable and available prenatal and postnatal information.
2. Cantonese women and their infants in Chinatown are at risk for fatigue, poor nutrition, and fitness related to lack of understandable and available information in Cantonese or simple English.
3. Mandarin women and their infants associated with the high-tech firm have the potential for improved health during the prenatal and postnatal period related to the interest of the firm in providing a support group.

Attachments: The following would be attached but are not included here: maps, questions used in progressive inquiry, questionnaire, tables of data, reference list.

CHAPTER 6

Planning the Collaborative Action and Evaluation

ELIZABETH DIEM

SCENARIO | *DAYTIME SHELTER FOR THE HOMELESS*

For the last four months, a four-member project team and a project leader have been working on the assessment portion of a project organized by several agencies providing services for the homeless. The organizations had received a small grant to improve the coordination of their services. The funding provided the salary for the part-time project leader, who is an experienced community health nurse, and for a few hours of administrative support each week from one of the agencies. Four other organizations each provide a person from their staff to work on the project one day a week.

The project team consists of the project leader, a nutritionist, a recreational therapist, and two nurses who usually work in a medical clinic. During the first part of their assessment, they mapped the downtown area to show all the organizations and services provided to the homeless, interviewed at least one staff member from each of the 15 agencies in person or on the phone, and attended two meetings of the Homeless Coalition. They found that the chronic homeless population consisted of approximately 200 people, 25 to 60 years old. Ninety percent were men. Later, they developed a 15-minute interview questionnaire and conducted 30 face-to-face interviews with homeless persons from several agencies.

The key informant interviews with the staff of agencies serving the homeless identified client issues of poor hygiene, medications, and anger management and mentioned possible reasons for the issues. Staff in the homeless shelters felt that they had too little time and resources to learn more about working with the homeless and about the other services available to their clients.

The client questionnaire developed by the team covered first aid, food, foot care, transportation, clothing, medical care, daily activities, and an open-ended question on what gave them satisfaction. The team found that the homeless spent a lot of time looking for food. If one place was out of food, everyone would rush to another place to often find the same situation. This early result was discussed at a Homeless Coalition meeting, and the agencies decided to try having a staff member phone ahead to make sure food was available before people left their establishment hungry.

After the overwhelming concern about finding food, the homeless talked about the sameness of the food, dealing with the cold, and having nothing to do for long periods of the day. They gained satisfaction from being able to survive each day and from the opportunity to help someone else who was on the street. Several had a story about consistently "looking out" for a friend or giving advice to someone new to the street.

The team had started to analyze the assessment data for a meeting with the coalition members. They were not able to have a meeting with everyone because of an upcoming holiday but were able to individually contact the people who had been the most involved.

Through their analysis and discussions, they defined three issues for action: food, shelter, and the support system. The issues and evidence are given in Table 6-1.

TABLE 6-1	Issues for Action
ISSUE	**EVIDENCE**
Amount of food	90% of homeless expressed difficulties obtaining sufficient quantities of food. 12 of 15 agencies talked about often having too much or too little food each day.
Quality of food	55% of homeless stated boredom with food choices. 14 of 15 staff identified that most of the food was donated bread, potatoes, doughnuts, and other sweet goods. The nutritional value of the food available most days was substandard compared with national standards.
Lack of shelter	50% of homeless had a concern about shelter from the cold, difficulty getting warm clothing, having no warm place to gather during the day, and lack of activities during the day. 3 people almost died from hypothermia in the previous winter (reports from staff). There were 20 incidents of severe frostbite (reports from staff).
Support system	45% of homeless stated that they gained satisfaction from passing on information or taking someone somewhere to get some help.

They developed ten possible action statements but were able to reduce them to four through discussions with their project leader. The following four action statements were felt to be the most relevant:

1. The homeless are at risk for poor nutrition related to no coordination of food supplies among homeless agencies.
2. The homeless are at risk for poor nutrition related to donated food that is low in protein and includes little fresh fruit or vegetables.
3. The homeless are at risk for hypothermia and frostbite related to insufficient daytime spaces and warm clothing and footwear.
4. The homeless have a mutual support system related to helping others to find food, shelter, or social events.

The team members were excited about the information that they had discovered. They could see that they had already made a difference and had a lot of ideas about what they would do when they returned from their holiday break.

OBJECTIVES   After reading this chapter and answering the questions throughout the chapter, you should be able to

1. Determine a priority action statement with a community group.
2. Identify appropriate strategies and related theories and research.
3. Determine a broad goal and specific objectives for the project.
4. Identify products and associated activities and resources.
5. Develop relevant evaluation indicators.
6. Document and communicate plans and results.

KEYWORDS   collaborative action ▪ evaluation measures ▪ Gantt chart ▪ goal ▪ objectives ▪ planning ▪ priority action ▪ products ▪ strategy ▪ theories

Collaborative action using the community health nursing process

Collaborative action involves a close working relationship with community groups and organizations to bring about a desired change that supports community health. If the team was involved in an assessment process with the community, the action builds on the assessment data and collaboration developed previously. If the team is starting at the action phase, the action must begin with forming a close working relationship with the community groups or organization. Collaborative action is the second phase of the community health nursing process. The community health nursing process was developed from three different sources: 1) traditional health planning models, 2) the nursing process in community health planning, and 3) Primary Health Care and planning models that incorporate the active participation of community members. The sources are discussed in Chapter 1.

Collaborative action is organized into four steps of the community health nursing process that build on or work in concert with each other. The first step, planning the collaborative action and evaluation, is provided in this chapter. The second step, discussed in Chapter 7, is to implement the planned activities and evaluation. The third step, found in Chapter 8, involves completing the project by reporting on results and providing recommendations. The fourth step on evaluation of individual and team roles occurs concurrently with steps 1 to 3 and is discussed in Chapter 2. Similar to the assessment phase, collaborative action has two forms for planning and documentation: the action timeline and workplan. Both are provided in Appendix C.

Table 6-2 depicts the approximate amount of time (shaded areas) that a team would spend on completing the collaborative action and evaluation, based on 7.5 hours per week for 12 weeks. The information in the table is based on the team organizing and preparing material with guidance from an experienced community health nurse or instructor.

Project teams have various options open to them in using the collaborative action of the community health nursing process in this text. If the teams have already completed an assessment with the same community group and have 90 to 100 hours spread over several weeks and easy access to the same or similar community group, all components of the community health nursing process can be used by teams of two to four. This timeframe has

TABLE 6-2	**Timelines for Collaborative Action**

TIMELINES FOR PLANNING AND TAKING COLLABORATIVE ACTION AND EVALUATION

Steps	Week or Number of Days Working on Project											
	1	2	3	4	5	6	7	8	9	10	11	12
1. Plan collaborative action and evaluation.												
2. Take collaborative action.												
3. Determine results/impact.												
4. Evaluate teamwork.												

been determined through the coordination of more than 100 community health nursing projects for undergraduate baccalaureate nursing students over a five-year period.

Teams that have less time, have fewer weeks, or have not completed an assessment with the community group have various options. They may decide to compress all the steps and focus on one type of activity. Another option is for project organizers to have preparations all ready for a team to implement and evaluate a planned activity such as workshops, a mall display, or an injury prevention presentation with schoolchildren. Teams that do a part of the process will still gain an understanding of the full process by following the information and scenarios in this text.

The importance of planning

Planning may not seem as exciting as quickly taking action to change a situation, but it can save the team from making costly mistakes. Consider the examples in Boxes 6-1, 6-2, and 6-3.

These examples identify the importance of various aspects of planning. The mall walking example emphasizes the importance of not jumping to conclusions and taking time to talk to people. The stress reduction program emphasizes the importance of

BOX 6-1	**Mall walking program**

A community health nurse was assigned to work with a seniors group that manages a shopping mall walking program. When she first attended one of their meetings, several people raised the issue that they can no longer walk as fast as they want. They discussed the increased popularity of the program, especially among seniors in wheelchairs and using walkers. A working group was organized to deal with the issue. At the first meeting of the working group, the nurse presented the group with a plan that placed people into walking periods according to how mobile they were. She had separate times for people with wheelchairs, walkers, or canes; for unassisted slow walkers; and for fast walkers. Her plan was met with stunned silence. She had not considered that people want to walk with friends.

BOX 6-2	**Stress reduction program**

In a case study titled "Why Do We Do What We Do," Kreuter, Lezin, Kreuter, & Green (1998) described the situation of a new health promotion practitioner implementing a stress reduction program for women working in a factory. The new practitioner felt that she had done a good job because the women enjoyed the program and learned how to relax. Later she learned that the geographical area where she worked had high rates of stroke, hypertension, infant mortality, and teen pregnancy, and that for each of these situations research had identified effective interventions. The case study emphasized the importance of having and following agency goals and objectives that address issues that will make a difference in the health of the population.

considering the major factors that affect the health of the people living in the community before embarking on a program. These factors include morbidity and mortality statistics for the region and the mandate of the agency. The examples from everyday life emphasize that although planning may be taking place, the right people need to be involved to make effective decisions.

Frequently in the community, health promotion depends on a variety of factors and requires input from people in different organizations. Planning brings together people with different views to work out feasible, worthwhile outcomes. In the process, the participants become collaborators in the project by forging a relationship that is important for the success of the project. With that relationship and a plan, the team and collaborators can stay on track through the many difficulties that are a natural part of working in the community.

The ability to plan and revise a project with the community is the most challenging aspect of working in the community. The community health nursing process has the same components of the nursing process as those used with individuals and families, but it is much more complex. Creativity, critical thinking, negotiation, teamwork, and clear written and verbal communication are some of the necessary skills for planning using the community health nursing process.

Step 1: Plan

Planning involves the team, collaborators from the community of interest, and stakeholders working together. Because project organizers and collaborators are the people who will know if the plan is thorough and feasible, they need to be included and their feedback should be sought at the end of the planning step.

The following are the substeps in planning. Although the substeps are numbered, the process is best represented by a dance of "two steps forward, one step back" rather than a "step-by-step" progress.

1. Plan:
   a. Assess/reassess.
   b. Set priorities.

    c. Identify goal.

    d. Identify strategies and associated theories and research.

    e. Identify products and activities with timelines.

    f. Identify administrative objectives for the pilot test and final products with associated evaluation measures.

    g. Identify specific objectives and associated evaluation measures.

Assess/reassess

A short assessment or reassessment may be necessary if the information on the community is not available or is out of date. The amount of time spent on assessment or reassessment depends on the previous involvement with the community of interest and stakeholders and the amount of change that has occurred since the previous involvement. This is the only substep that will vary according to the previous involvement of the team with the community. Teams who are continuing after doing an assessment will usually need less reassessment time than teams starting a new project at the planning stage.

Continuing a project

Teams that have completed an assessment with the community group need to take time to quickly reassess the situation. Although the team usually will have determined the present situation and preferred situation and compiled possible action statements, they will need to reassess this information to ensure that the action statements are still relevant.

Reassessment is particularly important if there has been a lengthy period between when the assessment was finished and planning was started, project members have changed, the particular people in the community of interest have changed, or a new issue has arisen. For example, the team may have done the assessment with a teacher and students in one class; however, the collaborative action is to be with teachers and students in other classes. In those situations, the team needs to establish new working relationships. Without the relationships or knowing what has changed in the situation, the planning would be like building on sand.

Starting a new project

If the team is starting a new project at planning, the beginning of Chapter 3 can be used for guidance in establishing relationships within the project and community. The project organizers will probably provide some potential issues and possible action statements that can be used in planning. Alternatively, issues can be determined from policy documents such as state documents based on "Healthy People 2010" (U.S. Department of Health and Human Services, 2000) or "Healthy Canadians: A Federal Report on Comparable Health Indicators 2002" (Health Canada, 2002). Chapter 5 explains how to determine the present health situation and preferred health situation and how to determine issues for action and possible action statements.

In addition to determining the issues, a quick assessment provides the team with the opportunity to learn about the community and to begin to establish a relationship with community members. A modified orientation to the community including a windshield survey, interviewing key informants, and attending meetings (Chapter 4) will provide connections to the community members and stakeholders that are invaluable in developing realistic plans to the community. The expectation is that community members will be recruited as project collaborators.

Set priorities

Planning must be based on a fairly thorough understanding of the barriers, the strengths, and the preferred health situation of the community of interest. That information is used to prepare a list of action statements that address the different issues, recognize the strengths of the community, and identify where nursing in collaboration with the community could provide assistance. From that list, one **priority action** must be selected for the project. Within the time allocated to the short-term projects in this text, only one priority is manageable. Having more that one could mean that very little is actually accomplished.

Although only one priority is set, more than one of the action statements can be combined, especially if one type of action could address more than one issue or if a smaller and more accessible community of interest is involved. Often the action statements indicating community strengths can be combined with one or more indicating an issue for action.

After clarifying the issues to develop or revise possible action statements, the team members are ready to present the action statements to the collaborators, composed of project organizers, community members, and other stakeholders who have shown a particular interest in the project. This is the one point at which collaborative decision making must occur. Although collaboration is encouraged throughout the community health nursing process, most of the day-to-day decision making may be left to the team. However, at this point, the decision must be mutual to ensure that the action is relevant and sustainable. Priority setting requires a consideration of who will be involved in making the decisions and what process will be used. The example in Box 6-4 identifies some of the factors to consider in decision making in the community.

Decision makers in priority setting

Although planning models and frameworks usually identify a method and criteria for determining priorities, the decision makers are not always clearly identified. Two categories of people will be affected directly or indirectly by the project. The community of interest is expected to benefit directly, and the stakeholders are expected to benefit indirectly and have the resources to continue with work on the project. Although the project may eventually affect more people, these two groups are the most pertinent to small-scale projects and must be included in the decision making, especially in identifying the priority action. Because it is not feasible for everyone to take part, a few people from each group must be actively recruited to become the collaborators in the project. The categories and descriptions of people associated with the project are given in Table 5-1 in Chapter 5.

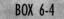

BOX 6-4	**Determining a community priority**

A small community needs to decide among building a playground, making sidewalks more accessible for wheelchairs and strollers, or expanding the municipal golf course. All have the potential to increase physical activity and social interactions and indirectly would have an impact on morbidity and mortality. Health practitioners could propose that the criteria could be the number of people in the community who would benefit and the number of people from outside the community who would find the change attractive. They could also suggest that most people in the community be given the opportunity to rate the three proposals rather than having the rating done by municipal politicians or a volunteer planning committee. The results would depend on the criteria selected, how the proposals are presented (e.g., accessibility for both strollers and wheelchairs greatly increases the numbers of people who benefit rather than if wheelchair accessibility alone was used), and the people doing the rating.

The community members who would be the recipients of the services developed by the project and the people closely associated with them, such as parents, friends, and caregivers, are best able to identify relevant action. The people who could use the results from the project in future work with the community group are able to identify useful and feasible action. These stakeholders would have been identified in your key informant interviews and could be teachers in a classroom, health professionals in community health centers, or an established coalition of people or agencies working on the issue. The inclusion of these people is important to ensure that the work done on the project continues or is sustainable after the project is completed. The two other stakeholder groups, the management of the agency or agencies sponsoring the project and the project team, are usually automatically considered part of the priority setting. All these people are important to include in some way to ensure that the decisions support action that can be sustained.

Process for priority setting

Both the process that allows people to have a say and the way information is presented are important in encouraging rational and equitable decision making. Team members have the potential to improve the health of many or of those most in need by framing the issues, providing criteria for determining priorities, and supporting a decision making process. The team develops a list of possible action statements so that the collaborators can choose one or a combination of statements that they think will make the most difference in the lives of the people in the community. The action statements can be presented at a regular or special meeting or distributed by email or through a phone call.

The team can also present criteria that can be used to determine a priority. Six criteria that take into account the community, administrators, and experienced community health practitioners have been consistently used to determine priorities (Brown, Morgan, & Burbank, 2001; Shuster & Goeppinger, 2003). Those criteria have been adapted and expanded to accommodate the use of recent action statements and to include the stakeholders, capabilities, and sustainability. Box 6-5 provides the criteria and process to consider when determining a priority.

BOX 6-5	Criteria for determining the priority for collaborative action

For each action statement, consider the evidence for the following:
1. The issues for action
2. The number (or percentage) of individuals in the community group who are or could be affected by this health problem
3. The severity of the barrier to health
4. The strengths or capacity of the community
5. The availability of potential solutions
6. Practical considerations such as individual skills, time limitations, available resources, and sustainability of the initiative as identified by the team and stakeholders

Along with the criteria, the team can present a decision-making process. When there are few possible action statements, the priority action statement may be quickly identified. When there are more possibilities and many people involved, the process requires more structure. Structure can be provided by determining that each criterion in Box 6-5 has equal weight, and each action statement will be rated on a scale from 1 (low) to 3 (high) for each criterion. All the scores for each action statement are compiled and compared. The one with the highest score becomes the priority. At this point, everyone may decide that two or three action statements could be addressed by similar action and could be combined. Examples of possible forms that could be used are provided in Application 6-1.

When planning immediately follows the assessment, validating the issues for action and determining the priority for collaborative action may seem to be the same. Both the issues for action and priority setting require that decisions be made by the people who will be affected, and both are part of the process of taking action. However, the purposes are different. The purpose of validating the issues for action is to determine whether all the important issues and strengths of the community have been identified. The purpose of priority setting, however, is to determine which action statement is most appropriate to address given the community concern and interest, impact on health, availability of feasible solutions within the available time, and sustainability.

DAYTIME SHELTER FOR THE HOMELESS SCENARIO (continued)

When the team returned from their break, several changes had occurred. The recreational therapist on the team had been replaced by a social work student, one of the agencies had closed because of lack of funding, several staff people in different agencies had changed, and a bylaw banning "loitering" on the street had been passed. With the changes, the team members felt discouraged initially because they felt that all the work they had previously completed was lost. Gradually, they started remembering the ideas and interest of the coalition members, staff people, and homeless who had worked with them during the assessment and realized that they still had those people to collaborate with them. They reminded themselves that the purpose of the project was to improve the coordination of services for the homeless. That purpose would not be achieved if they planned something that was not realistic for the actual situation.

Because they were no longer comfortable with their four action statements, they decided to do a quick reassessment of the situation. They learned that the Homeless Coalition was meeting in two weeks, and they wanted to be ready to identify the priority action statement and determine the goal and some objectives at that time.

Using the same process that they had used during the initial interviews with key informants, they fanned out to talk to as many agency staff and homeless persons as they could. They each had the list of four action statements, and for each action statement they asked if it was still important and how important it was in relation to the other three. By the second week, the team members had received responses from ten staff members and ten homeless persons using eight shelters and churches during the reassessment.

They found that the lack of food had been quite successfully addressed by phoning between agencies and by homeless persons spreading the word on the street. The food was still starchy, but little interest was shown in trying to change that at this time. The lack of warm clothing causing concern about frostbite and hypothermia was an ongoing issue that was a barrier to health. Evidence was reconfirmed by five of ten staff members and homeless participants.

The issue of greatest concern for the homeless and staff was finding places for them to be off the streets during the day because of the antiloitering bylaw. Present evidence for the issue was gathered from seven of ten staff members and seven of ten homeless participants who stated that there were ten arrests for loitering in the last week and poor attendance at daytime shelter activities. The staff explained that the homeless were required to leave most of the shelters during the day and were not admitted back in until evening because the space was used for other purposes during the day. Some agencies and churches did provide social and recreational events during the afternoon and evening, but these were poorly advertised and would not be sufficient to accommodate even a quarter of those using the night time shelters.

The strength that was identified during the original assessment was the support and communication system that the homeless developed among themselves, and this was reconfirmed by six of ten homeless participants. Based on this information and evidence, the team revised their action statements and reduced the number to three:

1. The homeless are at risk for hypothermia and frostbite related to insufficient warm clothing and footwear.
2. The homeless are at risk of arrest and social isolation related to insufficient number of daytime shelter spaces and communication about shelter opportunities during the day and early evening.
3. The homeless have a mutual support system related to helping others to find food, shelter, or social events.

At the planning session with the coalition members after the break, the team members took some time to bring each other up to date. At first everyone seemed quite discouraged, until the project leader stated: "Well, that makes the work we are doing all the more important!" Everyone agreed with that statement.

The project team presented the criteria and the priority process and their three action statements. The ten members agreed to utilize the priority process with the action statements using the form given in Application 6-1. The results of the scoring for the second action statement, which had the highest score, are also given in Application 6-1.

Once the scoring was completed, the group realized that risk of hypothermia and frostbite could also be addressed by increased daytime shelter opportunities. The priority action statement was: "The homeless are at risk of arrest, social isolation, hypothermia, and frostbite related to insufficient number of daytime shelter spaces and poor communication about shelter opportunities during the day and early evening."

DISCUSSION QUESTIONS

1. How important was the reassessment in this case?
2. If the team had not been involved previously with the community assessment, how could they determine fairly quickly the issues for action and possible action statements?
3. Could the priority setting be done without having a face-to-face meeting?
4. How could the homeless be involved in priority setting?

TABLE 6-3	Relationship of Collaborative Action Statement to Components of Plan		

PART OF ACTION STATEMENT	RELATIONSHIP	COMPONENT OF PLAN
Parts 1 and 2: Name of group and issue or strength	*provides*	Goal
Part 3: Related-to clause	*provides*	Specific objectives and activities for collaborative action
Evidence	*provides*	Evaluation measures

Identify goal

A **goal** is a broad term that provides direction toward improving the health of a particular population. The project goal, objectives, and evaluation evolve directly from the priority action statement and the evidence. The relationship among the parts of the collaborative action statement and the components of the plan (Anderson & McFarlane, 2000) are given in Table 6-3.

The goal is a revision of the priority action statement. It is the positive expression of the group's issue, barrier to health, or maintenance of a strength. A goal is simple and concise with two parts: who will be affected and what will change (McKenzie & Smelzer, 2001). A goal answers the question: How will this project provide future benefit for the population? For example, if the first two parts of the priority action statement are "Toddlers are at risk of being injured in the home," the goal would be "Toddlers are protected from home injuries." If a strength is the priority action statement, the goal is to maintain the strength.

There is a hierarchy in the order of the goal and **objectives** (McKenzie & Smelzer, 2001). The hierarchy means that the goal sets the criteria for the objectives. From another perspective, activities and objectives must be directly relevant to achieving the goal.

Identify strategies and associated theories and research

After the project goal is determined, the next decision involves identifying a type of **strategy** that could be used to achieve the goal. Strategies, theories, and research can all contribute to increasing the successful outcomes for the project. Strategies and the theories associated with the strategies tend to be consistently used to encourage change at either the individual, group (interpersonal), or community level (McKenzie & Smelzer, 2001). These levels can assist in determining a relevant strategy and associated theory.

BOX 6-6	**Health promotion strategies for short-term projects**

1. Mass communication activities
2. Educational activities
3. Counseling/tutoring and skill development activities
4. Connecting people for support (support groups, buddy system, social networks)
5. Environmental and organizational change activities
6. Community development or capacity building activities
7. Healthy public policy activities

Types of strategies

A variety of strategies can be used to promote health. For the purpose of planning, the strategies are introduced in this chapter; strategies are discussed in more detail in Chapter 7.

Strategies to promote health can be categorized in different ways. McKenzie and Smelzer (2001) identify 11 categories, The Health Communication Unit (2002) identifies 6, and the Public Health Nursing Section of the Minnesota Department of Health (2001) identifies 17. The seven categories most pertinent to short-term projects are provided in Box 6-6 and are listed at the bottom of the action workplan (Appendix C). Actions that can augment these seven strategies, such as incentives and social activities, are discussed in Chapter 7.

Mass communication activities

Mass communication involves the preparation and dissemination of health information to a large number of people. Communication strategies are implemented at the group and community level. The most simple form is a one-page poster or a fact sheet. The most complex is a multimedia campaign to change an attitude or behavior of an intended audience. The latter situation is part of social marketing, and the techniques used are not very different from those used to advertise a product on television. Mass communication strategies are important because they help a group to reach many of the goals and objectives of health promotion and reach the most people (McKenzie & Smelzer, 2001). Examples of mass communication activities are print and electronic formats such as newspapers, television, radio, newsletters, and magazines. Communication activities include billboards, pamphlets, posters, fact sheets, and product labels (McKenzie & Smelzer, 2001). Other examples are a poster display that could be used in a mall or lobby of a building and a health fair with information on various health topics.

Educational activities

Educational activities are formal or informal courses, seminars, or workshops and include educational methods such as lectures, discussion, and group work (McKenzie & Smelzer, 2001). Material can be delivered in various formats such as audiovisual, computerized, or written instructions such as a workbook. Educational strategies usually are implemented at the interpersonal or group level.

A particular type of education is called "train-the-trainer." This education involves training of and ongoing support for lay workers from the community to provide services in the community. Usually the trainers work with specific groups such as mothers and infants considered to be at risk. A specific form of train-the-trainer is called "child-to-child" and involves children in the assessment and planning process to improve their health and the health of the family or the community (The Child-to-Child Trust, 2003). Mothers have also been involved in supporting other mothers, particularly for breast-feeding.

Counseling/tutoring and skill development activities

Counseling/tutoring involves a professional or trained person working with individuals or groups to help them develop the knowledge and skills to change or learn a specific behavior and to provide them with ongoing support while they are learning (The Health Communication Unit, 2002). The counseling or tutoring may occur in a group or individually, but the purpose is individual behavior change. An example is individual or group counseling to reduce smoking or weight.

One type of counseling is called *behavior modification*, based on the stimulus response theory (McKenzie & Smelzer, 2001). An example is group counseling to reduce smoking by first identifying when people smoke the most and changing that environment (McKenzie & Smelzer, 2001). Counseling for skill development for a group would be similar to educational activities except that the counseling would have more flexibility to address individual needs and would include support.

Connecting people for support

Connecting people includes using support groups, the buddy system, and social networks. Connecting or bringing together people who share similar personal concerns or interests is a valuable strategy. Although the reason for connecting and the amount of time spent together may vary, the purpose is to provide social support. Social support involves interactions with family, friends, and practitioners who provide information, esteem, physical assistance, and emotional help (Stewart, 2000). These strategies are implemented at the interpersonal level.

Support groups form around a personally experienced concern that people want to address with others. Examples are Alcoholics Anonymous, parents of children with asthma, or newly separated or divorced women. In the buddy system, two people agree to what is expected to happen or change and what timelines will be used. A buddy system is useful for losing weight, quitting smoking, increasing exercise, or any habit that someone wants to start or stop.

Social networks link people with others who could assist them and who they could assist. To determine your own social support network, think about who you would call if your car broke down, you failed an exam, or you have just won an award. Social networks and support are especially valuable when people are new to a community, have been isolated from others, or are trying to cope with a problem or developmental change such as a new baby.

Environmental and organizational change activities

Measures taken to change the area "around" people can influence their awareness, knowledge, skills, or behavior (McKenzie & Smelzer, 2001). These changes help make the healthy choice the easy choice (Milio, 1976) and could involve the physical or social environment. These strategies are implemented at the organizational or community level.

Examples of forcing or encouraging a healthy choice in an organization are to provide only healthy food in vending machines and to allow extra time at lunch to exercise. Change can occur quickly if management decides on a new policy (McKenzie & Smelzer, 2001), such as allowing flexible work hours or providing workshops on dealing with stress.

Changing the social culture or environment can involve massive media campaigns or be as simple as recruiting the most popular youth to lead an initiative. For example, when the most popular people no longer smoke or if they start to exercise, others will eventually follow. Other environmental cues to move people in a healthy direction are posters extolling freedom in choosing a smoke-free environment or arranging transportation to a health promoting event.

Another way of starting a change in the social environment is identifying issues that affect the health of the community in a way that allows people to discuss the issues. This is often called "putting the issues on the table." For example, the number of teen pregnancies in a school might be higher than that in other schools, but no action is being taken. An initiative to encourage discussion could include a meeting with the school board, parents, or students to present the information and consider different options.

Community development or capacity building activities

Community development and capacity building activities bring people together to address issues in the community. Although the people themselves would benefit, the thrust is the benefit to a larger group or community. Organizations that work in community development bring community people and professionals together and support the development of organizational and management skills for projects (The Health Communication Unit, 2002). This is directed at community-level change.

Examples of community development are community residents working with a municipality to develop a community garden and a tenants association working with the police and a community developer to organize a neighborhood watch. Smaller community development projects are working with parents to identify the options of providing a safety barrier around a playground and working with seniors to petition for monthly health sessions with a public health nurse. Chapter 10 deals in depth with community capacity building.

Healthy public policy activities

Healthy public policy activities are focused on changing rules, guidelines, operating procedures, laws, bylaws, and legislation that impact health (The Health Communication Unit, 2002). The most common policy changes are those at the company, community, or regional level dealing with smoking. Others include the use of seat belts, bicycle helmets, speed limits, drinking and driving, air quality, and pollution. Nurses can work on policy change at all levels. For example, nurses may decide to band together through their professional associations to change policies regarding the promotion of milk formula in developing countries or the distribution of formula to all new mothers in hospitals.

Once issues have been determined, they can be reframed "into a policy issue by asking the question: What could or should be done about this issue?" (Public Health Nursing Section, 2001, p. 315). Smaller projects involved in healthy policy activities are working on changing the hours that a clinic is open, the type of services that are provided, or the cultural competence of the staff. Although most small projects would probably not start with a goal of changing policy, a small project or series of projects can initiate a change in thinking that could eventually lead to policy change. The evaluation of the outcomes of the projects is particularly useful in providing evidence to support a policy change. The implications for policy change would be included in the final recommendations section of the project report. For example, if the team found that college and university students wanted smoke-free events and participated in them, the report could recommend that their findings be presented to administration to consider changing smoking policies at events.

In addition to initiating a change in policy, small-scale projects may also be involved in implementing and enforcing a policy. The first step in enforcement is education about the policy, its rationale, and methods of complying with it (Public Health Nursing Section, 2001). For example once a no-smoking bylaw has been passed in a municipality, it must be implemented and enforced. A project could involve educational sessions for service staff in bars and restaurants on how to appropriately inform clientele about the no-smoking policy.

Naming strategies

Although seven categories are identified, there can be overlap of the activities among the categories. For example, assume that you are working with the women in a town who want to maintain a well baby clinic that has been quite popular. The public health nurse who has been running the clinic is employed by a public health agency that serves a large urban and rural area. The agency has decided to cut out all the well baby clinics. Because you are working closely with the women on an issue important to them, this could be called community development or capacity building. Because you are working to change a policy, this could be called healthy public policy activities. The activities will overlap because community capacity building identifies how you are working with the community, and healthy public policy identifies what you want to change. Because they are compatible with each other, they can be combined and the strategy can be called "community capacity building to change a public policy."

During this planning stage, all the various nuances and combinations of the strategies are not as important as identifying a strategy that will provide movement toward the goal and is at the appropriate level. The level is also very important in determining a theory that would be associated with the strategy.

Identify associated theories

Theories provide different lenses through which to view a problem and therefore different ways to address it. Theories prevent us from reinventing the wheel and allow us to improve the wheel by testing and altering the wheel for different situations (Budgen & Cameron, 2003).

TABLE 6-4	Levels of Influence and Related Theories for Health-related Behaviors

LEVEL OF INFLUENCE	THEORY OR MODEL
Community includes institutional, organizational, community and public policies	Community development, capacity building, or empowerment (explained in Chapter 10) Diffusion theory (as cited in McKenzie & Smeltzer, 2001) Population Health Promotion Model (Hamilton & Bhatti, 1996) Logic Model (explained in Chapter 13) Framework for developing health communications (National Institute for Cancer Research, 1989, explained in Chapter 7)
Interpersonal	Learning theories: Knowles' assumptions about adult learners, social learning, cognitive, humanistic, behavioral, and developmental (as cited in Meade, 2001)
Individual	Transtheoretical stages of change (explained in Chapter 7) Health Belief Model (as cited in Meade, 2001) Health Promotion Model (as cited in Meade, 2001)

When reviewing theories, consider how a theory or model could assist in accomplishing the goals and objectives of the project. The theory must also be at the same level as the strategy you have chosen. Table 6-4 provides a list of theories commonly used in health promotion, categorized by the level of influence.

Identify evidence-based interventions

During planning, appropriate databases need to be identified and searched for relevant evidence-based interventions. Considerable resources that identify best practice guidelines or that provide meta-analysis of published research in areas of great concern for researchers, such as tobacco, drinking, and injury prevention, now exist. You can find guidelines through government or public health association Web sites. Meta-analysis can be found by searching research databases available through universities or colleges. Searches for evidence-based interventions are discussed in more detail in Chapter 7.

Identify products and activities and resources with timelines

The **products** of the project are the expected results or outputs of your collaborative action. Health promotion products are usually categorized into three types: messages for communication, material that has been developed or identified, and the delivery of the messages and material (McKenzie & Smelzer, 2001). These categories also apply to the community health nursing process, with the addition of a fourth category:increased knowledge, skill, ability, and interest of organizations and community members in working together on issues that affect their health. The products include the tangible items such as written or electronic material, as well as abilities that have developed during the project.

Objectives and activities related to the products must first be determined to ensure that the products are completed by the end of the project. The development of objectives usually begins with the administrative activities and objectives (Anderson & McFarlane, 2000; McKenzie & Smelzer, 2001). Administrative activities answer the question: What tasks must be completed? (McKenzie & Smelzer, 1997, 2001). These activities are given in a time sequence to plan, implement, and evaluate the action. Sometimes these activities are called program activities (Anderson & McFarlane, 2000) or process objectives (Ervin, 2002). In this text, most of the tasks are designated as administrative activities and are listed according to a time sequence. Two administrative complex activities, conducting the pilot test and developing the final product(s), are termed administrative objectives and have associated evaluation measures.

Determine activities, timelines, and resources

During planning, the team will determine the timelines for the administrative activities and objectives and the specific people responsible for completing the activity. Two forms in Appendix C are used. The action timeline is used to plot out when the steps and substeps will begin and end. This timeline is also called a **Gantt chart** because it provides a sequencing of tasks and is easily understood by most people (Ewles & Simnett, 1999). The team can expand on the timeline given in Table 6-1. An example of a timeline for the scenario is given in Application 6-2.

Although it is useful to determine when the steps and substeps need to occur, planning the timing for activities or tasks associated with the steps is also important. The activities and tasks are described with dates and responsibilities in the right hand column of the action workplan. The planning using the timeline and right hand column of the workplan are expected to be completed in approximately five weeks and before a pilot test is conducted. If desired, the activities with times and responsibilities can be plotted on a separate Gantt chart. An example is given in Application 7-1.

The resources that are needed to complete the task also become apparent as the activities leading to the completion of the products are identified. For example, if the team is going to provide a workshop on child safety, the team will need to book a place for the workshop and find or develop education materials. One of the main reasons for developing a plan is to ensure that resources are in place when needed. Your team may have developed marvelous educational material for a workshop, but if a room has not been booked in advance, the intended audience will not receive any benefit.

Identify administrative objectives for the pilot test and final products with associated evaluation measures

Most of the administrative activities are tasks that are defined on the Gantt chart and evaluated with the results recorded in the workplan. That approach is not sufficient for the pilot test and the final product of the project. The pilot test is conducted to obtain invaluable feedback from the community of interest to help tailor the product to meet their needs. The pilot test and evaluation are discussed in more detail in Chapter 7.

The administrative objective for the pilot test needs to include criteria that indicate the number and characteristics of the participants and the type of information that they are expected to provide. For example, if you were developing information on healthy sleeping patterns for toddlers, you would probably want to test a draft of various aspects of the material with at least five mothers of toddlers. The objective would be stated as follows: "On February 14, conduct an interactive and enjoyable pilot test with at least five mothers of toddlers to determine the relevance of the content, possible layouts, and where and how the information should be provided."

The evaluation measures for the pilot test would indicate what data is collected and how it would be collected. In the example with mothers of toddlers, at least one person on the team would need a form to document the number of women who participated; their responses to questions on content, layout, delivery and location; and some measure of their enjoyment, such as asking them or documenting laughter and involved discussion.

The administrative objective of the expected products for the projects in this text have at least two criteria: 1) the products are relevant (useful) for the community of interest and stakeholders, and 2) the products have been developed collaboratively. To determine relevancy, evaluation measures would include questions on usefulness or observations of use by the community members and by stakeholders. Collaborative development could be substantiated by a summary from the workplan of the people who have been involved throughout the project.

DAYTIME SHELTER FOR THE HOMELESS SCENARIO (continued)

After determining the priority action statement with the Homeless Coalition members, the project team felt they now had a clear direction that dealt with the most pressing concern of the homeless. They were ready to convert parts 1 and 2 of the action statement "The homeless are at risk of arrest, social isolation, hypothermia, and frostbite" into the goal "The homeless are at decreased risk of arrest, social isolation, hypothermia, and frostbite."

The decision that needed to be made now by the project team and members of the coalition was the type of strategy that would address the related-to clause "an insufficient number of daytime shelter spaces and communication about shelter opportunities during the day and early evening." They felt they could work with the staff of the shelters to identify the events and accommodations that were available and determine the way to communicate the information. They decided that educational activities using a train-the-trainer approach was a good description for what they wanted to do.

They had some difficulty deciding on the level of influence for their project. An educational strategy is usually implemented at the interpersonal level; however, they were working with several organizations across the city to improve communication. They decided that they were working at both the interpersonal and community levels of influence. At the interpersonal level, Knowles' principles of adult learning and social influence theory would be useful; at the community level, the framework for health communication would be applied.

They attempted a literature search using the databases available through their organization. Based on the past experience of their project leader, however, they did not expect the search to be fruitful, and that proved to be the case. They expected that they would be relying on the theories and framework for health communication and the advice of their project leader.

The next decision was to determine the products that they would develop. They thought about how information on activities and daytime shelter could be easily displayed and updated. An electronic activity and shelter calendar was the answer. The shelter staff would need to learn about collecting the information and how to keep the calendar updated each month.

The team wondered if they would have sufficient time to complete the project. The project had ten weeks left. The team needed two weeks to complete the evaluation and report, so they had eight weeks to complete their activities. After discussing the issues among themselves and with their project leader, they felt that it would take them approximately a month to collect the information and develop a process and another month to work with the staff in the homeless shelters. Therefore, they proposed to the coalition *members that in two months they would collaborate with the staff of the agencies to deliver a calendar of daytime shelter and activities that would be updated monthly. The coalition members felt that the information and poor communication process would be very useful. Each coalition member said that they would ensure that the staff in their agencies would work with the team. As they discussed the products, they also indicated how the homeless could be included. The products of the project would include an electronic copy of an activity and daytime shelter calendar that would be updated monthly by shelter staff and the homeless.*

Now that the team had the final products identified, they started to work backward in time to determine what would need to be in place each week. They felt that they would need to have a workshop with the staff and homeless to pass on the information and therefore would need to book a room. At this point, they did not yet have a clear understanding of what they needed for the workshop or how they would involve the staff and homeless before the workshop. They had more details on what they needed to do immediately to collect the information on daytime activities. Their project leader assured them that this was usual, and they would develop more specific details once they started taking action.

As the team was working through all these decisions and documenting them in the timeline (Application 6-2) and workplan (Application 6-3) they felt frustrated by the paperwork. They eventually realized the usefulness of having things written down and distributed to coalition members when they had to change several activities and dates because of time conflicts. Their project leader explained that the amount of paperwork is heavy in a short-term project because everything happens within a short period of time and requires a coordinated effort. Documentation and activity in projects that occur over longer periods are more balanced.

As they were working on planning the activities, they also developed the administrative objectives and evaluation measures for the pilot test and final products. These were documented in the workplan. Although they defined the objectives and evaluation measures, they expected that there would be some changes by the time they developed and tested the evaluation measures. At the end of four weeks the team had completed the timeline shown in Application 6-2 and the workplan in 6-3.

DISCUSSION QUESTIONS

1. What is the purpose of having a goal for a project when it is something that is not measured?
2. Was there another theory or model that could have been used?
3. When they explained the project to family and friends, do you think the team members would talk about the goal or the products that were going to be developed?
4. Why was it important to develop a plan so early?
5. What was useful about planning activities in the workplan rather than just using the timeline?

Identify specific objectives and associated evaluation measures

A project objective is a measurable step toward achieving the goal. Project objectives build on the administrative activities and objectives and each other to bring about a change. They are milestones along the way to completing the activities that indicate what change is expected. Objectives used in planning large health promotion programs are 1) administrative activities and objectives, 2) learning objectives, 3) behavioral objectives, 4) environmental objectives, and 5) program objectives (McKenzie & Smelzer, 2001). All the objectives except program objectives, which are long term, will be discussed and applied in this chapter. However, not all will be relevant to every project. Just as the action statements took time and several revisions to improve clarity, the objectives are frequently revised.

TABLE 6-5	Comparison of Administrative Objectives to Other Types of Objectives

ADMINISTRATIVE ACTIVITIES/OBJECTIVES	LEARNING, BEHAVIORAL, AND ENVIRONMENTAL OBJECTIVES
The team will present information on the different methods to communicate information.	100% of the shelter staff will identify two types of communication methods (knowledge learning objective).
A team member, _____ (specify name), will book rooms for the workshop.	The percentage of the homeless attending day-time events will increase by 10% (behavioral objective).
The team will organize a meeting with agencies providing shelter spaces for the homeless to discuss how to increase the number of spaces.	The percentage of the homeless sheltered during the day will increase by 10% (environmental objective).

Parts of a well-written objective

A well-written objective has four parts (McKenzie & Smelzer, 2001):

1. *Who* is expected to respond or change?
2. *What* response or change is desired? (outcome)
3. *When* will the response or change occur?
4. *How much* change will occur?

The "who" in each objective must be specific to the community of interest. For example, the who could be defined by a geographical location, age, gender, and relationship to other people, such as "mothers of toddlers attending the East End play group."

To specify the desired change, the verbs used in writing objectives must be explicit. For example, precise verbs such as "to identify," "to state," "to list," or "to compare and contrast" would be used instead of less precise verbs such as "to understand" and "to realize" (Anderson & McFarlane, 2000; Ervin, 2002).

Some verbs are appropriate only for administrative activities. For example, verbs associated with activities that will be done by the project team, such as "to provide," "to develop," and "to perform" are not to be used in objectives defining impact or outcome (Ervin, 2002). A comparison of the administrative activities/objectives to the other objectives is given in Table 6-5.

Objectives also need to specify both a time deadline and the amount of change that is expected to occur. These dates and figures often are a "best guess" or a reasonable expectation and need to be determined through discussion with the project organizers and collaborators.

The SMART acronym presented in Box 6-7 provides an additional method with which to assess an objective. The parts of a well-written objective and the SMART criteria share some common features. Both identify time and require that who and what are specific and measurable. These parts of the objective can be assessed by people not familiar with the situation. However, the SMART criteria have two additional terms, *appropriate* and *reasonable,* that may be determined only by people familiar with the actual situation. For

BOX 6-7	**SMART criteria for a well-written objective**

Specific—clear
Measurable—provides sufficient information to determine if a change has occurred
Appropriate—relevant for the situation
Reasonable—sensible and realistic
Timed—deadline for expected change

example, the following objective has all the parts and is specific and appears measurable: "By January 30, 20% of the youth attending South Bend School will be aware of the February workshop on combating media advertising targeting youth." The objective would be inappropriate and unreasonable if the situation at the school did not permit a simple way to count the number of students who knew about the workshop.

Types of project objectives

Six types of objectives build on each other to bring about change. The first four are learning objectives, which detail the educational or learning needed to achieve the desired behavior change and are based on the educational and organizational assessment of the PRECEDE-PROCEED model (as cited in McKenzie & Smelzer, 2001). They answer the question: What learning factors must be considered to prepare people to make the change? Learning objectives build from 1) awareness objectives, to 2) knowledge objectives, 3) attitude or appreciation objectives, and finally to 4) skill or ability objectives (McKenzie & Smelzer, 2001).

The behavioral/accomplishment and environmental objectives build from the learning objectives. These objectives answer the question: "What behaviors must be learned to deal with the problem and how must the environment be changed?" (McKenzie & Smelzer, 1997, p. 154).

The six project objectives are awareness, knowledge, appreciation, ability, accomplishment, and environmental. Each of the objectives is written to include what, who, when, and how much. The sequence of the objectives is displayed in Figure 6-1.

The sequence displayed in Figure 6-1 indicates that an awareness objective would be completed before a knowledge objective, a knowledge objective before an appreciation objective, and so on. In practical terms, this means that the time deadline in the lower objective is earlier than the time deadline in the next higher objective. This time sequence is used to allow time for higher objectives to build on earlier ones, rather than expecting that all objectives can be accomplished on one day or at one event.

To build toward the goal, the "who" in the awareness, knowledge, appreciation, ability, and accomplishment objectives must include some of the same people. For example, if the awareness objective is that mothers of toddlers are aware that safety measures exist, the ability objective must talk about the ability of mothers of toddlers, not the ability of health educators to teach mothers.

When there are two different groups who could benefit from the project, the team, community members, and stakeholders need to carefully consider their focus. In most short term projects, there is not sufficient time to address the needs of two groups separately. For

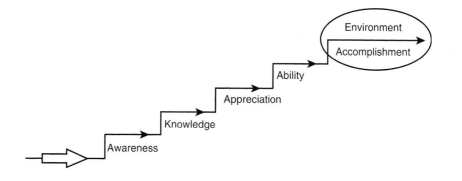

FIGURE 6-1. Sequence of six project objectives.

example, if a team is placed with an organization providing outreach services to a community comprised mostly of newcomers to the country, they may have found that the community has need of health information written in plain language and that the practitioners do not understand the particular needs of the newcomers. Each action on its own could consume the time available to the project. The team can decide to work mainly with one group or to combine the two groups in all the objectives. If the needs of one group are not addressed in the project, a recommendation could be that those needs could be addressed in a subsequent project. Another option is to include the provider group in the environmental objective. In the latter situation, the collaborative development of health information written in plain information could be the focus and the acceptance of the need to use and distribute the health information by the practitioners could be the environmental objective.

Not every project will use all six objectives. For example, mass communication strategies using social marketing may work only at the levels of awareness and knowledge. However, the project would be able to reach a great number of people. In other situations, people may already have gone through the steps of awareness, knowledge, and appreciation and want to gain some skill and ability. Although the initial objectives may not require a lot of time or effort, they should be included to ensure that people are ready to make changes.

Awareness objective

Awareness is the least complex of the objectives in terms of time, effort, and resources (McKenzie & Smelzer, 2001). However, unless people are aware of an issue, they will not be interested in learning more about it. For people to become involved in your plan, they need to know about the topic and what the team expects to do.

Because awareness is the first step in all action for change and takes little effort by participants and few resources from the team, every project should include an awareness objective. This objective would have the highest percentage of involvement of all the objectives. For example, if your team was working with 30 mothers of toddlers in a parent resources center, a reasonable objective would be that by January 30, 100% of mothers are aware that a workshop on safety issues is being planned. Activities with which to achieve the awareness objective could include information spread by word of mouth, posters, a media campaign, or a short speech.

Knowledge objective

Once people are aware of a health concern, they must expand their knowledge about the concern (McKenzie & Smelzer, 2001). The knowledge should contain information on various options or aspects of the concern that could be addressed. Using the previous example, a knowledge objective could be that by February 14, 50% of mothers are aware that the workshop will include different types of safety issues and where and when it will occur.

Similar to the awareness objective, every project should include a knowledge objective. Usually people are not interested in just being aware of an issue; they want to have some details. Activities to achieve the knowledge objective include those for the awareness objective, plus pamphlets, a fact sheet, or a newspaper article.

Appreciation objective

Appreciation means that people have developed an attitude that encourages them to deal with the concern (McKenzie & Smelzer, 2001). To develop an appreciation that they can take action on a concern, people need to think that action is possible and will be worthwhile. An appreciation objective for the previous example could be that by February 28, 40% of mothers will attend the safety workshop. This objective implies that the women think the workshop will provide them with something that will be beneficial to them and their care of their children.

Appreciation requires more commitment from participants and more resources from service providers. Therefore, communication projects using social marketing would not be expected to reach the appreciation objective or beyond. Also, projects that have only short, one-time contact with different people would be unlikely to have an appreciation object. However, both types of projects can reach many people and move some of them toward healthy behavior change.

Ability objective

To engage in health-enhancing behavior, people need to have the necessary skills and ability (McKenzie & Smelzer, 2001). For most people the development of skills and ability is difficult but can be greatly enhanced by learning with others under the direction of an experienced instructor. The level of skill and ability can vary, as anyone who has learned how to give an injection or to ski can attest to. For this objective, people would be expected to demonstrate their ability. In the example, an appropriate ability objective would be that by February 28, 30% of mothers demonstrate the ability to follow child-proofing procedures.

Accomplishment objective

Accomplishment is a behavior incorporated by the community of interest or the stakeholder that will resolve the health problem and indicates a definite move closer to the project goal (McKenzie & Smelzer, 2001). Accomplishment is at a higher level of competence than the ability objective and encourages people to include the change in their daily lives. Changes include those related to maintaining the new behavior, coping, prevention, self-care, and utilization (McKenzie & Smelzer, 2001). In the example, the accomplishment objective could be that by March 14, 20% of mothers are accomplished in incorporating more safety measures into their daily routine.

Environmental objective

Environmental objectives are changes that indicate a reduction of the social, physical, and/or psychological factors contributing to the health problem (McKenzie & Smelzer, 2001). This objective identifies that the environment needs to support healthy behaviors. The "who" in the environmental objective is probably different from that in the other objectives and could include the project team. In the example, an environmental objective could be that by February 28, the Parents' Resource Center provides bus passes for the safety workshop, or the team identifies resources or a process that could provide transportation or incentives in the future.

At a broader level, environmental change includes the area surrounding people, such as air and water quality, access to healthcare, and the social climate (McKenzie & Smelzer, 2001). An example of the latter situation could be intensive social marketing that leads to less tolerance for smoking. At the community or system level, the environmental objective usually requires a change in policy, such as designating a portion of cigarette taxes for social marketing or establishing parenting resource centers according to the number of families in the population.

Develop associated evaluation measures

Evaluation measures are developed at the same time as the objectives. This ensures that the objective is measurable and that feasible evaluation measures are available. Impact evaluation is used with the six short-term project objectives (McKenzie & Smelzer, 2001) described earlier. Evaluation measures include both the data that is required to measure whether the change occurred and a process to collect the data. In comparison to objectives, descriptions of evaluation measures do not include any numbers or percentages. Evaluation is discussed in more detail in Chapter 7.

In Table 6-6, possible evaluation measures for the example of mothers of toddlers are given.

DAYTIME SHELTER FOR THE HOMELESS SCENARIO (continued)

After the team had completed the goal and administrative activities, they looked at the objectives, which are also based on the related-to clause. The first question they needed to consider was who would be doing the learning and making the behavior change. Because they had decided that the homeless could be included, they would be working with volunteers from the shelter staff and the homeless who use the shelters. For the environmental objective, the "who" would be the agencies providing new daytime spaces.

As they were developing the objectives, they kept checking their ideas with coalition members and the data from their assessments to be certain that they were consistent with the issues from the community. After numerous changes, they developed the following list of their objectives and associated evaluation measures and documented them in their workplan in the fifth week of their project.

Awareness: *By February 8, at least one staff member and homeless person in each agency will be aware that daytime shelter opportunities and activities for March and April are being collected.*

Evaluation: Document from phone call or visit to each agency whether each person knows about the collection of daytime shelter information.

| TABLE 6-6 | Examples of Evaluation Measures for Objectives |

OBJECTIVE	POSSIBLE EVALUATION MEASURES
Awareness: By Jan. 30, 100% of mothers will be aware that a workshop on safety issues is being planned.	Ask each mother in turn whether she is aware of safety issue and document response, or Ask the group of mothers to indicate by a show of hands whether they are aware of safety issues and document response.
Knowledge: By Feb. 14, 50% of mothers will be aware that the workshop will include different types of safety issues and will know where and when it will occur.	Develop a short questionnaire on the three types of issues and distribute the questionnaire before and after information sessions.
Appreciation: By Feb. 28, 40% of mothers will attend the safety workshop.	Document the number of women attending the workshop.
Ability: By Feb. 28, 30% of mothers will demonstrate the ability to follow child-proofing procedures.	Prepare a checklist of the most important items. As part of the workshop, arrange an actual situation in which women demonstrate child-proofing ability. Alternatively, ask each woman which child-proofing procedures she already does and which she needs to do. In both situations, check off items that were addressed.
Accomplishment: By March 14, 20% of mothers will be accomplished in incorporating more safety measures into their daily routine.	Use the same checklist from evaluation of the ability objective. After the workshop, contact the women to determine whether they are using more safety measures. Indicate additional safety measures being used.
Environmental: By Feb. 28, the Parents' Resource Center will provide bus passes for the safety workshop.	Document whether the bus passes were available and how easy it was for the women to get the bus passes.

Knowledge: *By February 8, at least one staff member and homeless person in each agency will* know *why the daytime shelter and activities are being collected and who is involved.*

Evaluation: Document from phone call or visit to each agency whether each person can answer the following question: Why are the daytime shelter and activities being collected and who is involved in the collection?

Appreciation: *By February 15, at least one staff member and homeless person in 75% of the agencies will agree to participate in the daytime shelter/activity calendar project, and one person will agree to coordinate the project.*

Evaluation: Document from phone call or visit the name and status of the people who are volunteering as contacts for the agency and coordinator for the project.

Ability: *By March 7, at least one staff member and homeless person in 75% of the agencies will know which daytime activities to collect from other staff members and where to submit the list.*

Evaluation: Both volunteers in each agency can answer the following questions: Which activities need to be collected? What information on each activity needs to be collected? When will the information be available? How is the information passed on?

Accomplishment: *By March 21, at least one staff member and homeless person in 75% of the agencies will submit their daytime shelter and activities for April, and the coordinator will prepare a draft of the updated calendar for April.*

Evaluation: Document the number of agencies submitting information. Have the coordinator demonstrate/explain how the information was obtained and how the calendar was updated. Document the explanation and attach a copy of the draft.

Environmental: *By March 14, 75% of agencies will have posted the activity calendar for March, and 20% of staff members and homeless persons will know about the calendar.*

Evaluation: Visit each agency and document the number with calendars posted and the number of staff members and homeless persons viewing or knowing about the calendar.

The team found that when they were working on one set of objectives or evaluation measures, they kept having to return and revise previously written ones. They knew that the percentages they were using were just an educated guess. If they had been working in an area with a considerable research base, such as smoking reduction, they could possibly have used figures that were based on evidence.

Because the identification of the specific objectives is the last substep in planning, they were ready to complete the step by summarizing the results for the planning. The project leader was pleased with their plan because the team had developed all the components by consulting with coalition members and referring back to their reassessment data from the staff and homeless. They documented the comments they had received in the results column across from step 1 in the workplan.

At first they felt frustrated with the development of the objectives and evaluation measures. They really just wanted to get started. However, by the time they were working on the objectives for appreciation and accomplishment, they realized that the objectives provided a base for material that they had to develop for the workshop and training for the coordinator. As they kept working on their plan, they found that certain team members developed expertise in different areas and kept them on track.

DISCUSSION QUESTIONS

1. How important is the "who" in each objective?
2. Why were the percentages in the awareness and knowledge objectives greater than those in the higher level objectives of appreciation and ability?
3. Explain why having knowledge about something does not also mean that you have the ability to use the knowledge.
4. Are there other measures that could be used to evaluate the objectives?
5. How is each objective linked to the previous and following objectives?

Teamwork during planning

The team dynamics during planning can be quite difficult because of the number and types of decisions that must be made. Decisions during planning must be made in a relatively short period of time on the basis of a minimal amount of information. Another difficulty is maintaining timely communication while decisions are being made. Although there is a tendency to avoid evaluation when relationships among team members could be strained, this is when a team evaluation could get the relationship into working order.

Decision making

Often during planning, teams will think that they are being pushed to make decisions when they are not ready. Their project leader could be telling them to book a room in two months, before they even know what they will be doing in the room. Although the project leader is aware of the scarcity of rooms, the team is wondering whether they will be holding a workshop or a health fair. A similar situation involves booking agenda time into a meeting that occurs once every month or two. The best decision is to follow the advice of people who have done this before. Initially the team may not be aware of the limited resources or the importance of having time to present at a meeting.

Your team may also be pushed to make planning decisions simply to allow you more time to take action. Although planning is important, it can consume a considerable amount of time. Even with carefully considered plans, a change or an event in the community can make plans redundant. For example, a bus strike, a hurricane, an epidemic such as severe acute respiratory syndrome (SARS), or a cut in funding could mean that the plans would need to change. Again, follow advice and the suggested timetable shown in Table 6-1 to determine the amount of time you should devote to planning.

Another aspect of the initial planning decisions is that they can be changed. Sometimes inconsistencies or conflicts become apparent only after decisions are made. Also, difficulties can occur while taking action. In both situations, everyone reviews the plans and makes adjustments.

Communication

While you are planning, you are often making decisions based on a limited amount of information. Although your team may feel uncomfortable distributing tentative ("half-baked") decisions, communication of what your team is thinking is important to alert others to provide you information on possible conflicts or opportunities. Questions that you want to pose to the people on your distribution list can be put at the end of the weekly summary (Appendix C).

The workplan (Appendix C) can be attached and distributed with the weekly summary as early as the second or third day of work on the plan. Be certain to change the revision date at the top of the workplan. You will also find it useful to include the date with the page number.

After you receive feedback on your workplan, be certain that all team members are aware of the feedback and are involved in making changes based on the feedback. Interruptions in communication can occur if a person replies only to the person who sent the email or other communication document rather than replying to all who are involved in the project.

Team evaluation

An evaluation of the team members' roles and responsibilities and the functioning of the team should occur at least halfway through the collaborative action project or sooner if designated in your team agreement. You will note that the team working on the homeless project evaluated their teamwork every second week (see Application 6-3). If the team has just started to work together, by this point the members may be busy trying to avoid any confrontation with each other. However, to effectively carry out the project and especially to be able to work with people in the community, the team members need to develop a working relationship with each other. That means bringing up differences, listening to each other, and probably finding new ways to relate that allow the team to function effectively.

Chapter 2 explains in detail, with examples, how to deal with the storming process. Without storming to bring out differences and free up energy for the project, the team and the project will only limp along. Teams that have unresolved issues also have a tendency to blame other people for their problems. A steady litany of complaints can be a clue for the need to go through conflict resolution described in Chapter 2. The results of the team evaluation are included in step 4 of the workplan (Appendix C).

Summary

Planning is not optional when one works in the community; it is a necessity. As Benjamin Franklin said, by failing to prepare, you are preparing to fail. Planning with others for activities that will occur over weeks or months lays the groundwork not only for what will be done but also for how you relate to each other. The process of planning provides both direction and flexibility to deal with unforeseen barriers and to capitalize on unexpected opportunities. Most important of all is the fact that planning provides the team with a shared vision to achieve the desired outcomes during action and evaluation.

PRACTICE AND APPLICATION

1. In the homeless scenario, what evaluation forms and processes are used in more than one objective?

2. Using action statements that you have developed from a community assessment or from the information in Chapter 5, determine and document the following in a workplan:
   a) A priority action statement with the community group
   b) The project goal
   c) The administrative activities
   d) The project objectives and associated evaluation measures

3. Using available Internet sources, determine a relevant theory and research for the following:
   a) Smoking initiation by teens
   b) Weight reduction

REFERENCES

Anderson, E., & McFarlane, J. (2000) *Community as partner* (3rd ed.). Philadelphia: Lippincott.

Brown, D., Morgan, B., & Burbank, P. (2001). Community health planning, implementation and evaluation. In Nies, M. & McEwen, M. (Eds.). *Community health nursing* (3rd ed.) (pp. 102-126). Philadelphia: W.B. Saunders.

Budgen, C., & Cameron, G. (2003). Program planning, implementation, and evaluation. In J. Hitchcock, P. Shubert & S. Thomas (Eds.) *Community health nursing: Caring in action* (2nd ed. pp. 369-412). Albany, NY: Delmar.

Child to Child Trust, (2002). The child to child approach. Retrieved June 4, 2004 from http://www.child-to-child.org/about/approach.html.

Ervin, N. (2002) *Advanced community health nursing practice.* Upper Saddle River, NJ: Prentice Hall.

Ewles, L., & Simett, I. (1999). *Promoting health, a practical guide.* London, UK; Bailliere Tindall.

Hamilton, N., & Bhatti, T. (1996). Population health promotion model. Retrieved June 4, 2004 from http://www.hc-sc.gc.ca/hppb/phdd/php/php.htm.

Health Canada. (2002) Healthy Canadians A Federal Report on Comparable Health Indicators 2002. Retrieved June 4, 2004 from http://www.hc-sc.gc.ca/iacb-dgiac/arad-draa/english/accountability/indicators.html.

Kreuter, M., Lezin, N, Kreuter, M., & Green, L. (1998). *Community health promotion ideas that work*. Sudbury, MA: Jones and Bartlett.

McKenzie, J., & Smeltzer, J. (2001). *Planning, implementing and evaluating health promotion programs* (3rd ed). Needham Heights, MA: Allyn and Bacon.

McKenzie, J., & Smeltzer, J. (1997). *Planning, implementing and evaluating health promotion programs* (2nd ed). Needham Heights, MA: Allyn and Bacon.

Meade, C. (2001). Community health education. In M. Nies & M. McEwen (Eds.). *Community health nursing: Promoting the health of populations*. (3rd ed., pp. 129-169) Philadelphia: W.B. Saunders.

Milio, N. (1976). A framework for prevention: changing health-damaging to health-generating life patterns. *American Journal of Public Health, 66*, 435-439.

Public Health Nursing Section (2001). *Public health interventions-Applications for Public Health Nursing Practice*. St. Paul: Minnesota Department of Health.

Shuster, G., & Goeppinger, J. (2003). Community as client: Assessment and analysis. In M. Stanhope & J. Lancaster (Eds.), *Community and public health nursing* (6th ed, pp. 342-373). St. Louis: Mosby.

Stewart, M. (2000). Social support, coping, and self-care as public participation mechanisms. In M. Stewart (Ed.), *Community nursing: Promoting Canadians' health* (2nd ed., pp 83-104). Toronto: W.B. Saunders.

The Health Communication Unit. (2002). *Health promotion planning*. University of Toronto, Centre for Health Promotion. Retrieved June 4, 2004, from http://www.thcu.ca/infoandresources/planning.htm.

U.S. Department of Health and Human Services. (November 2000). Healthy People 2010: Understanding and Improving Health (2nd ed.). Washington, DC: U.S. Government Printing Office. Available at: http://www.healthypeople.gov/.

WEB SITE RESOURCES

The Child-to-Child Trust: http://www.child-to-child.org. Provides a description of the child-to-child approach and lessons that are appropriate for children of different ages.

Community tool box. http://ctb.lsi.ukans.edu. KU Work Group on Health Promotion and Community Development. Lawrence, KS: University of Kansas.

The Health Communication Unit: http://www.thcu.ca/infoandresources.htm. Provides documents on health planning and links to other sites in the United States and Canada.

FORMS AND SCORING IN PRIORITY SETTING

Instructions for Scoring Each Action Statement:

Please rate each item: 1, low; 2, moderate; 3, high.

CRITERIA	#1 RISK FOR HYPOTHERMIA	#2 RISK OF ARREST AND SOCIAL ISOLATION	#3 HAVE MUTUAL SUPPORT SYSTEM
1. Issue for action evidence			
2. The number (or percentage) who could be affected			
3. The severity of the barrier to health			
4. The strengths or capacity of the community			
5. The availability of potential solutions			
6. Sustainability			
Comments			

Total Score on # 2, Risk of Arrest Action Statement from Ten People

CRITERIA	RATING OUT OF 30	COMMENTS
1. The issue for action evidence	25	Concern about being arrested for loitering was the most important at the moment.
2. The number (or percentage) of individuals in the community group who are or could be affected by this health problem	28	At least 70% of the homeless had difficulty finding shelter during the day and evening and would be at risk of arrest.
3. The severity of the barrier to health	20	After arrest, often the homeless became quite depressed.
4. The strengths or capacity of the community	25	The homeless took considerable responsibility in spreading the word about food sources.
5. The availability of potential solutions	20	A communication system identifying daytime shelter and activities would 1) provide an inventory, 2) encourage more effective use, and 3) encourage development of more shelter space.
6. Sustainability	27	If a communication system is set up and shelter staff is trained, shelter staff could continue the system.
TOTAL	145/180	Score for #1 was 120 and for #3 was 130

APPLICATION 6-2

ACTION TIMELINE

Revision date: *Feb. 8, 2005*

Daytime Shelter for the Homeless

STEPS AND SUBSTEPS IN PROCESS	J 11	J 18	J 25	F 1	F 8	F 15	F 22	M 7	M 14	M 21	M 28	A 5
1. PLAN	■	■										
a. Assess/reassess	■		■									
b. Set priority	■		■									
c. Identify goal	■		■									
d. Identify strategies, theories, and research	■			■								
e. Identify products and activities with timelines in step 2	■			■								
f. Identify administrative objectives for pilot and final products with associated evaluation measures	■				■							
g. Identify project objectives and associated evaluation measures	■				■							
2. TAKE ACTION		■			■							
a. Prepare for action		■			■							
b. Conduct pilot				■	■	■						
c. Complete action						■	■					
3. DETERMINE RESULTS/IMPACT						■	■	■	■	■	■	■
a. Collect and analyze data for project objectives						■	■	■				
b. Present findings to community										■		
c. Show appreciation to collaborators											■	
d. Complete project report								■	■	■	■	■
4. EVALUATE TEAM WORK	■	■	■	■	■	■	■	■	■	■	■	■

COLLABORATIVE ACTION WORKPLAN HOMELESS EXAMPLE*

Revision date: *Feb. 1, 2004 (4th week of project)*

Daytime Shelter for Homeless

STEPS, SUBSTEPS AND ACTIVITIES (list activities under sub-steps, number and date activities across columns)	SUMMARY OF RESULTS WITH DATES
I. PLAN *Jan. 11–Feb. 8*	[complete Feb. 8]

a. Reassess
 1) Determine questions and means of reassessing situation, Jan. 11
 2) reassess, Jan. 18
	1) Decided to use action statements and same process as assessment
	 2) Developed new 3 action statements:
	   i) The homeless are at risk for hypothermia, frostbite related to insufficient warm clothing and footwear
	 Evidence: 50% have difficulty getting warm clothing, and shelter staff cite a total of 3 people almost dying from hypothermia in the previous winter, and more than 20 incidents of severe frostbite (reconfirmed by 5 of 10 staff members and homeless)
	   ii) The homeless are at risk of arrest and social isolation related to insufficient number of daytime shelter spaces and communication about shelter opportunities during day and early evening.
	 Evidence: 1) 10 arrests for loitering in last week though statements and 2) poor attendance at daytime shelter activities from 7 of 10 staff members and 7 of 10 homeless in 8 shelters and churches during re-assessment
	   iii) The homeless have a mutual support system related to helping others to find food, shelter, or social events
	 Evidence: 45% stated how they gained satisfaction passing on information or taking someone somewhere to get some help. (reconfirmed by 6 of 10 staff members and homeless)

b. Set Priority 1) determine criteria and process for priority setting, Jan. 18 2) identify priority action statement with Coalition, Jan. 25	1) Used criteria and process in text. Priority process displayed on flip chart, each person rated each action statement 2) The homeless are at risk of arrest, social isolation, hypothermia and frostbite related to insufficient number of daytime shelter spaces and communication about shelter opportunities during day and early evening
c. Identify goal Jan. 25	Goal: The homeless are at reduced risk of arrest, social isolation, hypothermia and frostbite
d. Identify 1) strategies, Jan. 25, all 2) theories, Jan. 25-Feb. 1, all and 3) research, Jan. 25-Feb. 8, Mai	1) Strategies: Education activities using a train the trainer approach 2) Theories: Learning theories and social influence (as cited in Meade, 2001), framework for health communication (National Institute for Cancer Research, 1989) 3) Feb. 1 Research: Search using key words of "communication" and "homeless" on a sociology and nursing data bases [provide specific names] provided no results. Will follow other leads and review best practice guidelines

e. Identify *1) products, 2) activities and resources with timelines, Jan. 25-Feb. 1*	*1) Product: An electronic copy of an activity and daytime shelter calendar that would be updated monthly by shelter staff and the homeless* *2) Activities for taking action identified with dates and responsibilities assigned (see step 2)*
f. Identify administrative objects for *1) pilot, and 2) final products with associated evaluation measures* *Feb. 1*	*1) Administrative objective: Pilot and evaluation measures: On Feb. 15 conduct a pilot test of the calendar with at least 3 staff and 2 homeless to determine how to depict the activities on the calendar and the size of the calendar. Evaluation: Document the number present. Prepare a check list of various symbols that could be used to depict activities and check the ones that each person likes. Record the most desired size for the calendar.* *2) Administrative objective: Product and evaluation measures: By Mar. 21, provide an activity and daytime shelter calendar that can be updated monthly by staff and homeless that was produced collaboratively and is relevant. Evaluation: Review workplan to identify collaboration and request and document comments about the collaborative effort in producing the calendar and its usefulness from the staff and homeless*
g. Identify specific objectives and associated evaluation measures *Feb. 8*	
2. TAKE ACTION *Feb. 1–Mar. 21*	

a. Prepare for action
  1) Determine information needed about daytime activities and make forms, Feb. 1–8
  2) Book rooms for workshop and final presentation, Feb. 1. Les
  3) Prepare and document procedure for collecting and recording data on monthly calendar, Feb. 8, Jan & Les
  4) Determine resources and source of resources for producing a calendar, Feb. 8–15, Jan & Les
  5) Determine and contact all agencies to obtain time, location and description of any daytime shelter, Feb. 8, Mai & Tom
  6) Identify staff person for calendar in each agency and the agency who will continue to coordinate calendar, Feb. 8–15, Mai & Tom
	1)
	
	2) Training room booked for Mar. 14, board room for presentation Mar. 21

b. Conduct pilot on calendar with at least three staff and two homeless people *Feb. 15, Mai & Tom*	

c. Complete action
  1) *Revise calendar based on feedback from pilot, Feb. 22, Jan & Les*
  2) *Record regular & occ. shelter and activities on calendar for Mar., Feb. 22–Mar. 7, Jan & Les*
  3) *Present workshop on calendar to staff, homeless and coordinator, Mar. 14*
  4) *Work with coordinator to collect updated information on shelter and activities for Apr., Mar. 7–21 Mai & Tom*

*Note: Specific information for scenario is in italics

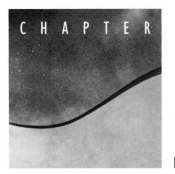

C H A P T E R **7**

Taking Collaborative Action

ELIZABETH DIEM

SUPERMARKET BACK HEALTH

Four community health nursing students were assigned to work on an injury prevention project at a large supermarket. The supermarket employed many college and university students on a part-time basis. The Health and Safety Committee of the supermarket had asked for the project because they had figures indicating a high number of work-related injuries. The store manager had agreed.

The team members had 1 day a week for 12 weeks to work on the project. For the first two weeks, the student team spent time meeting with the Health and Safety Committee and the instructor, becoming familiar with the store, and reviewing the statistics on injuries and days off work. The team found that the "stockers," the employees who moved cases of food goods and stocked shelves, had the highest number of days off work due to back pain. The stockers all worked on the night shift. A woman from the committee, Letecia, was available to work with the team members on a regular basis. By the end of the fifth week, they had produced the following elements of the plan:

Priority action statement: *Stockers have the potential for improved back health related to the interest of the Health and Safety Committee in using effective measures to reduce back injuries. Evidence: 1) Injury statistics for previous three years showing back pain as the most common cause for days off work, 2) stockers having the most days off work due to back pain, 3) no back injury prevention training available to staff working nights, 4) the Health and Safety Committee's interest in providing training and support to reduce back injuries.*

Project goal: *Stockers have improved back health.*

Final products: *By November 30, locate back injury prevention video, provide workshop on back injury, train Health and Safety Committee members to provide workshop, and conduct store contest.*

Strategy and related theory and research: *Educational activities and framework on health communication. Search Cochrane databases on back injury prevention. The* **Cochrane databases** *are housed in the Cochrane Collaboration, an international not-for-profit organization that collects and maintains regularly updated databases on health and evidence-based healthcare.*

Activities: *See Gantt chart (Application 7-1).*

Awareness objective: *By October 7, at least 75% of stockers know that they have the highest rate of time off work due to back pain and that a workshop is being planned. Evaluation: Team and Health and Safety Committee members ask stockers about the prevalence of back pain and their awareness of the workshop. Document results on a checklist.*

Knowledge objective: *By October 21, at least 50% of stockers know that the workshop will cover the prevention of back injuries and how they can attend the workshop. Evaluation: Team and Health and*

Safety Committee members ask stockers if they know what will be covered in the workshop and how and when they can take part. Document results on a checklist.

Appreciation objective: By October 28, at least 40% of stockers sign up for injury prevention workshop. Evaluation: Tally number who sign up for each workshop.

Ability objective: By November 14, 50% of participants in back injury prevention workshop for stockers have demonstrated safe lifting techniques. Evaluation: Develop checklist with each type of lifting technique. Document number in each workshop who are able to demonstrate safe lifting techniques.

Accomplishment objective: By November 21, 40% of stockers demonstrate safe lifting techniques during work. Evaluation: Observe stockers on different nights and document use of correct and incorrect lifts, use of flexibility exercises, and use of lumbar belts.

Environmental objective: By November 14, 75% of Health and Safety Committee members are trained to provide back injury prevention workshop to all shifts on a regular basis. Evaluation: Number of Committee members able to demonstrate presentation of workshop at end of training.

At the end of four weeks, the team members were quite pleased with their plan and had started on some of the activities. The Health and Safety Committee felt that the workshop was going to make a difference for the stockers and were looking forward to learning how to conduct the training. Their comments were documented on the workplan.

SCENARIO   *COLLEGE STUDENTS' SMOKING KNOWLEDGE*

The four team members were setting up their smoking display for the fourth and last time. They could not believe that they were actually doing this in a bar. The Full Jug was a bar near the college that was staffed and frequented almost exclusively by college students. Nothing in their original plans mentioned a bar. That original plan had gone through a lot of changes in the past four weeks—not in what they were to do, but in how they would do it. They would still be producing a list of topics and approaches related to smoking that interested college students for the health clinic at the college. The clinic was planning to use the list and approaches in a health-related Web site and in fact sheets.

The team had originally planned to identify the information through a display booth set up at various locations within the college. Their pilot display had been in the great hall of the college with about 20 other health-related displays. They also planned to identify topics using a questionnaire. Both the location and methods had changed, but they were still on track.

OBJECTIVES   After reading this chapter and answering the questions throughout the chapter, you should be able to

1. Apply relevant theory and evidence-based interventions in the action.
2. Develop evaluation measures.
3. Take effective action using process evaluation to adjust plans.
4. Involve collaborators in the action.
5. Document and communicate action.

KEYWORDS   Cochrane databases ■ framework for health communication ■ marketing strategy ■ recruiting ■ sustainability ■ Transtheoretical Stages of Change Model

Step 2: Take Action

The exciting part of community projects is working directly with people taking action to bring about change. Often this is the time when collaborators have more interest in becoming directly involved and become motivated to start taking over. This changeover, if it has not already happened, is necessary to sustain the actions initiated by the project. Taking action is the reward you receive from planning well. Taking action is also the "acid test" for your plan. When you are taking action, you will find out whether you planned well or whether there were situations that you did not consider or events beyond your control.

Taking action involves performing the activities you listed in your workplan. You may also choose to list these activities in a Gantt chart similar to the one in Application 7-1. You will start working on these activities even before your plan is complete. Initially, there is an overlap in planning and taking action, and then, at the end of action, an overlap with evaluation.

In the community health nursing process applied to projects, taking action on planned activities is the second step in collaborative action. The following is the second step and substeps given in the workplan (Appendix C).

Step 2: Take action

- Prepare for action.
- Conduct pilot test.
- Complete action.

As team members move into action, they need to decide what indicator of success they will use for this step. The team is expected to be working collaboratively, so an indicator of success could be that designated community members or stakeholders feel that appropriate action has been taken. Most actions will have three overlapping phases: prepare for action, conduct pilot test, and take action.

Preparation

The first activities in your plan would indicate some time to prepare for action. The first part of preparation involves completing a more extensive review of relevant theory and evidence-based interventions, making organizational arrangements, and recruiting people or marketing for the action. The second part is the development of material and evaluation measures.

Review theory

During planning in Chapter 6, you learned to identify a theory according to the level of influence of the strategy that you were planning to use (Table 6-4). During the preparation for action, you need to look more closely at the theory or model to determine what guidance it can provide to your action. Two models commonly used in health promotion practice are described in the following sections and applied in the scenarios. You can obtain

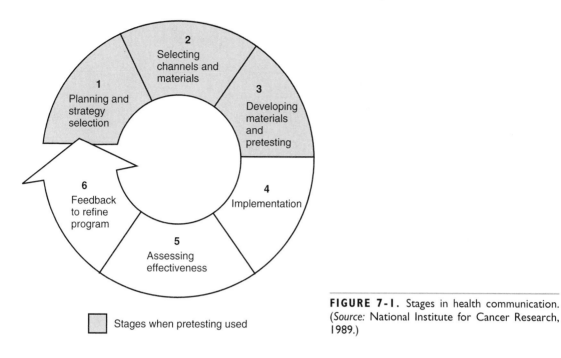

FIGURE 7-1. Stages in health communication. (*Source:* National Institute for Cancer Research, 1989.)

□ Stages when pretesting used

further explanations for the two theories by following the instructions given in the References or Web Site Resources. Sources for other theories are given in Table 6-4 in Chapter 6.

The framework for health communication

The National Institute for Cancer Research (1989) has provided a **framework for health communications** that has been used by many organizations and texts in recent years. The framework consists of six stages, which are depicted in Figure 7-1. The use of the framework fit well with projects using mass communication and educational strategies.

The first three stages of the framework represent development and the last three represent implementation. Many of the stages are similar to the community health nursing process as it would be applied to the development of health communication. The key factors included in stages 2 and 3 (National Institute for Cancer Research, 1989) are particular to health communication. The six stages are outlined in Box 7-1.

Transtheoretical Stages of Change Model

The **Transtheoretical Stages of Change Model** explains how individuals progress over time through predictable stages when adopting and maintaining health behavior change (McKenzie & Smelzer, 2001). The model uses the stages of change to integrate the processes and principles from major theories of intervention (Prochaska, Redding & Evers, 1997). The model has previously been applied to a wide variety of individual problem behaviors. These include smoking cessation, exercise, low fat diet, radon testing, alcohol abuse, weight control, condom use for HIV protection, use of sunscreens to prevent skin cancer, drug abuse, medical compliance, mammography screening, and stress management (Velicer,

BOX 7-1	**Framework for health communication**

Stage 1: Planning and Strategy Selection
Determining where to start:
- Conduct assessment to determine where to start, what data is available, what activities are presently occurring, and what is missing.
- Write goals and objectives.
- Gather new data from key informants or others who have experience in the area.

Determine the priority community of interest:
- Conduct focus groups or surveys to determine the specific community of interest and the baseline data for the tracking system.
- Determine resources.
- Draft communication strategies.
- Prepare program plan and timetable.

Stage 2: Selecting Channels and Materials
- Search for existing material that could be adapted.
- Consider what channels, such as workplace bulletin boards or email, face-to-face, or media, are most appropriate to reach the community of interest.
- Consider what formats, such as pamphlets, workbooks, or videotapes, will best suit the channels and the messages.

Stage 3: Developing Materials and Pretesting
- Consider different ways that the message can be presented.
- Determine whether the audience understands the message, recalls it, accepts it, agrees with it, and responds to the message format.
- Decide whether changes need to be made in the message or the format.
- Determine how the message could be promoted, the materials distributed, and progress tracked.

Stage 4: Implementation
- Prepare to introduce the program.
- Continue to track progress through measures such as focus groups or surveys.
- Establish process evaluation measures.
- Work with other organizations and consider working with businesses.
- Review and revise program components.

Stage 5: Assessing Effectiveness
- Consider various evaluation options according to resources.
- Determine what evaluation to do.
- Conduct outcome or impact evaluation.

Stage 6: Feedback to Refine Program
- Apply what has been learned.
- Revise program.
- Write an evaluation report.
- Share what has been learned.

Source: National Institute for Cancer Research (1989).

Prochaska, Fava, Norman & Redding, 1998). The model would be appropriate with strategies to change individual behaviour in areas such as smoking, weight control, exercise, sexual health, use of sunscreen, and other preventive behaviours.

The importance of the Transtheoretical Model is the direction that it can provide during the implementation stage. The direction is provided by finding the appropriate processes for the stage of development. This matching increases recruitment, retention, progress, process, and outcome during implementation (Velicer, Prochaska, Fava, Norman & Redding, 1998).

The Model has four constructs: 1) stages of change, 2) decisional balance between pros and cons, 3) self-efficacy between confidence and temptation, and 4) processes of change (Redding, Rossi, Rossi, Velicer, Prochaska, 1999). A detailed explanation and application in smoking cessation and stress management is provided online on the web (Cancer Prevention Research Center, 1998).

The key organizing constructs of the Model are the stages of change which allow the action to be tailored (Prochaska, Redding, Evers, 1997). Change occurs over time during specified time periods. Five stages are used: precontemplation, contemplation, preparation, action, and maintenance. The five stages are described in Box 7-2.

The second construct of the Model is decisional balance between the pros of continuing the behavior and the cons against the behavior change in relation to the stage of change. This is explained in terms of smoking (Velicer, Prochaska, Fava, Norman & Redding, 1998): In precontemplation, the pros for smoking far outweigh the cons against smoking. In contemplation, these two scales are more equal. In the advanced stages, the cons outweigh the pros. In application, this would mean that in precontemplation and contemplation the emphasis would be on providing information and processes to encourage an increase in reasons to change the behavior.

The third construct is self-efficacy related to the level of confidence and temptation that a person has to deal with different challenging situations (Prochaska, Johnson & Lee, 1998). Self-efficacy is low and temptation is high in the early stages (Prochaska, Redding, Evers, 1997).

BOX 7-2	**Transtheoretical model stages of change**

Precontemplation: Has no intention of taking action within the next six months. May be underinformed or demoralized about ability to change. Needs specialized material.

Contemplation: Intends to take action within the next six months. Aware of pros of changing but also of the cons. Can be stuck here for long periods of time. People at this stage are not ready for traditional action-oriented programs.

Preparation: Intends to take action within the next 30 days and has taken some behavioral steps, such as developing a plan, talking to a counselor, or buying a self-help book.

Action: Has changed overt behavior for less than six months. Vigilance against relapse is crucial.

Maintenance: Has changed overt behavior for more than six months. Less tempted to relapse and becoming more confident in maintaining behavior.

Source: adapted from Prochaska, Redding, & Evers (1977), Velicer et al. (1998)

The fourth construct of the Model, processes of change, are particularly applicable to implementation. The ten processes of change are the psychological and physical activities that people use to progress through the stages (Prochaska, Redding, Evers, 1997).

The Model has identified that the great majority of people are in the early stages of change. In American samples of smokers, 40% were in precontemplation, 40% in contemplation, 20% in preparation; in Europe 70% were in precontemplation, 20% in contemplation, and 10% in preparation (Velicer, Prochaska, Fava, Norman & Redding, 1998). These figures indicate the need to develop appropriate material for people in the early stages of change. Most action-orientated health programs are only appropriate for a small proportion of the population that is already preparing to change (Prochaska, Redding, Evers, 1997).

A simplified application of the Model is demonstrated in the situation of the early stages of smoking cessation with adults. Four processes—consciousness raising, dramatic relief, environmental reevaluation, and self-evaluation—are associated with the early stages (precontemplation and contemplation) (Prochaska, Johnson & Lee, 1998). Since smokers in the earlier stages are ignoring or are not immediately concerned about quitting smoking (Box 7-2), they are not drawn to situations where they can obtain information or advice. For this large group of smokers, they need to practically trip over the information or be confronted by family and friends. Tripping over the information means having it available on the media so everyone is exposed or placing it where they are likely to see it. Another approach is to provide the information to family and friends.

Media approaches and involvement of family and friends are useful for all four processes associated with the early stages (Velicer, Prochaska, Fava, Norman & Redding, 1998). For example, advertisements that show children concerned about parents' smoking followed by sources of help for smoking cessation are encouraging dramatic relief, and self and environmental reevaluation. Media strategies for environmental and self reevaluation would include using documentaries and providing healthy role models. Family and friends can be involved in increasing awareness through feedback, educational material, and confrontation. For dramatic relief, family and friends can be involved in role playing and personal testimonials. Both self and environmental reassessments can be fostered by questions posed by family or friends related to empathy, positive imagery and values clarification. As well, health practitioners have a role in asking questions, and providing information and approaches that could appeal to smokers and their families and friends.

The Transtheoretical Stages of Change Model provides direction in the design of interventions for individual behavior change both directly and through media campaigns. To effectively use the Model in long term programs, an indepth understanding of the four constructs and the desired behavior change is required. The web sites at the end of the chapter provide further resources.

Evidence-based interventions

Systematic reviews of literature on a particular topic or best practice guidelines can provide valuable direction during collaborative action. The amount of research available on a particular topic varies greatly according to the number of people who are or could be affected, the availability of research funding, and a variety of other factors. Certainly, considerable research has been done in smoking cessation. For example, in a search of all

Cochrane databases using the keywords "smoking cessation" on February 15, 2003, 1651 references were provided. In contrast, the keywords "back injury" with the limitation of "prevention" on the same databases on the same date provided 35 references.

Cochrane databases use specific criteria and a defined process to evaluate research studies in a particular topic area to arrive at conclusions relevant to practice and research. The Web Site Resources in this chapter provide sources for systematic reviews of research. Often the project organizers can provide search strategies to find relevant evidence-based interventions.

"Best" or "better" practice guidelines, which usually include an evaluation of research available in a practice area, are another source of direction for collaborative action. Often best practice guidelines can be found on the Internet on government sites, professional sites, or disease-specific sites. Potential sites are provided in the Web Site Resources at the end of this chapter.

For some projects, no appropriate systematic reviews or best practice guidelines may exist, or the research may be inconclusive. Inconclusive research includes a single study with minimal rigor or controls. When research is lacking, you can rely on a relevant theory or a framework and the advice of experienced community health nurses. Even if you do find a relevant systematic review, the information usually needs to be adapted to suit the particular situation.

Making organizational arrangements

At the same time as the theory and research are being reviewed, resources need to be organized. The first items to consider are what locations will be needed and when they will be needed. Those arrangements can take some time, especially if various people need to be reached. Often email can be used rather than the telephone to avoid "telephone tag." Project organizers often can assist with arranging accommodations.

Other considerations are the material and technology that will be needed to take action. For example, a computer, paper, and a printer are needed to produce fact sheets, pamphlets, and displays. Other resources such as a video camera could also be useful. The source and availability of these resources need to be determined. A budget for the project may be provided by the sponsoring agency, or teams may need to request funding for resources or special services such as translation or marketing. Often teams have little or no resources to develop products and feel that they may need to use a considerable amount of their personal funds to develop something that is worthwhile. Usually that is not required. There are a variety of alternatives, such as using relatively inexpensive material, seeking funding, or asking for donations of material.

Recruiting people or marketing for the action

For some projects, **recruiting** sufficient people to take part in the action can be a major part of the task. Unless the team has a group of people with whom they have been working with all along, they will need to employ some marketing strategies. **Marketing strategies** to attract people to participate in a short-term action include using social support, social activities, advertising, incentives, or competition (McKenzie & Smeltzer, 2001 are described in Box 7-3). Some of these strategies are similar to the strategies for taking action described in Chapter 6.

| BOX 7-3 | **Strategies to recruit people for the action** |

■ *Advertising:* Use of advertising requires decisions on what message will attract people and what channel will reach the community of interest. Timing also needs to be considered. Messages that will attract people include information from the remaining strategies: social support, social activities, incentives, or competition. Messages can be delivered through local or neighborhood newspapers, bulletin boards at churches or schools, the Internet, or posters in local businesses or organizations.

■ *Social support:* People can be encouraged to participate in the action because they will be with others who want to make the same changes as they do. Explanation of the support they can expect to receive needs to be in the advertising information.

■ *Incentives:* Incentives to attend could be the opportunity to win a donated door prize or each person receiving some token prize. To be effective, the incentive should be available to anyone who attends, be meaningful to the participants, and not conflict with health promotion goals (McKenzie & Smelzer, 2001). The availability of incentives needs to be clearly indicated in the advertising.

■ *Social activities:* Social activities include time when people can interact freely either with or without food, music, or entertainment. Although social activities are a form of incentive, they are likely to attract different people than those wanting a prize. The opportunity for social interaction, food, and music must be apparent on the advertising material.

■ *Competition:* The attraction for the action can involve contests between groups of people. The rules for the contest and the prizes need to be clear and fair. To be effective for recruitment, the contest needs to be described in the advertising.

Often the team already has ideas on how to attract people based on the assessment or discussions with key informants. Team members need to discuss their ideas and the strategies in Box 7-3 with collaborators to ensure that people will take part in their action. Often the marketing plan will simply be that the action takes place where the community of interest is located. In that case, the appropriate locations need to identified and booked. In other situations, the people in the community of interest may not normally congregate together. In those situations, more work in terms of advertising and other strategies is needed to attract people.

Developing or locating resource materials

Before developing any original resource material, thoroughly investigate through the project organizers, community members, and stakeholders any possible material that could be used or adapted. Resource material could include videos, fact sheets, pamphlets, computer programs, games, or electronic files with material that has been used in the past. Another source of materials is the Internet. If a relevant resource is found, the agency sponsoring the project may decide to purchase it.

Theories and research can contribute to the development of resources. Stages two and three of the framework for health communication provide some key points to consider. Other theories can also identify the type of information that should be developed. Systematic reviews and best practice guidelines can assist the team in determining what material to develop and what processes to use. However, the information from theory and research needs to be relevant to the community of interest. Include the collaborators when determining what material and processes to develop. Otherwise, the team may spend considerable time developing a resource that has not been successful in the past.

When material is developed, there will always be a trade-off between the time required to develop something that is comprehensive and something that is useful. Initially only develop material for a pilot test. After the material has been tested, more effort can be put into development if it will be used again in the future.

Even if you can obtain resources that have been developed, your team will still need to work with the material to support the use of the resources and to evaluate them. The developed material could include the schedule of events for a workshop, the groups who will be invited to participate in a health fair, and the structure of feedback sessions.

Developing evaluation measures

Both quantitative and qualitative measures are useful to indicate whether and how a change occurred or an objective was met. Many of the same tools used in the assessment (Chapter 4), such as interviews, focused discussions, questionnaires, and observation, are used in evaluation. Evaluation can include measures as simple as counting the number of people attending a session or something more complex, such as using a pre- and posttest questionnaire to determine a change in knowledge or attitude. Evaluation occurs in conjunction with the collaborative action, and therefore the evaluation measures must be identified during planning and developed during preparation for action.

Most of the evaluation measures will be collected by you or others as you document your work on the project so they should be fairly easy to record and analyze. People are usually more willing to respond verbally rather than by filling out a lengthy questionnaire, but they may not be as truthful as they would be if the evaluation were anonymous. When other people will be involved in collecting the evaluation data with you, you need to include time to provide them training and check with them often to determine whether they are collecting the data in the manner that you expected.

Similar to collection of assessment data, the collection of evaluation data for program planning requires that people are informed about who you are, the project which you are working on, how the data will be used, and the fact that they have a right not to contribute. For verbal evaluation methods, provide an explanation at the beginning of the session. For a written evaluation, provide an information letter explaining who you are, who you are working with, why you are collecting the information, and how the information will be used in planning or evaluating programs. People need to be assured that their names or specific information about them will not be asked. This is part of ethical practice.

Two types of evaluation measures are used with short-term projects. Process evaluation is used with administrative activities and objectives. Impact evaluation is used with the six project objectives.

Process evaluation

Process evaluation occurs during action to monitor and adjust the delivery (McKenzie & Smeltzer, 2001). Two types of measures are used and need to be developed in the preparation period: those based on determining quantity and those based on determining

TABLE 7-1	Example of Form to Collect Evaluation Data			
NO. FOR PARTICIPANT (DO NOT USE NAMES)	**COVER ELECTRICAL OUTLETS**	**SAFETY GATE FOR STAIRS**	**REMOVE FIGURINES**	**CLEANING MATERIAL OUT OF REACH**
1	Missed	Yes	Yes	Yes
2	Missed	Yes	Yes	Missed
3	Yes	Yes	Yes	Missed
4				

quality. The quantity measures include the number of sessions held, the number who attended, and the completion of tasks on schedule. These measures could be collected by recording the information on a simple checklist.

The quality measures involve obtaining feedback from community members or service providers on factors such as how interested they are in what you have prepared, how useful they expect it to be, and what suggestions they have to improve what is being planned. A measurement for participation could involve an observer recording on a checklist items such as the number of questions asked, people's willingness to volunteer for role playing, or tasks completed in group work. See step three in the framework for health communication for more suggestions.

As forms are developed and the data collection becomes more specific, usually the original evaluation measures need to be changed. This is expected. However, collaborators need to be consulted about the changes to ensure that the process evaluation data will be useful to them.

Impact evaluation

The data and processes to collect the evaluation measures for the six project objectives were identified during planning. In collaborative action, you need to develop the forms to collect the data and organize the procedures.

In the example from Chapter 6, the ability objective was that 30% of mothers attending a Parents' Resource Center demonstrate the ability to follow child-proofing procedures. The evaluation measures were to prepare a checklist of the most important items and, as part of the workshop, arrange an actual situation in which women demonstrate their child-proofing ability. Table 7-1 is an example of a performance checklist after three people have completed the demonstration.

SUPERMARKET BACK HEALTH SCENARIO (continued)

Shortly after they had started to work on the activities listed in their Gantt chart (Application 7-1), they wanted to make changes and put in results, but quickly realized that the chart was not designed to be an ongoing working document. They listed the activities they were working on under step 2 (take action) of the right-hand column of workplan (Appendix C). They made no changes to the Gantt chart after the fifth week of the project.

When the team members had determined that they would be using an educational strategy, they also decided that the framework for health communication (National Institute for Cancer Research, 1989) steps 2 and 3 would assist them in developing their resource material.

From their search of the Cochrane databases, they found two studies that were directly relevant to back injury prevention in the workplace: "Back Injury Prevention Interventions in the Workplace: An Integrative Review" (Karas & Conrad, 1996) and "Lumbar Supports for Prevention and Treatment of Low Back Pain" (van Tulder, Jellema, van Poppel, Nachemson, & Bouter, 2002). The first study on back injury prevention provided evidence that back school (educational sessions about back health) and exercise flexibility training programs decreased back injuries; the second study showed no consistent evidence for the use of lumbar supports. The team decided to provide information and a demonstration on preventing back injuries and increasing flexibility. They would not be recommending any back support belts. They changed each of their objectives that had "safe lifting techniques" to "safe lifting techniques and flexibility exercises."

From the framework, research, and advice from the Health and Safety Committee, they determined that they would search for a resource, probably a video no longer than 40 minutes, that demonstrated safe lifting techniques and flexibility exercises and did not include a lumbar belt. They contacted the occupational health departments of major firms and the Occupational Health Nurses Association in the city and obtained three different videos which they reviewed using their criteria. They made up a form with their criteria down the left side and the names of the videos along the top. After viewing the videos, they identified one which had all the right elements and was only 25 minutes long. However, it showed a lumbar belt. They went on the Internet and found that they could get a version without the belt. They had sufficient funds in their budget to order a copy.

While Denny and Maria were reviewing the theory and research and beginning the development of the resources, Stephanie and Jose had responsibility for the administrative arrangements and evaluation measures. Letecia worked with them. From the Gantt chart in their plan (Application 7-1), they knew that they needed to talk to the store manager about the arrangements for the workshops. They found it difficult even to arrange a meeting. Eventually, when they did and asked about a TV with a video player for the staff room, he became quite angry. He said that the stockers would be watching TV instead of doing their work. Letecia spoke up at that point and said that the Health and Safety Committee would take responsibility for ensuring that the stockers were not off work for more than two hours for the workshop. The manager calmed down and stated that they could have an hour and a half for each group, maximum, for the workshop. He was not prepared to buy a television but was willing to allow a Health and Safety Committee member to bring in one from home for the duration of the workshops. The staff room could accommodate about 20 people and could be used for the workshops and final presentation.

The subteam also had responsibility for observing and documenting the present lifting and carrying behaviors of the stockers to determine which lifts and demonstrations were needed in the workshop and to develop the evaluation form for the accomplishment objective. They did not start immediately as planned, because they wanted to include the results of the systematic reviews. Because of the research, they added the use of flexibility exercises and a lumbar (weight-lifting) belt to determine whether either was being used. They needed this information to know whether they had to concentrate on promoting flexibility exercises or discouraging the use of lumbar belts. They made up a form that collected information on 1) the number of times they saw someone lifting while bent over, 2) the observed use of lumbar or weight-lifting belts, 3) anyone seen doing any flexibility exercise, and 4) where lifting and carrying occurred.

Each person on the subteam used the form to observe the stockers during a different hour of the night shift. Staff had been told that this would be occurring and were self-conscious initially. One person asked not to be observed, and his request was respected. The subteam met to review their results and made changes to the form to include where the incorrect lifts occurred. They each spent an additional hour observing, questioning, and documenting the results.

After these separate activities were completed, the full team met to determine the material that would be included in the workshop, the administrative objectives for the pilot workshop and final products, and the evaluation measures. After considerable discussion, they realized that their objectives provided a direction for content for the workshop. To recruit for the workshop and address the awareness and knowledge objectives, they decided to prepare one-page posters on colored paper and distribute them about the work area. The Health and Safety Committee would also help by "talking up" the statistics and workshop with the stockers.

For the workshop itself, they knew they had an hour and a half to deliver a 25-minute video, a pretest and probably a posttest, and a demonstration. Because they wanted the participants to enjoy the workshops as well as learn useful techniques, they included an opportunity for them to share their experiences with back pain before the video and to have an open feedback session on their whole strategy at the end of the workshop. Team members were assigned different tasks. Stephanie and Jose, who had done the observations, were assigned to prepare the demonstrations and develop a demonstration checklist. The person working on the pretest was also to complete the posttest. The person who would be leading the workshop would develop a schedule and script.

They moved on to elaborating what they wanted to achieve during the pilot workshop. They had written in their Gantt chart that they would conduct two pilot workshops with at least seven participants in each. That still seemed to be reasonable. After reviewing stage 3 of the framework for health information, they decided that they wanted to obtain the following information from the pilot workshop: 1) clarity of pre- and posttest questions, 2) appropriateness of video, 3) timing, 4) enjoyment, and 5) suggestions about how back health could be promoted, such as the contest, or situations in the store that seemed particularly hard on backs. The pilot activity that they wrote under "taking action" in the workplan (Appendix C) was "Conduct pilot with two groups of seven people to obtain feedback on clarity, relevance, timing, enjoyment, and suggestions for other strategies." The evaluation measures were the following:

- Document comments made about pre- and posttest questions and the number of questions that were not answered.
- Include a question about the video on the posttest.
- Observe and document the ability to cover all the material in the allotted time.
- Observe and document participation in the discussion and demonstration.
- Document suggestions.

By this time, the team was quite adept at developing forms to collect data and drafted one on the spot. They decided that the same person, Maria, would lead the two workshops to provide consistency and to learn from the experience. She would then tutor others for the remaining workshops.

To evaluate the relevancy of the final products, which included the video, workshop, training of Health and Safety Committee members, and the contest, the team determined that they would have figures and responses from all the workshops. They also felt that they would have no difficulty showing that the products were developed collaboratively because the Health and Safety Committee, especially Letecia, had been working with them from the beginning.

The time for the pilot test was fast approaching. All the team members working on back injury prevention were working overtime to get things ready, but they were excited about finally taking action.

COLLEGE STUDENTS' SMOKING KNOWLEDGE SCENARIO (continued)

The team working on the smoking knowledge of college students were overwhelmed at first by all the concepts in the Transtheoretical Model. Their instructor pointed out to them that the main application for practice is that the stage of change of the smoker must be matched to the most effective processes for that stage.

Veena, one of the team members, asked, "Does that mean that people in different stages will get different information?" "Yes, that's what it means," responded the instructor. "Okay," Veena continued, "I guess that means that we look at the theory to see the type of information to provide." "Well, you can," stated Georgio, "but I think that will be a lot of work. I think that other people have already done that and tried it out. Let's look at the systematic reviews of research."

The team were able to quickly find systematic reviews relevant to their project when they checked the reviews listed by the Tobacco Addiction Group, as well as those listed under "Tobacco" in the Health Promotion and Public Health Field within the Cochrane databases (see Web Site Resources). Table 7-2

TABLE 7-2	Example of Three Systematic Reviews Relevant to Smoking Cessation Displays	
SYSTEMATIC REVIEW	**PRACTICE CONCLUSIONS**	**APPLICATION**
Lancaster, T., & Stead, L. (2002). Self-help interventions for smoking cessation.	Materials tailored for individual smokers increase effectiveness of self-help material.	Use material specific to stage of change.
Sowden, A., & Arblaster, L. (1999). Mass media interventions for preventing smoking in young people.	Work with representative samples of population to develop messages. Messages should be guided by behavioral theory. Channels must be preferred by audience and at a time when they are available.	Find places to interact directly with college students. Use Transtheoretical Model. Include questions about use of Web site.
University of York, NHS Centre for Reviews and Dissemination. (2001). Smoking cessation: What the health service can do.	Identify people who smoke and encourage them to stop. Provide advice about quitting. Increase cessation rates. Encourage use of nicotine replacement therapy in those ready to quit.	Seek out people who smoke. Provide material that gives advice about quitting. Include information about nicotine replacement for people at appropriate stage of change.

depicts the three most relevant studies and how the team expected to apply the information. They determined that the three systematic reviews supported the use of the Transtheoretical Model and the use of displays through which participants could assess their smoking.

When they searched all the Cochrane databases using the keywords "stages of change smoking," three randomized, controlled studies were identified, and two were relevant: The Stages of Change Model was found to be useful for giving brief advice (Goldberg et al., 1994) and in a computer-administered intervention program for young adults (O'Neill, Gillispie, & Slobin, 2000).

They decided to seek advice and information from agencies in the city that might be providing smoking cessation information. They discovered that the Lung Association and Public Health had developed a display and information using the Transtheoretical Model. The organizations were very happy to loan the display and would provide the material for the team to use at the college. They had used the display in malls with adults but had not used it with younger people.

The other aspect of their project was to identify the topics on smoking that interested college students. The health clinic staff had been collecting questions posed by students and had recently conducted focus groups on smoking behaviors. The team members reviewed the data and identified issues such as the cost of cigarettes; differences between male and female smokers; social or occasional smoking; changing from social smoking to being a smoker; smoking and drinking; parents, friends, and roommates who did or did not smoke; smoking and pregnancy; smoking and impotence; and the effects of working in a smoky environment. With the assistance of the health clinic and the Web sites of national associations concerned about reducing smoking (see Web Site Resources), they were able to find best practice guidelines, pertinent systematic reviews of research, and resources.

From the issues and resources they identified, they developed a list of topics for a questionnaire to be used with the display. In the questionnaire they asked whether the person was interested, somewhat *interested, or not interested in the topic. They had prepared a background document to assist team members in answering questions.*

Just before they conducted their pilot display, they were feeling very nervous. They started throwing questions about the Transtheoretical Model and smoking among college students back and forth to each other as if they were studying for an exam. They were amazed at how much they all had learned.

DISCUSSION QUESTIONS

1. What information from the framework for health communication was used by the back injury prevention team?
2. What were the various benefits of doing the observations of the lifting techniques before the workshops?
3. What aspects of the information from the systematic reviews were consistent with the Transtheoretical Model in the smoking project?
4. What aspects of changing behavior are not addressed in individual models of change such as the Transtheoretical Model?
5. When a display in a public area is used with a changing group of people, what would be the highest level of project objectives that the team could expect to reach?

Conduct pilot test

Conducting the pilot test or pretest is exciting because you finally have a chance to see whether your ideas work. Often you may feel that you are not ready to pilot test your material or that you have not done sufficient research to determine everything that could be used. For some topics such as smoking cessation, you could prepare for a year and never find all the information that could be relevant.

The pilot test provides you with an opportunity to obtain feedback on your direction before you have spent a lot of time or resources. If you are going in the wrong direction, the results of a pilot test allow you to change direction and save the project without losing too much time and energy.

The pilot test is definitely the time to consult with the community members. Most people cannot absorb a lot of new material at one time. The pilot will give the team a sense of how much the participants can absorb and what interests them.

The scope of a pilot test can range from testing partially developed resources to a full dress rehearsal for which only minor changes are expected. The team should have prepared at least one fairly well developed item, as well as samples or descriptions of what else might be included for the pilot. Some teams may have been working with collaborators all along and with resources that have been used previously. Those teams would be able to have a pilot test that is a dress rehearsal to determine the timing and reactions of an audience.

The pilot phase involves recruiting the people, preparing and conducting the pilot test, and evaluating the results.

Recruiting participants for the pilot test

The best people for the pilot test are people from the community of interest who have not yet been involved in the project. People who have been involved may not notice gaps in information that is presented because they already know the information or may feel that they should not say anything because they do not want to offend the team.

Often the project organizers or key informants can assist you in finding a group for your pilot test. Once you have a group of people identified, consider what would increase their willingness to attend. They will certainly need to know what the pilot test is about and why it applies to them. Your team may need to prepare a short information letter that can be distributed to potential participants.

Just like every other activity in the community, you also need to aim for convenience for the participants. Perform the pilot test at the beginning or end of another meeting that they are already attending. You team may also be able to offer an incentive such as refreshments.

The number of people for the pilot test can vary. Usually between four and ten people are sufficient. In other situations, such as a workshop, it may not be the number of people, but the number of sessions that need to be considered. Often, two sessions of a workshop are needed to determine the need for modifications.

Preparing and conducting the pilot test

Preparing for the pilot test is similar to preparing for a presentation except that a pilot test is usually more informal. Review the information on collaborative presentations (Appendix A) for aspects that could be relevant to your pilot. For example, prior to the presentation check out the room and audiovisual equipment (if used) to ensure that everyone will be able to view the material at the same time. Also review the criteria for the pilot test that the team developed during preparation to ensure that the criteria are still relevant and all the team members agree on what you want to accomplish. If you feel that you have too many items, list them in order of priority and deal with them one at a time as you have time. The next step is to prepare an outline. Box 7-4 provides a sample outline that can be adapted to suit different projects.

Along with the outline, consider how your team will help the participants feel comfortable in making comments and providing feedback. A very good method of obtaining feedback is to provide people with more than one option. For example, consider your options when given the following two situations: 1) a friend asks you what you think of the outfit she is wearing, 2) a friend holds up two outfits and asks which she should wear. In the second situation you have more options and freedom to state your true thoughts without offending your friend. Options can be used for semideveloped ideas or resources or for placement of completed components.

Another aspect of the pilot test is that it provides an opportunity for the team to learn how to work together. Each team member needs to be assigned a role. The common roles are leaders (including facilitators or demonstrators) and observers or evaluators. All team members must know the responsibilities of their role and when they will be performing it. The team may decide to practice what each person will do in a time sequence before the pilot test. This rehearsal is used to identify whether each person is prepared to perform his or her assigned role. The rehearsal also will allow the team members to get a sense of timing to know when they should be quiet and when they should be interacting with the participants. A rehearsal before the pilot test can help calm some feelings of stage fright.

BOX 7-4	Sample outline for the pilot test of an action

Introduction:
- Who you are
- What you are doing and why it is important
- Why their involvement is important
- What you hope to accomplish

Participants introduce themselves:
- Name
- Why this pilot would be useful to them (e.g., I have a son who is a toddler, I work as a stocker in a grocery store, I smoke and want to quit)

Presentation of material
- Deal with one item or group of items at a time. Allow them time to read or view material before posing questions.
- Encourage the idea that all comments are worthwhile.
- Allow discussion to continue until the same ideas are repeated. At that point, summarize the points and relate the points to another item that needs to be discussed.

Summary:
- Identify what has been accomplished.
- Identify how they have contributed.
- Ask them what they liked about the pilot and what they would change.
- Ask for final comments or questions.

In preparation for the pilot test, the team can consider what they will do if fewer people than expected attend. For example, the participants can be asked whether their views would be similar to those of others in the situation. Usually people volunteer examples of how they share the views of others. If fewer people than you expected show up for the pilot test, try not to give any indication that you are disappointed. If that sense is picked up by the participants, they can start to feel that there is something wrong with them because they did attend. Remind yourself that the people who are there are the right people and the right number because they will contribute in a way that would not be possible if more or different people were present. If you want to attract more people for subsequent parts of the action, ask these participants at the end how you could attract more people and if they would assist you.

During the pilot test, all team members should be monitoring the reactions of the participants. If the participants remain interested and involved, the pace should be maintained. If they look bored, the pace could be increased. If they appear confused, the pace needs to be slowed. If the participants are having difficulty grasping the information, the list of items that will be presented needs to be reduced. Usually, teams who are presenting for the first time have prepared far too much information. Although team members may feel disappointed, what they are observing is realistic. This is an appropriate occasion at which to have a "listen-to-learn" attitude and a readiness to start where the people are (Nyswander, 1956). Both attitude and action assure participants that their views and involvement are important.

All team members should also have some awareness of all that is occurring during the pilot test, even if it is not their particular responsibility. By remaining open to what is happening, the team members will produce a much more comprehensive evaluation.

With adequate preparation, time, and an atmosphere that encourages interaction, the pilot test will provide invaluable information. During evaluation, everyone's views will be used to make the products more relevant to the needs of the community.

Evaluating the results

As well as appropriately presenting your material and ideas during the pilot test, the team also needs to consider how the feedback and evaluation data will be collected. Although forms will have been developed during preparation, they need to be tested to see how easy or difficult they are to use and whether they are comprehensive. A rehearsal before the pilot can provide an opportunity for this testing.

During the pilot test, the people assigned to observe and evaluate need to be constantly attentive to the actions and comments of the participants. However, they also need to take notes in a way that does not interfere with the interactions. Some community members may feel suspicious or intimidated by anyone taking notes. If that is the case, all team members need to take mental notes on what was said or done during the pilot and contribute to reconstructing the feedback immediately after it ends. For some pilot tests, the observers and evaluators could be responsible for providing the summary at the end and handling any comments about the summary.

Evaluation of the results is best done in two stages: a debriefing immediately after the pilot test and an evaluation meeting to determine changes.

Debriefing meeting

The team must plan to meet immediately after the pilot test for a debriefing. The debriefing should have three parts. The first is an appraisal of the emotions of both the team members and participants that prevailed during the pilot. Because emotional involvement is important in engaging community members, the team needs to assess whether it was present and, if so, what encouraged it.

The second part of the debriefing is the collection of evaluation data from all team members. Evaluation measures that are qualitative, such as enjoyment or interaction, require everyone's input to ensure that information is are complete and validated by others.

The final part of the debriefing is an evaluation of the team and each member's performance. A way to structure this evaluation to reduce confrontation is to use the brainstorming method. Someone needs to be designated to take notes. During the first round, without interruption, all members can describe their evaluation of their own role, including what they liked about what they did and what they would change for next time. Once everyone has had his or her say, discussion can ensue about how each team member could improve his or her contribution to the team's performance.

Although team members may start talking about the changes they feel will need to be made to the material or format used in the pilot test, save these revisions for the next meeting. Participation in a pilot test can have a fairly emotional impact on people, either positive or negative, that could obscure their judgment. Also, time and distance from the event give people different insights. Plan a meeting that will be strictly devoted to making changes to the material and format based on feedback from the participants. End the debriefing meeting on a positive note by identifying what the team was able to accomplish and the valuable feedback you received.

Evaluation meeting

Before the evaluation meeting, usually the team members who collected the data should complete a preliminary analysis. Because they are familiar with the information, they will be able to do this fairly quickly and can explain it to the others.

In the evaluation meeting, first look at the number of people who participated and determine whether they represented the community of interest. If different people attend than those expected, consider the views that they can provide from previous experience or knowledge of others. For example, if the pilot test was for mothers of children who are two or three years old, and mothers of older children attended or if the pilot test was on sleep problems and the mothers who attended had few sleep problems with their children, you may feel the feedback was not relevant. However, in both situations the mothers may have learned from their experiences and may have been able to provide valuable insights. This part of the evaluation is to determine how much weight the team will give to the feedback. For example, if the expected number of people participated and represented the community of interest, you would probably give full weight to their feedback unless the team feels that the presentation was not done well.

When reviewing the analysis of the evaluation data, carefully consider how to apply the information. Sometimes there can be a clear indication that something needs to be changed. For example, in Table 7-4, two of three people have missed two of four items. If this trend continued with more people, the presentation of the missed items would need to be strengthened. There can be a tendency to "throw out the baby with the bath water" for situations in which major changes are needed. Before drastic changes are made, discuss the changes with the project leader and others associated with the project. They may have an entirely different and less emotional perspective.

On the other hand, only a few people could be involved or only one comment could have been made. These situations are more ambiguous and do not provide a clear direction. Discuss the situation with others associated with the project before making changes.

The evaluation of the pilot test is the main opportunity for the team to tailor the action to the needs of the community of interest. It can be a disconcerting experience because the team may need to give up cherished ideas that did not work. On the other hand, changes as a result of feedback are a measure of how responsive the team is prepared to be to address the community's issues.

SUPERMARKET BACK HEALTH SCENARIO (continued)

The supermarket team and Letecia met to decide who should be involved in the pilot workshop. They wanted people who would be representative of the stockers and decided to have one pilot during the week with full-time stockers and one on the weekend with part-time stockers. They picked a date for each pilot and decided that they would hold each workshop at the beginning of the shift at 11:30 pm. Letecia felt that there would be no trouble getting people to attend because everyone in the store knew about the workshop and wanted to find out more. The Health and Safety Committee members would be responsible for recruiting people for the pilots on the actual dates.

BOX 7-5	Timeline outline for pilot workshop for back injury

1900–1930
Introduction and pretest (5 minutes)
Introduction of participants (5 minutes)
Presentation on the effects and causes of back pain from work injury (10 minutes)
Discussion about personal experiences of back pain (10 minutes)

1930–2000
Show video on lifting techniques and flexibility exercises (25 minutes)

2000–2030
Demonstrate lifting and flexibility exercises (5 minutes)
Volunteers perform techniques and exercises (10 minutes)
Feedback session (5 minutes)
Posttest (5 minutes)
Summary (5 minutes)

They drew up an outline for the pilot workshops with a timeline. They decided to divide the time into three one-half hour blocks. Their outline is given in Box 7-5.

The team decided that they were closer to the dress rehearsal stage rather than the idea stage for their pilot workshop because they had been working consistently with Letecia and the Health and Safety Committee. However, they did not know how all the parts of the presentation would be managed by the team members. After all team members had prepared their parts, they held a rehearsal. They followed the outline using a stopwatch. They quickly realized that the outline did not indicate who was to do what. When they stopped and wrote in names beside each activity, they found that the activities of the observers and evaluators were not specified. The evaluators said that they would distribute and collect the pre- and posttest and, in between, would position themselves in different parts of the room so they could observe and document responses. After that issue was resolved, they started the stopwatch again and went through to the end. They found that the demonstration took ten minutes rather than five and reduced the number of techniques and exercises to those that were determined to be most relevant to the stockers during the observations. They went to the first pilot workshop feeling quite confident that everyone could perform his or her part.

At the first pilot workshop, only four stockers were available. The others were involved in unloading a delivery van that had to be emptied immediately because the refrigeration unit was not working. The team members were able to minimize their disappointment by feeling that the participants might find it easier to speak up with fewer people present.

The workshop went according to schedule until they reached the statistics about work injuries. The stockers looked bored and started shifting in their seats. The other difficulty was getting them to demonstrate the exercises in front of others. However, they enjoyed the video and had a lot of comments about how to promote back health. They did not feel that a contest involving competition between departments would be useful. They started to talk about how they could remember to remind each other about safe lifting and flexibility exercises.

The team met immediately after the workshop and quickly decided that the participants were emotionally involved and that their involvement started when they talked about themselves or people they knew who had back pain. It also continued when they were asked their views about how back health could be promoted. The participants mentioned three areas of the store that were cramped and did not have the space to permit use of safe lifting techniques. The team decided that those two elements of the pilot were important.

The team members then gave their views to the evaluators on the pre- and posttests, the video, timing of the presentation, enjoyment by the participants, and suggestions for improvement. Denny stated that the participants seemed very uncomfortable about being asked to demonstrate an exercise by themselves in front of the others.

Everyone then described what they felt that they did well and what they would want to improve next time. Maria, who was the leader, said she felt good about the way she presented the material because people easily provided feedback. She was not happy with how she managed the discussions. She felt she had trouble getting people back on track. The others described their performance. Once everyone was done, Stephanie commented that maybe the length or handling of the discussions was not a problem, but that priorities and the amount of time allocated to priorities needed to be changed. The others felt that this was a good point to bring up at the evaluation meeting after the second pilot workshop. Overall they were pleased with the first pilot.

At the second pilot workshop on the weekend, they had similar results that were more pronounced because they had eight participants. At the evaluation meeting, they made some changes to the confusing wording of a question in the pre- and posttest. They decided that the first discussion on back pain, the video, and the feedback discussion were priority elements based on comments from the participants. The demonstrations by the participants needed to be retained because it was an evaluation measure, but the team would need to consider other ways of getting people to participate. Those elements became the priority and were allotted more time. The times for nonpriority elements were reduced. Instead of the presentation on back injury in the workplace, a fact sheet would be prepared and distributed. The idea of the contest between departments was not supported, but other ideas were being considered and would be explored in the upcoming workshops.

When they presented these changes to their instructor and the Health and Safety Committee, everyone agreed to the revisions. They felt that the team had made the changes based on good evidence without losing the essential elements of the workshop.

COLLEGE STUDENTS' SMOKING KNOWLEDGE SCENARIO (continued)

At the debriefing session after their pilot display in the great hall of the college, the universal word used by everyone was "disaster." They tried to outdo each other in describing what did not work. Finally, Georgio had had enough.

"Now look," he said, "this was a pilot! We didn't have goodies to give out, we didn't have flashing lights or a video with half-naked dancers! So what if we only talked to 50 out of the hundreds who were there. The display board with the Transtheoretical Model went well!"

"Yeah," responded Francine. "I talked to one guy who was really wanting the information that I gave him because he intended to quit on the weekend."

"Well, I only talked to people who wanted to force it on someone else, like their mother, or boyfriend," said Veena.

"You were lucky that you got to talk to someone. Someone else always nabbed a person before I got close. I just got to talk to you guys and I'm tired of doing that!" complained Habib. "Okay, okay," said Georgio. "Let's get down some thoughts now, and book another meeting to work on changes before the next display in two weeks."

At the evaluation meeting, the team quickly determined that the display with the stages of change appealed to the people who used it. People could quickly identify what stage they were at and appreciated receiving the information that was geared to their needs. However, only ten people who approached the display were smokers, and they were in the preparation and action stages.

The questionnaire with the list of topics did not work. Only two were completed. More were distributed but were not returned. If someone wanted information on a topic, it was a scramble to try and find it. They needed to find another way to determine what issues interested college students.

The next two locations were in the foyers of residences. The team did not feel that they would be competing with so many other distractions there. However, they felt that four people were two too many for the display. They decided to work in pairs for the next displays.

DISCUSSION QUESTIONS

1. Why was the back injury team able to have a dress rehearsal for their pilot workshop, and the college students smoking knowledge team only tested partially completed material?
2. What are some ways that would help people feel more comfortable practicing the techniques and exercises in the back injury workshop?
3. In the smoking display in the great hall of the college, were the participants representative of the community of interest for the project?

Complete action

Completing action is putting all your promised products in place. In the action stage, the importance of the involvement of collaborators becomes apparent. That involvement can mean that a disastrous pilot program is saved or that the project will be carried on by others. Before the team can take action, modifications usually need to be made to the messages, material, delivery method, or evaluation measures based on the evaluation from the pilot. You will also need to consider how to recruit people and to prepare people to take over the project.

Modifications to products

After a team has determined what modifications need to occur as a result of the pilot, these need to be completed. The messages may have been confusing, written material or props may have been ineffective, or the situation or skills of people may need to be improved. As discussed previously, carefully evaluate what items or issues showed some promise and what can be eliminated. If you change too much, you will be conducting another pilot test rather than taking action.

Collaborators are crucial in assisting the team identify what is important and what is not. They can also help the team members recognize that revision and modification are part of the work of health promotion. As long as team members are prepared to listen and work with the community members, they will produce something that is beneficial. Collaborators and other stakeholders can also assist with providing ideas or new props to deal with difficulties identified in the pilot. Teams are encouraged to request advice and help from everyone. They will usually be amazed by the people who come to their assistance.

If changes have been made to the products, those changes will need to be carried through to the evaluation measures. Often this will simply mean changing or adding a heading on a form. In other situations, a new type of evaluation measure that is more appropriate to capture the effect of the action may need to be developed. For example, if the mothers of toddlers did not want to do the demonstration on safety features during the pilot project, the team could decide to collect information by offering the women tea and cookies after the workshop and asking them to explain how they might (or might not) use the safety information at home. The data collection tool for this would be recording the statements that they made rather than using the checklist for the demonstration.

Review of recruitment or marketing

The pilot test will have given the team some idea of how easy or difficult it will be to attract a greater number of people for the action. For teams who are working closely with community members, recruitment for the action may be done by the community members. In other situations, the attendance of people in the community of interest will need to be negotiated. For example, if you were planning a health fair in a school, the team would need to negotiate with the principal and teachers to determine a time when the students could attend.

Recruitment is more challenging for projects that need to attract people from the public. People who want to quit smoking or lose weight do not necessarily congregate together. Often for these projects some form of advertising is necessary. Box 7-3, provided earlier, includes some messages and means that can be used to attract people. Review these strategies with people in community organizations who have worked on these issues in the past. For some issues, strategies might be found on the appropriate Web sites. For some projects, the main challenge will be to reach the right people.

Preparing people to take over the project

Although these community team members' projects were designed to be time-limited, they are not designed to end when the students' time was up. The projects are expected to have some measure of **sustainability.** One component of sustainability is that the material produced by the team is relevant to the community of interest and stakeholders; another is that the community members or stakeholders are prepared to use the material.

Relevance for the community can be achieved by including community members in the decision being made. Preparation of the community can be achieved by providing them opportunities to gain the necessary knowledge and skills. The preparation can simply take the form of having community members work alongside team members as action is taken. This is an extension of team building.

Another type of preparation is more formal and would involve specified training or education sessions. If materials and a process have been pilot tested for use with community members, but not necessarily tested for people who will use the materials and process to teach others, some modifications will be needed. The modifications will include the knowledge and skills each trainer will need to teach this material to others. Because the team members have just been through this process themselves, they will be able to impart the "lessons learned" to others.

In addition to changes in how the information is presented, material that will be used by others needs to be considerably more detailed than that used by team members. Often even though team members could work from a simple outline, people who have not been previously involved with the development of material and process will need far more information. For example, an item in a workshop may state "do demonstrations." The written material to be used for others would need to indicate exactly what would be demonstrated and for how long. Tips on how to make the demonstration clearer, such as standing sideways to the audience, would also be included.

Usually training or education sessions will be held with people who have already been involved with the project. During the training, they will be know what information they would need to carry on the project. The necessary information could be brought together in an instructor's manual.

SUPERMARKET BACK HEALTH (continued)

In preparing for action, the problem facing the back injury team was how to deal with the demonstration of the lifting techniques and exercises. They included members of the Health and Safety Committee in trying to decide what approach would be acceptable to the participants. As they were thinking about it, Letecia asked if the demonstrations had to be done by one person at a time. They realized that that was not necessary. They also felt that if the movements were done by everyone at the same time or in two small groups, participants would naturally join it. They decided that if there were six or more people they would have two groups; otherwise, they would use one. They would also have two evaluation forms for the demonstration so that two people could collect the data.

The other question that they had was how to promote safe back practices throughout the store. The contest idea between departments was not accepted. One of the Health and Safety Committee members mentioned that the store was in the process of ordering work aprons that had a front and a back panel to protect clothes. The store logo would go on the front, but maybe something could be put on the back? All kinds of ideas were offered until someone suggested that they could have a back slogan contest that they would promote in the remaining workshops. They felt the store would be willing to offer a prize for the winning slogan. They decided that they did not need to make any changes in how they would recruit for the remainder of the workshops. Everyone seemed to be talking about them and wanted to take part.

They had originally planned to do the training with three members of the Health and Safety Committee after the two pilot workshops. Now, they felt that the training would work better if it followed the revised workshop. The potential trainers would first take part in that workshop, and then the team and the trainers could sit down together and determine what information and practice that they would need to continue the workshops.

The remaining workshops and training went well, and several slogans for the back contest were submitted. Staff other than stockers started to complain that they were not getting any training and wanted more information on the contest. The Health and Safety Committee was scrambling to arrange workshops for the other departments. They liked those kinds of complaints!

Because the Health and Safety Committee was pleased with the work of the team, the team filled in the following statement in the results column across from step 2 in the workplan: "All Health and Safety Committee members have indicated individually and collectively that the workshops are working well." Note: This scenario continues in Chapter 8.

COLLEGE STUDENTS' KNOWLEDGE OF SMOKING SCENARIO (continued)

The team working with the college students had two pressing issues when they completed their pilot. They needed a better way to present the information on smoking topics and a better way to attract people who smoked. They felt that they had strong evidence from the systematic reviews that it was important to actually talk to smokers about their smoking.

To deal with the presentation on smoking topics, they contacted people in the college health clinic, the Lung Association, and Public Health. A Public Health nurse remembered that they had used a roulette wheel a few years ago with high school students and it was a big hit. She would find it for them. That seemed to be the answer they were looking for. Now they needed to figure out a way to link the wheel and the questions and revise their evaluation measures.

At the next display in the foyer of a residence, the roulette wheel attracted a lot of attention. However, only one person at a time could use it. Once again, they attracted mainly nonsmokers, especially because it was a nonsmoking residence.

The next residence had smoking floors, so they felt it would be useful to go there. The final location was to be outside the college cafeteria. They felt that a display at the cafeteria would not attract smokers because people would be rushed and would not want to be separated from their friends.

Veena said: "We really have not considered a recruitment strategy. We have just gone where the health clinic has arranged for us to go."

"Yes, I think we should go where people smoke, like in a bar," stated Habib.

"Who would let us in a bar?" asked Francine. "They make money by selling smokes and drinks."

Well I think we could get in where I work. The manager has really come down on smoking since his brother died of lung cancer last year," explained Veena.

The team got into quite a heated discussion about going to the bar. The bar would certainly have smokers. They finally found out that Francine was reluctant to go to a bar because she did not think it was professional. The others quickly informed her about the places that public health nurses go to deal with sexually transmitted diseases and tuberculosis. Francine agreed that it did make sense to go to a bar.

Veena talked to her manager, and he was willing to allow them to come for one shift, as long as they would not disturb the service and the customers. On a busy night, more than 500 people could be served. The team really started thinking about what information they would like to get at this last site. They felt that they had already established that the display board using the Transtheoretical Model was useful for college students and did not need to include it this time. They decided to focus on how or where smokers would like to get information and what topics on smoking interested them.

Before they made the final decisions about how to obtain their information, they decided to visit the bar. After the visit, they knew that they could not ask anything that took more than 10 to 15 minutes or a lot of thinking. The bar was very busy and crowded. They had 60 topics and 5 questions on where and how smokers wanted to receive information on smoking. They knew that that was too much information for one questionnaire.

They also knew that some type of incentive would help to recruit people to complete the questionnaire. The bar manager mentioned that a new video store had just opened in the same block as the bar, and the manager would probably be willing to provide discount coupons for the team to give to people who participated.

The team chose a Friday night to conduct the survey. They had dealt with the number of topics by having three different questionnaires with a variety of topics on each. The participants were to pick their top five topics and identify a source they would use. There was room to offer a topic if they wanted. The questionnaire included two demographic questions: age and number of cigarettes smoked in the past seven days.

Once customers were seated, one of the team members would approach them and offer them the opportunity to take part in the survey. If they agreed, they were given the questionnaires and an envelope. When they were done, they were instructed to put the questionnaires in the envelope and put the envelope near the edge of the table. When the envelope was picked up, the customers were offered the discount coupon for the video shop. Although some customers refused and some questionnaires were not completed, the team received more than 100 from customers who smoked. Note: This scenario continues in Chapter 8.

DISCUSSION QUESTIONS

1. How would you decide whether to have a formal or an informal training session?
2. Why did some workers feel that they were not learning about the back slogan contest?
3. Do you think an earlier recruitment or marketing strategy would have helped the project with the college students?
4. Why were the bar customers asked to put their completed questionnaire in an envelope?

Teamwork

The two new challenges for the team during action are maintaining morale and expanding the team membership. Leadership, decision making, and communication can still be problems if they have not been resolved earlier, but by this stage, most teams have learned to work together.

Maintaining morale

Team members usually devote a lot of time and effort to promote the material and resources used in their pilot test. When the response is not totally positive or things do not go as planned, they can feel demoralized. That is a normal reaction, and team members should have the opportunity to express their frustration.

People can be frustrated because they feel that they may not have performed as well as expected or that some idea of theirs led the team astray. Others may feel that the participants just did not appreciate all the time and effort that the team had put into the project. These types of thoughts might be the same as those experienced when you receive a low grade on a paper or exam. The difference here is that this situation is more public, and sometimes people are unrealistic about their responsibility for a poor result. When these thoughts come out, people can be reassured that this was a team effort, and everyone can learn from their mistakes. After team members start repeating the same statements during venting, the leader can suggest that each person can use the experience for their critical reflection (Appendix C). Even if the team determines from the pilot test that they were on the wrong track, the team deserves praise for conducting a pilot that provided sufficient information to save them from a continuing disaster. At the next meeting, they can concentrate on looking at the lessons that they have learned from the experience.

One valuable lesson to be learned when things do not go well in a pilot test is that more consultation is needed with community members and stakeholders. Sometimes team members feel that they must do this project on their own without advice from others. In other situations, maybe no one was available or had ever done this before. Whatever the reason, the lesson to be learned is that success depends on the involvement of people who know the community.

Expanding team membership

If up to this point community members or stakeholders have just been involved in making decisions, now is the time to fully include them in what you are doing. This is the same process that was used in building the original team.

Although some community members are quite comfortable with the planning and documenting required in community health nursing practice, others are not. However, community members are likely to enjoy taking action. As an example, I was working with a group of women in a small town who decided to put on a healthy living festival at their community center. Very few ever came to the planning meetings. The women explained that the information was passed along at the food store check-out or the post office as they went about their daily business. Their communication system worked well, and the festival was a great success.

Community members bring expertise from living in the community and many other resources that you may not know about. By enlisting them in your action, your team will suddenly have a greater wealth of resources and a much better chance for success.

Just as team members in the initial stage of group development needed a defined task to feel comfortable, the same is true of community members who are joining the team. All the tasks that need to be done can be presented, and everyone can indicate what they would like to work on. If new members do not offer to take on a task, team members can invite them to work alongside them. If a complicated task is taken on by a new member, a team member can volunteer to work with the new person. Everyone should have something to do, and all the tasks need to be addressed.

During the final stages of collaborative action, it may be reasonable for a community member to take over the lead of the team. This will allow the team members to complete their documentation for the project and the community members to learn the various aspects of the project before everyone has left.

Summary

Taking action is the reward for working diligently and collaboratively with community members during assessment and planning. The diligence and collaboration do not stop during action but are more meaningful because they are directly related to interactions with people in the community. Taking action also lays the groundwork for evaluation and expanding the number of collaborators. Both evaluation and increased involvement of the community are important for the sustainability of the project or products produced by the project. These ideas are discussed in more detail in Chapter 8, which details the final stage of the project.

PRACTICE AND APPLICATION

1. For the supermarket back health project, document the action and results in the taking action section of the collaborative workplan (Appendix C).

2. For the college students' knowledge of smoking project, identify the products and objectives, and design the evaluation forms.

3. For the college students' knowledge of smoking project, devise a marketing strategy to reach college students who smoke.

4. Based on your experience with a community group, identify the preparations needed to take action and conduct the pilot test.

5. Using an issue such as weight reduction, increasing exercise, or safe sexual practices, indicate the following:
   a) How would you define and use a relevant theory?
   b) What databases or Web sites would have systematic reviews of relevant research?
   c) What community groups or organizations would be interested in the issue?
   d) How you would involve community members in the action?

REFERENCES

Cancer Prevention Research Center. (1998). *Detailed overview of the Transtheoretical Model.* Retrieved July 21, 2003 from http://www.uri.edu/research/cprc/transtheoretical.htm.

Goldberg, D., Hoffman, A., Farinha, M. Marder, D. Tinson-Mitchem, L, Burton, D, & Smith, E. (1994). Physician delivery of smoking-cessation advice based on the stages of change model. *American Journal of Preventive Medicine.* 10(5): 267-74.

Karas, B. & Conrad, K. (1996). Back injury prevention interventions in the workplace: An integrative review. American Association of Occupational Health Nurses Journal, 44, 189-96.

Lancaster T., & Stead L. F. (2004) Self-help interventions for smoking cessation (Cochrane Review). In: *The Cochrane Library,* 2. Chichester, UK: John Wiley & Sons.

McKenzie, J. & Smeltzer, J. (2001). *Planning, implementing and evaluating health promotion programs* (3rd ed.). Needham Heights, MA: Allyn and Bacon.

National Institute for Cancer Research. (1989). *Making health communication programs work.* Retrieved July 21, 2003 from: http://oc.nci.nih.gov/services/HCPW/HOME.HTM.

Nyswander, D. (1956). Education for health: Some principles and their application. *California's Health, 14,* 69-70.

O'Neill, H., Gillispie, M., & Slobin, K. (2000). Stages of change and smoking cessation: a computer-administered intervention program for young adults. *American Journal of Health Promotion, 15*(2), 93-6.

Prochaska, J., Redding, C., & Evers, K. (1997) The transtheoretical model and stages of change. In K. Glanz, F. Lewis, & B. Rimer, (Eds.), *Health Behavior and Health Education: Theory Research and Practice* (2nd ed. pp 60-84). San Francisco, CA: Jossey-Bass Publishers.

Prochaska, J., Johnson, S., & Lee, P. (1998). The transtheoretical model of behavioral change. In S. Shumaker, E. Schron, J. Ockene, & W. McBee (Eds.), *The handbook of health behavior change* (2nd ed., pp. 59-84). New York: Springer.

Redding, C., Rossi, J., Rossi, S. Velicer, W., & Prochaska, J. (1999). Health behavior models. In G. Hyner, K. Peterson, J. Travis, J. Dewey, J. Foerster, & E. Framer (Eds.), *SPM handbook of health assessment tools* (pp. 83-93). Pittsburgh, PA: The Society of Prospective Medicine.

Sowden A. J., & Arblaster L. (2004) Mass media interventions for preventing smoking in young people (Cochrane Review). In: *The Cochrane Library,* 2. Chichester, UK: John Wiley & Sons.

University of York, NHS Centre for Reviews and Dissemination. (1998). Smoking Cessation: What the health service can do. *Database of Abstracts of Reviews of Effectiveness, 2, 2004.*

van Tulder, M., Jellema, P., van Poppel, M., Nachemson, A., & Bouter, L. (2002). Lumbar supports for prevention and treatment of low back pain (Cochrane Review). In: *The Cochrane Library,* 1, 2003. Chichester, UK: John Wiley & Sons.

Velicer, W. F, Prochaska, J. O., Fava, J. L., Norman, G. J., & Redding, C. A. (1998). Smoking cessation and stress management: Applications of the Transtheoretical Model of behavior change. *Homeostasis, 38,* 216-233.

WEB SITE RESOURCES

Framework for development of health communications

National Institute for Cancer Research: Making health communication programs work: http:// cancer.gov/pinkbook. A variety of resources are available, including a method to calculate literacy level.

Systematic reviews and best practices

Cochrane Collaboration: http://www.cochrane.org. This site identifies the different groups and fields within the Cochrane Collaboration. Groups include the Tobacco Addiction Group. The most relevant field is Health Promotion and Public Health. Each group and field provide a list of reviews relevant to its area. A full search of Cochrane databases is available through institutional libraries. Some abstracts are available at the following web site: http://www.update-software.com/cochrane/abstract.htm.

PHRED (Public Health Research, Education and Development): www.phred-redsp.on.ca. Systematic reviews of the effectiveness of public health practice.

EPHPP (Effective Public Health Practice Project): http://www.hamilton.ca/PHCS/EPHPP/EPHPP Research.asp. The EPHPP initially focused on public health nursing practice.

Scottish Executive—Nursing for Health: http://www.scotland.gov.uk/library3/health/ephn/eph-00.asp. A review of systematic reviews of the effectiveness of public health nursing.

Registered Nurses of Ontario: http://www.rnao.org/bestpractices/faq.asp. Best practice guidelines.

Search strategy: Use the keywords "best practices" and then limit the search to "nursing" or "community health."

Smoking/tobacco reduction associations

American Lung Association: http://www.lungusa.org/tobacco/

American Public Health Association: http://www.apha.org/index.cfm. APHA links to tobacco control and prevention are found at http://www.apha.org/public_health/TobacConPrvnt.htm.

Canadian Public Health Association: http://www.cpha.ca

National Clearinghouse on Tobacco and Health: http://www.ncth.ca/NCTHweb.nsf

Transtheoretical model

Cancer Prevention Research Center: http://www.uri.edu/research/cprc/transtheoretical.htm. Detailed overview of the Transtheoretical Model.

Search strategy: Use the keywords "Transtheoretical Model" or "Stages of Change Model."

APPLICATION 7-1

GANTT CHART FOR SUPERMARKET SCENARIO— REVISED OCTOBER 21, 2004

ADMINISTRATIVE ACTIVITIES OBJECTIVES	RESPONSI-BILITY	WEEK OF MONTH									
		Sept 22	Sept 29	Oct 6	Oct 13	Oct 20	Oct 27	Nov 3	Nov 10	Nov 17	Nov 24
Product: A package of education/awareness material* to reduce back injuries											
Conduct literature search to determine best practices for back injury prevention.	Denny, Maria	▪	▪								
Locate appropriate video on back injuries.	Denny, Maria	▪	▪								
Observe and document lifting/carrying behaviors.	Steph, Jose, Letecia	▪	▪								
Contact/negotiate with store department managers on timing for workshop.	Steph, Jose, Letecia	▪	▪								
Book or locate rooms for workshop and final presentation.	Steph, Jose, Letecia	▪	▪	▪							
Prepare workshop material (e.g., the cost of back injuries) plus evaluation measures.	Maria, Steph		▪	▪	▪						
Conduct pilot workshops (two groups of seven stockers).	Maria					▪					
Conduct training for employee workshop instructors (three).	Jose					▪	▪				
Develop contest between departments.	Denny					▪					
Conduct two workshops (seven to eight stockers each).	Jose						▪	▪			
Evaluate change in back prevention behavior.	All								▪		
Prepare presentation.	Denny								▪	▪	

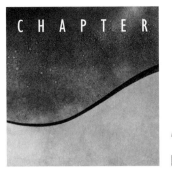

CHAPTER 8

Ending Well

ELIZABETH DIEM

SCENARIO   *SUPERMARKET BACK HEALTH*

The four nursing student members of the supermarket back health team had three weeks to go before their final presentation. The back injury prevention workshops were going well, and the training for members of the Health and Safety Committee had been completed. After the training, they decided that the student team and the Health and Safety Committee would join and share the final tasks, and they had a meeting planned to organize this. They identified two co-chairs for this last stage: Letecia from the store and Stephanie from the nursing students. These two people would need to be in constant communication to ensure that everything was completed.

SCENARIO   *COLLEGE STUDENTS' SMOKING KNOWLEDGE*

The team members working on the smoking project felt that they would be able to provide the expected products now that they would be going to a bar during the next week to talk to smokers. With that concern off their mind, they realized that they had better start planning their presentation and project report.

OBJECTIVES   After reading this chapter and answering the questions throughout the chapter, you should be able to

1. Complete an evaluation of the products and objectives.
2. Present the project and findings to community members and stakeholders.
3. Prepare a concise project report.
4. Involve collaborators in final plans.
5. Show appropriate appreciation for people who supported the project.
6. Document and communicate action.

KEYWORDS   analysis of evaluation data ▪ collecting evaluation data ▪ consultative presentation ▪ ending well ▪ limitations ▪ recommendations ▪ showing appreciation

Ending well

During the project, the team has built a working relationship with collaborators, composed of community members and stakeholders, and now needs to consider how to end that relationship in a fitting manner as well as completing the project tasks. Balancing relationships and tasks is the challenge in ending the project well. **Ending well** means that the participants on the team and the collaborators from the community feel that the best job was done within the time allotted and with the resources that were available.

Step 3: Determine results/impact

The determination of results/impact is the third step of collaborative action in the community health nursing process. The substeps from the workplan (Appendix C) are listed here:

Step 3: Determine Results/Impact
a. Collect and analyze data for project objectives.
b. Present findings to community.
c. Show appreciation to collaborators.
d. Complete project report.

Before the team members start determining the final results, they need to decide how they will know that it has ended well. Consider which people the team would like to satisfy by the results of the project. If this project has an educational component, a person serving as an educational supervisor would need to be satisfied. Also consider people in authority and the team collaborators.

There can be a tendency to wait until the evaluation data is collected and analyzed before starting work on the presentation and report. Avoid that tendency and begin planning for the presentation and report during the completion of the evaluation.

Collecting and analyzing the data for the project objectives

 Each project will have products to evaluate and at least three objectives. Evaluation includes both the collection and the analysis of data.

Collecting evaluation data

Before starting to **collect evaluation data,** review each objective, the evaluation measures, and the forms that were developed in Chapters 6 and 7. Now that the team members have spent more time on the project, they may find that the criteria used in the objective or the process to collect the data are unrealistic. Moreover, the forms that were developed during implementation may now need to be changed because adjustments have been made since the pilot test. The final preparation measure is to ensure that a fairly consistent data collection method is used. This would involve how the data is to be collected and what follow-up methods will be used.

These points will be explained using examples from the homeless project in Chapter 6 in which the following environmental objective and evaluation measures were identified in the plan.

> *Environmental:* By March 16, 75% of agencies will have posted the activity calendar for March, and 20% of staff and homeless will know about the calendar.
> *Evaluation:* Visit each agency. Document the number of agencies with calendars posted and the number of staff and homeless viewing or knowing about the calendar.

The team knew that there were 14 agencies involved in the homeless coalition; however, they did not know how many staff these agencies had or the number of homeless people they sheltered. Once the team started to ask for information on staff from the coalition members, they quickly discovered that few staff were directly involved with the homeless. They also found that the best time to contact both the staff and homeless was between 7 a.m. and 9 a.m. That period was when most of the homeless would be present. Because often only one or two people were involved, they changed the objective from "20% of staff" to "75% of agencies have staff who know about the calendar." They obtained the average number of homeless sheltered each night by each agency, but were informed that the number could vary greatly.

The procedure for collecting the data also needs to be developed in more detail. For the project with homeless people, two team members decided to visit one of the large and one of the small agencies to test the data forms a week before the evaluation date. They found the atmosphere in each place to be quite different. In the larger agency, the homeless seemed to be rushed through breakfast and out the door. They would have little chance to view the calendar. In the smaller agency, the homeless were standing around talking to each other and the staff both before and after breakfast. The staff in the smaller shelter said that this was the one day in the week when they did not need to get people out quickly before another activity started in the building.

After considering these different situations, the team members decided that they would count the number of homeless at breakfast, and ask the homeless during breakfast whether they knew where the calendar was posted. Because there were only 4 team members and 14 agencies, they decided that they could not visit every agency in the time they had left. They divided the agencies into two categories of large and small, and randomly selected two large agencies and four small ones to collect the data from the homeless. Each team member had either a large shelter or two smaller shelters to visit. The remaining shelters would receive a call to identify whether the calendar was posted and whether the staff member knew about a particular event on the calendar.

Every team will have some adjustments to make before actual evaluation data collection begins. The adjustments are expected because the team usually knows little about the functioning of organizations when the team is in the planning stage. Changes are also necessary because of the pilot test. Adjustments and changes are necessary, but must be done after consulting with the project organizers and collaborators.

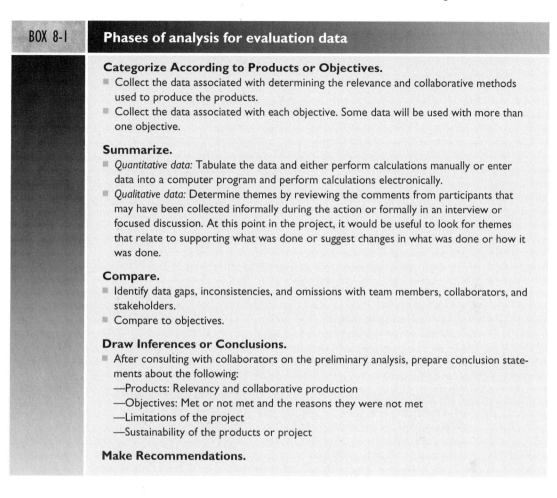

BOX 8-1

Phases of analysis for evaluation data

Categorize According to Products or Objectives.
- Collect the data associated with determining the relevance and collaborative methods used to produce the products.
- Collect the data associated with each objective. Some data will be used with more than one objective.

Summarize.
- *Quantitative data:* Tabulate the data and either perform calculations manually or enter data into a computer program and perform calculations electronically.
- *Qualitative data:* Determine themes by reviewing the comments from participants that may have been collected informally during the action or formally in an interview or focused discussion. At this point in the project, it would be useful to look for themes that relate to supporting what was done or suggest changes in what was done or how it was done.

Compare.
- Identify data gaps, inconsistencies, and omissions with team members, collaborators, and stakeholders.
- Compare to objectives.

Draw Inferences or Conclusions.
- After consulting with collaborators on the preliminary analysis, prepare conclusion statements about the following:
  - —Products: Relevancy and collaborative production
  - —Objectives: Met or not met and the reasons they were not met
  - —Limitations of the project
  - —Sustainability of the products or project

Make Recommendations.

Analyzing evaluation data

The **analysis of evaluation data** follows a process similar to that followed for the analysis of the assessment data, as explained in Chapter 5. However, the analysis of the evaluation data is usually less complex because the comparison is designated by the criteria in the objectives.

After the data have been collected, difficulties in collection must be assessed first to determine whether the difficulties could compromise any conclusions. If the data collection could not be completed or if the data may not be accurate, these facts need to be documented and included in the **limitations** (barriers to achieving the desired results) to the project. For example, if you were collecting observational measures of a group of people when a fire drill forced them to leave the building, your observations would be accurate only up to the point that the drill was announced. The limitation would be that there was insufficient time to conduct a full evaluation. Box 8-1 identifies the phases of analysis for the evaluation data. For additional explanations and examples of analysis, refer to the analysis in Chapter 5.

■   **SUPERMARKET BACK HEALTH SCENARIO (continued)**

With three weeks to go in the project, the members of the supermarket back health team held a joint meeting with the Health and Safety Committee to organize what had to be done in the remaining time. The following is a list of the tasks that they identified:

FINAL TASKS FOR PROJECT (WITH THREE WEEKS TO GO)

1. *Evaluations*
   - *Product*
   - *Objectives*

2. *Presentation*
   - *Prepare*
   - *Rehearse*
   - *Invitation list*

3. *Thank yous*
   - *List people who have contributed.*
   - *Determine how to show appreciation for each.*
   - *Show appropriate appreciation.*

4. *Project report*
   - *Summarize assessment.*
   - *Summarize plan and action.*
   - *Summarize findings.*
   - *Finish remainder of report.*
   - *Distribute to store and instructor.*

As they looked at the list, they were amazed at how much needed to be done in just three weeks. Then they realized that some of the tasks would overlap with others. For example, the people completing the evaluations could put their findings in that section of the project report.

The expanded team started to assign people to the tasks. The co-chairs, Stephanie and Letecia, would coordinate the tasks and be responsible for the invitation list for the presentation and the thank-yous. Denny and two people from the Health and Safety Committee would start to organize the presentation. The remaining two student team members, Maria and Jose, would start preparing the project report. All would take part in collecting the remaining evaluation data and analyzing the data.

The data for the first four objectives—awareness, knowledge, appreciation, and ability—had been collected at the workshops, and three members of the Health and Safety Committee had been trained and had already conducted another workshop on their own. The remaining evaluation measures were to determine whether 20% of the stockers were using the lifting techniques and flexibility exercises during work and whether the workshop and contest were relevant. Each of the seven people (four students and three staff) took a different one-hour period over the three shifts to observe the stockers. They modified the form developed by Stephanie, Jose, and Letecia to count the number of people observed, the number doing incorrect and correct lifts, flexibility exercises, and using a lumbar belt. The team decided to determine relevancy by reviewing the comments made by the participants in the workshop.

To prepare for the analysis, they developed a table to collect the information from each pilot and workshop. They had been told that there were 40 full- and part-time stockers. Table 8-1 presents the data collected from the evaluation forms used for each workshop.

They decided to list the data that they had collected so far. They had been told that there were 40 full- and part-time stockers. They had found that on Oct. 7, twenty-seven stockers, or 68%, had met the awareness objective and on Oct. 21, twenty-eight stockers, or 70%, had met the knowledge objective (see first page of Chapter 6). To evaluate the objectives for appreciate and ability, they recorded the information from the workshops in a table. Table 8-1 presents the data that was collected from the evaluation forms used for each workshop.

TABLE 8-1	**Example of Categorizing Data**					
MEASURES OF PARTICIPATION	**PILOT 1**	**PILOT 2**	**WORKSHOP 1**	**WORKSHOP 2**	**WORKSHOP 3**	**PROPORTION**
Attendance/ Appreciate	4	8	6	7	6	31/40 78%
Ability	0	0	3	5	5	13/31 42%

Once they had the figures in the table, they easily completed the calculations. When they compared the percents to the criteria in the objectives, they determined that they exceeded every objective so far except ability. For ability, 50% of the stockers who attended the workshop were to demonstrate the techniques; however, only 42% did because few were willing to demonstrate until the format was changed to a group demonstration.

To determine the relevancy of the workshop and video, they reviewed the comments made at the end of each workshop. The following is a sample of some of the comments:

- They made the lifts look easy.
- It makes sense to do the flex exercises, but I would feel silly doing it.
- The video covered the kinds of lifting that I do.
- Maybe we could have a stretch break!
- I don't know if I will lift right when we are busy.

The team members determined that the video and workshop showed techniques and flexibility exercises that were relevant to the stockers. However, they realized that more work was needed to reinforce the continued use of the information from the workshop.

For the accomplishment objective, the team first collected the data from each team member's observation period and tried to put it in a table. They quickly realized that some had counted the number of incorrect lifts, rather than the number of stockers doing the incorrect lifts.

When they revised the results from these two members, 22 stockers had been observed. Of the 22, 10 had not done any lifting during the observation, 8 had lifted incorrectly, and 2 or 20% of the 10 lifting had lifted correctly. No one was observed doing flexibility exercises or using a lumbar belt.

The team was disappointed. The percent was the same as the baseline data. When they discussed reasons for the poor results, staff members said that the stockers were very busy during the week of observation because they were getting ready for a big promotion. The team realized they were probably expecting too much in a short period of time.

Stephanie went on to explain that during their observations, they had found two particular areas in the store where staff consistently used the incorrect technique. When they tried to use the correct technique themselves, they realized that there wasn't room. In the feedback sessions, these two areas and another similar area were consistently mentioned as problems. The team felt that these areas needed to be mentioned. On a positive note, the meeting ended with Letecia describing how she had come across three stockers in the middle of the night practicing the lifting techniques in the loading dock.

COLLEGE STUDENTS' SMOKING KNOWLEDGE SCENARIO (continued)

The team working on college students' knowledge of smoking were very pleased by their night spent in the bar. There was a response rate of approximately 60% to the questionnaires. There were more than 100 responses from smokers and more than 200 from nonsmokers. The manager said that he had had no complaints about the questionnaires. The team's job now was to figure out how to organize the analysis in the short time they had until the presentation.

They decided to concentrate on the returns from the smokers in the 18- to 25-year-old age category. That left them with 90 responses. By working in pairs and using a large form that contained all the items, they found that they could quickly collate the data. The results were compared with the team's objectives on college students' awareness, knowledge, and response to material related to smoking.

Those results, along with the results from the use of the display, would provide the evidence to guide the selection of certain approaches and topics as relevant to increasing college students' knowledge about smoking. The team at first felt that those products were not produced collaboratively. Then they realized that they had certainly collaborated with people in the college health clinic, the Lung Association, and Public Health. Veena added that the bar manager had also helped. Although these agencies and people, other than the health clinic staff, had not worked closely with them all along, they had all contributed to the results.

DISCUSSION QUESTIONS

1. What benefits does a table provide for collating results?
2. What preparation would have been necessary to ensure that everyone collected the observations on the incorrect lifts in the same way?
3. Was the amount of collaboration appropriate for each type of project? Explain.

Presentation

The presentation provides a finale for the project. The presentation is the opportunity to display what was learned and who contributed and is also an opportunity to discuss how the work could be continued. The best gift that could be given to the project team at the end of their final presentation would be the collaborators declaring through word or action that they had taken over.

As with any presentation, the first consideration is to determine the main purpose for the presentation. Some possible purposes could be

- To show that the team members were able to do what they said they would
- To show what the team was able to do with the help of others
- To show what the team and collaborators did and what still needs to be done
- To show what doesn't work

Although all of this information can be included in one presentation, the purpose is a theme that is emphasized throughout the presentation.

Appendix A describes and details the development and delivery of a **consultative presentation.** Chapter 5 explains and includes examples of presentations at the end of assessment. Both sources provide the basics for preparing a presentation. The following discussion will concentrate on aspects of final presentations that are different from presentations done earlier in the project. In the final presentation, there will probably be differences in the audience, objectives, preparation of the speech, promoting of the value of the products, interaction, and follow-up.

Audience

The audience at a final presentation could include quite a few more people than those who have been involved throughout the project. For the final presentation, the project organizers may want to include people who can ensure that the work is carried on or that the work is disseminated to other groups or organizations in the community. The team members would want to include the people who contributed to the success of the project. The collaborators may want to include others who can benefit from the information. Suddenly the list of invitees can grow quite large.

Similar to deciding on the number of guests to invite to a wedding, negotiations need to occur. Usually the size of the room will limit the number of people that can be accommodated. For some groups, other sessions or a different means of providing the information would be more appropriate than a presentation.

Invitations to the presentation can be sent informally, such as by email, phone, or in person, or formally in the form of a letter at least two weeks before the event. The invitation would include the date, time, place, and parking and child care arrangements. If space is limited, people should be asked to confirm their attendance.

Objectives for the presentation

The final presentation is the last chance the team will have to consult with the people in the community. This requires special consideration of what message you want to leave with them. Although the team wants the audience to know what was accomplished, they also want to know that others can use the work that was started. To be effective, a presentation needs to meet the following four objectives: 1) to inform, 2) to entertain, 3) to touch the emotions, and 4) to move to action (Bender, 2000). In the final presentation, the move to action will be independent action, without reliance on the team.

Preparing the speech

The actual content that is prepared for the final presentation can be more complex than basic presentations because more people are involved both in the presentation and in the audience. Similar to basic presentations, an outline must be developed first. Then different people, including the collaborators, can be assigned to prepare different parts of the presentation. Box 8-2 provides an outline for a final presentation.

BOX 8-2	Proposed outline for a final presentation

1. An introduction (start with something to grab the attention of the audience such as a picture or a story from the action) to tell them what you are going to discuss
2. A background to the issue or situation
3. A description of what was done—the action
4. The results of the action
5. Your proposed options for what could be done now (recommendations)
6. A summary to tell them what you have discussed
7. A final point that you want to leave with the audience

Source: Adapted from Health Communication Unit, 2000; KU Work Group (2000).

Promoting the value of products

During the presentation, the team will want to make the case that the products they produced are relevant and can be continued through collaboration. One way to do that is through your own conviction; the other is by involving collaborators. At the end of a project, there usually is no difficulty finding some aspect of the project to get passionate about, which is expected when you have put a lot of effort into what you have been doing. When presenting the information, however, focus on a range of options or actions that could be taken, rather than promoting only one. When only one action is promoted, the audience may feel that the team is too directive. Recommendations can include teaming up with other community organizations with similar interests. When the project is organized by an educational institution, one option can be that arrangements are made for another student group to carry on with the project.

Both the relevance of and collaboration involved in the products and project can be demonstrated by including the collaborators in the presentations. Their inclusion sends a strong message that the action was relevant and that collaboration was productive, even before anything is said. Not all collaborators will want to get up in front of an audience; however, they may be willing to assist in some other way, such as preparing material or assisting with small group discussions.

Interaction

As in the basic presentation, interaction increases the chances of emotional involvement. In the final presentation, the interaction could be as simple as asking for comments about the findings to involving the audience in trying some aspect of the action, or working in a small group to decide on "next steps."

Interaction allows the audience to take some ownership for the information that you are presenting. When they have a chance to interpret the information in terms of their own circumstances, they are more likely to make a commitment to continue with the work that was started.

Follow-up

The follow-up for the final presentation is for the benefit of those who will be carrying on. At the end of the presentation, you can refer people to the collaborators if they have questions or want to become involved. This interaction can be assisted by having the collaborators hand out information on the products, project, and contacts and having them wear a certain name tag or T-shirt. Alternatively, another meeting might be announced and people asked to sign up with their name and phone number.

The team shows support for the collaborators by using the presentation as an opportunity to recruit new people to the continuing project. Team members may find it much easier to advocate on behalf of others rather than for themselves. This gesture and the response to it can provide the impetus for the collaborators to continue on their own. The scenario in Chapter 1 demonstrates this approach.

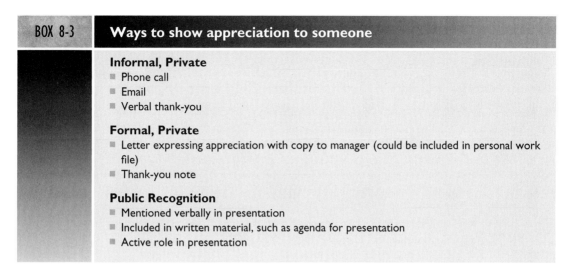

| BOX 8-3 | **Ways to show appreciation to someone** |

Informal, Private
■ Phone call
■ Email
■ Verbal thank-you

Formal, Private
■ Letter expressing appreciation with copy to manager (could be included in personal work file)
■ Thank-you note

Public Recognition
■ Mentioned verbally in presentation
■ Included in written material, such as agenda for presentation
■ Active role in presentation

Show appreciation

Although **showing appreciation** is a normal part of nursing practice as well as good manners, in community health nursing it is especially important. Most of the people who you contact during your project have no particular obligation to work with you or to help you. However, they do so because they want to support what you are doing or the people who could benefit. Recognizing them reinforces their continued support for community health.

As you are organizing for the end of your project, you must determine the people that you want to recognize and how you will show your appreciation. To determine the people, simply start listing all the people who have been involved and the contribution that they have made. Next consider the various options that you have for showing your appreciation. Box 8-3 provides some options to consider. Discuss the options with others who are familiar with the situation or people to determine which option would be the most appropriate.

Usually teams do not have any difficulty identifying people who should be recognized. They do have difficulty, however, ensuring that people are thanked appropriately in the final rush to complete the project. The thank you's must be a designated task to ensure that the project ends well.

SUPERMARKET BACK HEALTH SCENARIO (continued)

The three people who had been working on the presentation were excited about the plans they had made. They had taken the outline given in Box 8-2 and adapted it to their situation. Table 8-2 shows the outline of the presentation and the people responsible.

The expanded committee really liked the ideas for the presentation. However, they had learned from doing the pilot workshop that they would need to gather all the needed information and then rehearse. At that point, Letecia asked who would be coming to this presentation. She and Stephanie had started a list

TABLE 8-2	**Sample Outline for Final Presentation on Back Health**

OUTLINE ITEM AND TIME	DETAILS	RESPONSIBILITY
1. Introduction: 5 min	Pictures from the supermarket showing "before" and "after" shots of staff lifting and flexing	Health and Safety Committee (H&S)
2. Background: 2 min	The facts and figures on days off work due to back pain	Stephanie
3. The action: 10 min	The workshops—description The video—short clips Demonstrations	Denny H&S H&S
4. The results of the action: 2 min	Ability and accomplishment objectives	Jose
5. Options: 5 min	Options on how to increase use of techniques and flexibility exercises	Stephanie and Letecia
6. Summary: 2 min	What worked and what needs more work	Stephanie and Letecia
7. A final point: 4 min	Announcement of the winner of the slogan contest	Stephanie and Letecia Manager

that already had ten names. The store manager had presented them with a list of other supermarket managers in the city and the district manager he had invited. The list also included people who had provided the videos on back health. Letecia said that representatives from the Health and Safety Committees in other stores wanted to come. The staff room had space for only 20 people, and the supermarket staff had not been included yet.

They started to consider what they would do. They felt obligated to the people who had provided the videos and to the supermarket staff. However, they knew that if they wanted support from the manager to make more changes, his guests needed to be included. The Health and Safety Committee members conferred and proposed that they would set up a display in the staff room with the pictures and material from the presentation. That way everyone on each shift would have a chance to see it. They could also invite the representatives from different Health and Safety Committees at different times during the week. The team felt that this was the best solution under the circumstances.

Now that the audience for the presentation was determined, the team became more concerned about what message they wanted to convey with to audience. They had come to realize from doing the workshops and the follow-up observations that the training was not sufficient by itself. There had to be more changes in the environment and ongoing encouragement for the staff to adapt safe back health measures into their work routines. From what they had observed they could make some recommendations. They did not want the workshops either dismissed or considered as the only solution to back health.

Another preparation for the presentation was to select the winning slogan. Fifteen had been submitted, and Maria and the Health and Safety Committee members had looked through them all. They had narrowed them down to five finalists: "We back each other," "Back your future," "Be good to your back," "I'm backing you," and "We watch our backs." Everyone had a different favorite until they decided that the criteria would be that it had to indicate back health and to promote each other's back health. With those criteria, "We watch our backs" was selected as the winner. That slogan came from two night stockers, after one yelled to the other, "Hey, watch your back," as the other person bent over to lift a heavy carton.

The team realized that the presentation would be a good opportunity to recognize the people who had helped with the project. They decided to call the people who had contributed "sponsors" and to list them at the end of the agenda for the presentation. They recognized the participants in the two pilot workshops by including their names in the staff room display under the title of "Thanks to the workshop guinea pigs!" They would thank the manager for his support during the presentation.

The expanded team held two rehearsals for the final presentation. They knew that because of the greater number of people in the presentation and the short timeline, everyone needed to know exactly what they and the other team members were doing. As the room was filling up for the presentation, they were feeling excited but not especially anxious.

The audience was enjoying the presentation and were ready to get into discussions on how to promote a "back health culture" in the supermarket. Stephanie and Letecia proposed three options: 1) offer rewards for people "caught" lifting correctly, doing flexibility exercises, or helping a co-worker maintain back health; 2) have certain areas of the store assessed to determine necessary modifications for safe work movements; and 3) distribute posters throughout the store demonstrating techniques pertinent to that area. After some discussion recognizing the value of each of the options, the district manager got up and asked how they could implement the workshops and the three recommendations in each of the supermarkets in the district. The quick response from the store managers was that they needed more staff time and money devoted to health and safety. The district manager said, "Okay, we'll do that then. It will pay because of less sick time and better health for our employees!" This was first greeted with stunned silence, and then everyone burst into applause.

After that announcement, rewarding the two stockers for their winning slogan seemed like an anticlimax. The student team had also arranged to have three of the new work aprons with the new slogan on the back finished early so that they could present them to the members of the Health and Safety Committee.

The team members were quite overwhelmed by the response to their presentation. After the presentation, several of the managers asked how they could get nursing students to work on a project in their store.

As a final gesture, the team worked with their instructor to write a letter commending Letecia for the work she had done on the project and gave it to the store manager. They hoped that she would get a full-time job working on health and safety.

COLLEGE STUDENTS' SMOKING KNOWLEDGE SCENARIO (continued)

When the team working on smoking made arrangements for their final presentation, they booked a small room at the health clinic during the day. As their agency representative at the clinic started telling the rest of the staff what the team was doing on the project, more people expressed an interest in attending, but could not attend during clinic hours. The team also wanted to invite the people from the Lung Association and Public Health who had helped them. They were able to find a bigger room at a more convenient time.

The team decided that they wanted to emphasize the lessons they had learned during the project. Although they gained some valuable information from the experience, the display in large public areas just did not attract smokers, especially smokers in precontemplation and contemplation stages of change. The other aspect that they wanted to emphasize was the need for organizations to work together in the area of smoking. They felt that the amount of information on smoking was too vast for everyone to have up-to-date information. Certainly the Lung Association and Public Health worked together, but the health clinic staff seemed to be working on their own.

After coming up with these two purposes for the presentation, they discussed them with their agency representative from the health clinic. She felt that it would be a great opportunity to let the clinic staff know what factors influenced smoking by college students and how the clinic could improve their smoking *cessation services. The involvement of people from the Lung Association and Public Health could help to reinforce the messages.*

Because this was a professional audience and they had an hour for the presentation, the team decided to deal with their purposes by having two interactive components in the presentation. In the first part, they compared and contrasted the different approaches that they had actually used and the approaches identified by smokers in the bar. In the small group discussion, they asked the participants to identify the approaches that they felt would be the most effective for college students. In the second part of the presentation, they used the display of the Transtheoretical Model and provided information on the systematic reviews of the literature on smoking they had found. In the small group discussions, they asked the participants to identify how the effective approaches could be implemented for college students.

They soon found out that either discussion could have taken the whole time. However, it did stimulate considerable interest in looking at different approaches for individual counseling of college students and in the material that would be available in the clinic. The health clinic, Lung Association, and Public Health had also started talking about working together on a Web site with a chat room that could deal with issues such as smoking.

During the presentation, the team identified the people and organizations who had assisted them. After the presentation, they met with their instructor and the agency representative from the health clinic to discuss the presentation.

"Well," said Veena, "We certainly engaged them! But we had too much. They would hardly stop talking so we could present the stuff for the second half."

Their agency representative immediately responded, "Too much was okay. It was great. Just the kind of thing the staff needed to hear!"

Georgio said, "Yeah, I heard one of the doctors say to another that he hadn't thought that it was worthwhile even to ask about smoking."

"And the nurses working in the clinic said that they wanted to have the display using the Transtheoretical Model in the waiting room," added Habib.

Francine said, "I can't believe that a Public Health nurse and a woman from the Lung Association actually came up and thanked me just for inviting them. This was just a student presentation!"

"I also can't believe that because of us they will be working together on a Web site," said Veena. "Who would have thought this could happen after our disastrous pilot?"

The instructor and agency representative exchanged a telling glance that said, "We kept telling them that they were doing good work, but they had to hear if from others to believe it!"

DISCUSSION QUESTIONS

1. Why was it important for both teams to clarify their objectives for this final presentation?
2. Why did the audience need to be determined before the objectives could be clarified?
3. Would the presentation be considered a way to validate the findings and recommendations?

Project report and portfolio

The project report and portfolio are contained in a binder or folder that includes a title page, a table of contents, the two page project report, and sections for the different attachments. Attachments can vary according to the project, but usually include references, the products that were produced, data collection measures, and tabulations of the evaluation data.

At this point in the project, the team will have a sizable amount of written work including the timelines, workplans, evaluation data, and material prepared for the presentation. The final task for the team is to collate this information into the project report and portfolio. The project report form in Appendix C identifies the elements that are to be included. The project report serves the same purpose as an abstract for a journal article or an executive summary for a lengthy report.

Purpose of the report and portfolio

Teams may feel that since they have already conveyed their information in the presentation to the people who matter and have lengthy workplans, that there is no need to have a written report. The workplans provide a plan and summarize the daily or weekly activities and results. The presentation summarizes what was done and found, but also seeks validation for sustainability and recommendations. The report brings the findings from the workplan and presentation together in a concise way. The project report provides an opportunity for others who were not present for the event to quickly learn from what you have done and build on it. The report can reach many people over a longer period of time and contributes to the sustainability of the project.

Project reports are a valuable asset for community organizations. Often community groups and organizations do not have the time or finances to allow staff providing services time to write reports. Other groups may not have people with experience in writing reports. In both situations, the project report provided by the team contributes to the history of the group or organization. This written history is important because there can be a frequent turnover of staff and a less frequent change in problems and issues. When the issue arises again or when more work is needed, the project report can serve as a base and save valuable time and effort.

From another perspective, teams may feel that a two-page project report does not fully reflect all the work that was involved in the project and that a full report should be written. There are two main arguments against doing a full report, which is a paper written in paragraph format rather than point form. The first is that a full report is not structured to quickly provide practical information. Because the project is a collaboration between the team and people in the community, the report must be useful to the community. The second argument is that writing a full report is a very difficult and time-consuming task for a group. This means that time would be taken from completing the project and the report could be done poorly or by only one person in the group. The two-page project report does maintain important elements of academic writing: a logical flow from initial issue to recommendations, and referencing of sources. The attachments to the project report provide the details of the work that was done.

Sections of the project report

The two-page project report has six main sections: assessment, plan, action, findings, conclusions, and attachments.

Assessment section

The first part of the report provides the information on the project's assessment. This part of the report can be completed as soon as the issues for action have been determined. For teams that have completed an assessment report (Chapter 5) this section will be a condensed version of that assessment. The assessment section includes the following items:

- Importance of issue/problem:
- Agency mandate:
- Agency priority or issue:
- Community of interest:
- Collaborative assessment goal:
- Assessment methods and timeline:
- Validated key results/findings and supporting evidence:
    Present health situation (barriers and strengths)
    Preferred health situation
    Issues for action

The importance of the issue or problem is a statement referenced from a reputable source or sources that indicates that the issue causes hardship, illness, or death and deserves to receive attention. If the project issue was safety of toddlers in the home, the statement on the importance of the issue would include statistics on the number of toddlers injured in the home locally, regionally, or nationally. As a rationale for working with specific groups, the importance statement could include statistics related to the group, such as women living in poverty having a high rate of low-birth-weight infants. Although the team may have many statistics at this point, choose two or three that are the most pertinent and make the point that it is worthwhile to work on this issue or problem.

The agency mandate or mission statement is included to indicate that the project will contribute to the work of the agency. The mandate is usually written in broad terms. If the agency provides health or social services, the mandate usually relates to the health and well-being of people living in a certain area. Sometimes the people are defined by gender, age, ethnic group, or financial resources. If the mandate is long, you may need to use a shortened version. If you are working with the workers or staff in a business, you would use the mandate or policy statement of the human resources or personnel department.

The priority or issue is the reason that the agency or community group wanted to have the team work on a project. Once the team has done the assessment, the priority or issue might change, but the original one should be used here. The inclusion of the original priority indicates that further refinement has occurred during the assessment.

The community of interest for the project might also have become more specific during the assessment. In this situation, the original community of interest should be given as well as the revised community of interest, with the dates for each.

The assessment for the project report has two parts: the methods, which include a description of the participants, and the findings. For teams that completed an assessment report, both parts have extensive detail and timelines. For the project report, the information can be condensed by first indicating only the total period for the assessment. Further condensing would remove specific details that do not comprise an understanding of the assessment process.

Table 8-3 provides an example of how to condense information from a detailed account without losing the important elements. The example used in Table 8-3 is an excerpt of the assessment report given in Application 5-1 in Chapter 5.

TABLE 8-3 Example of Condensed Version of Assessment Me~

ORIGINAL INFORMATION IN ASSESSMENT REPORT	CONDENSED INFORMATION~

Assessment methods:
    —Collect and review secondary data, Sept. 10–24.
    —Community mapping, Sept. 17–24.
    —Interviews with key informants: Sept 24–Oct. 8;
    five people including multicultural worker and
    executive, Cantonese community leaders.
    —Progressive inquiry: Oct. 15–Nov. 12, 22 women
    speaking Cantonese and Mandarin attending ESL
    class and church meeting.
    —Questionnaire: Oct. 29–Nov. 12, 20 women
    speaking Mandarin associated with the Com-
    puter Age firm.
	Assessment methods: Sept. 10–N~
	    —Review secondary data and map ~
	    —5 key informant interviews.
	    —Progressive inquiry with 22 Cantonese ~
	    Mandarin speaking women for 5 weeks.
	    —Questionnaire with 20 Mandarin speaking
	    women.

Validated Key Results/Findings: Present health situation Barriers to health: no information available on pre and postnatal health care services in Cantonese, Mandarin or written in simple language. No informa- tion on nutrition, exercise and sleep. Evidence: pro- gressive inquiry with 22 women over five weeks, 15 out of 20 responses to question in questionnaire, no prenatal classes in Cantonese or Mandarin, most unable to understand written information in English.	Validated Key Results/Findings: Present health situation Barriers to health. No written information nutri- tion, exercise and sleep for pregnant and new mothers that is intelligible to community. Evidence: progressive inquiry, 15 out of 20 responses in ques- tionnaire, no prenatal classes in Cantonese or Man- darin, most unable to understand written informa- tion in English.
Strengths: anxious to learn English and ways to keep themselves and their children healthy. Evidence: re- sponses in progressive inquiry and 20 question- naires. Cantonese women organized ESL classes held in church. Mandarin speaking women experi- enced in using internet and interested in support group. Evidence: responses in 18 of 20 question- naires. Supports available: meeting rooms available at church in Chinatown, Public Health Department has mandate to support child-bearing families and is willing to tailor information, Computer Age firm has mission statement which includes promoting the health of employees and their families and manage- ment is willing to organize a support group for preg- nant and new mothers. Evidence from key informant interviews, meetings, and policy documents.	Strengths: anxious to learn English and ways to keep themselves and their children healthy. Evidence: progressive inquiry and 20 question- naires. Cantonese women organized ESL classes Mandarin speaking women experienced in using internet and interested in support group. Evidence: responses in 18 of 20 questionnaires. Supports available: meeting rooms at church, Public Health Department mandate, Computer Age firm. Evi- dence from key informant interviews, meetings, and policy documents.
Preferred health—have energy from good food, exer- cise, and sufficient sleep. Evidence: progressive inquiry.	Preferred health—have energy from good food, ex- ercise, and sufficient sleep Evidence: progressive inquiry
Issues for action: need for pre- and postnatal infor- mation in Cantonese and Mandarin or simple lan- guage, especially on nutrition, sleep, and exercise.	Issues for action: need for pre- and postnatal infor- mation in Cantonese and Mandarin or simple lan- guage, especially on nutrition, sleep, and exercise.

Plan section

The plan for the project report includes the items covered in Chapter 6. This section can be completed near the end of implementation. The items in the plan section are as follows:

- Priority action statement
- Project goal
- Products
- Strategy, theory, evidence base
- Ability objective (or the second highest objectives achieved)
- Accomplishment objective (or the highest objective achieved)
- Environmental objective

The action statement, goal, and objectives simply need to be transferred from the workplan to the project report. Often the products and strategies have gone through some revision or expansion during the implementation and evaluation. Products are both tangible items and process that have been developed and evaluated. The products that were expected at the end of planning could be quite different by the end of the project. For example, assume that one of the products for toddler safety was to be a pamphlet that would be available at a medical clinic. During the pilot test, the women inform the project team that the medical clinic is difficult to get to and that they want information that is accessible, either on the Internet or in the local shopping mall. This would require a change in where the product will be delivered and how it will be delivered.

Another thing that will require a change in the description of the products is that some aspects may not have been considered relevant or were taken for granted. For example, although one of the products of your project may be a health fair for seniors, another invaluable product would be a documented process to organize a health fair for seniors that details what worked and what did not work. The evaluations that were done for the pilot test and at the end of the project mean that the team is able to provide tailored products and a process that could be adapted for use elsewhere.

Although the strategy, theory, and source of evidence will probably remain the same from the plan, certain applications from the theory or findings from the systematic reviews may have been used to make a difference during implementation. The most important to identify would be the titles of the evidence-based studies or reports that made a difference in how action was taken.

Five possible types of objectives could be used in a project. If all were developed, only the top three—accomplishment, environmental, and ability—need to be mentioned in the final report. If only two learning objectives, such as awareness and knowledge, were developed, they would be included instead along with the environmental objective. For example, if the project was to develop a marketing strategy to determine what interested a particular population, only awareness, knowledge, and environmental objectives would be relevant and be included in the final report.

Collaborative action section

Collaborative action is an updated summary of the activities from the timeline or Gantt chart completed in Chapter 6 and revised during implementation in Chapter 7. Rather than listing separate activities according to date, the activities could be grouped into preparation, pilot test, action, and evaluation, with a time period indicated for each. You may find that what you planned to do and what you actually did do, changed after your pilot. For each activity, include the actual number of participants who were involved.

Key findings section

Key findings include the results from the process and impact evaluation; these can be completed before the presentation. Process evaluation is used to determine whether the activities and products were relevant to the needs of the community of interest and stakeholders. Although the achievement of target numbers and deadlines can be important during the process, for the project report, the adjustments made after the pilot test and the relevance and collaboration used to develop the final products are more important.

Impact evaluation is the comparison of the results with the criteria given in each objective. Only the top three objectives need to be presented and discussed, unless the results from other objectives compromised the achievement of more important ones. Explanations of discrepancies between what was planned and what was achieved can be provided in the impact or limitations.

Conclusions section

Conclusions are the interpretation of the findings. Conclusions can be completed only after the findings have been presented to the community members and stakeholders. Their feedback provides validation for the conclusions. The conclusions include the following items:

- Limitations
- Sustainability
- Recommendations

Limitations are the barriers encountered that reduced the ability to achieve the desired results. Time and resources can often be a barrier in these short-term projects. Other barriers might have been revealed during the project or even during the presentation. For example, the purpose of a project may have been to market a certain health promotion Web site. During the project, it may be discovered that the Web site had several nonfunctioning links that frustrated people or that the computers provided for use by the public were often nonfunctional. The analysis of why objectives were not met can be just as beneficial to community groups as identifying what worked. Limitations used in research studies usually identify factors known to the researchers that would limit the generalizability of the results. Although these projects are focused on improving practice rather than on conducting research, there may be some weaknesses in the measures and comparisons that need to be qualified. For example, results of pre- and posttests might not be totally comparable because the questions were changed.

Although sustainability for the products and project has been considered from the beginning, sustainability may not be realized until some time after the project. All that can be reported at the end of the project is what training has been provided, what reception the products have received, and what has been promised.

The **recommendations** are based on what you found during the project and what was confirmed at the presentation. Similar to conclusions for papers or reports, the recommendations must be a logical conclusion from the findings. In other words, each recommendation would either propose the continuation of what worked well or suggest a means to address areas identified in the findings or limitations that did not work well.

For example, if the project showed that women who were learning English were comfortable learning in groups of four to six using pictures and plain language, you would recommend that scenario. If at the same time, you found that they had difficulty concentrating in a noisy environment, you would recommend a quiet one.

One caution must be made about the limitations or recommendations that are made in the report. These project reports and recommendations survive much longer than the feelings and experiences of the team members. At times, miscommunication or personality differences may have created friction. These types of situations are not to be reported in the project report. Other approaches to dealing with the difficulty need to be taken. To ensure that statements are appropriate, they should be discussed first with the agency representative and supervisors.

An important purpose of the recommendations is to identify policy changes that could improve the health outcomes of the people involved in the project. These recommendations would deal with the barriers to health that still remain because of socioeconomic determinants, such as poverty, or the added resources and legislation that could extend the outcomes of the project to others. For example, the project might have involved working with low-income women to address their concerns related to poor nutrition. Although during the project the women learned about the nutritional content of food and worked together to buy food in bulk, they will continue to be concerned about adequate food unless policy on the amount of income they receive or the availability of low-cost food is changed. Recommendations on which type of action to take based on the experience of working with the women would be useful to decision makers.

Policy change can also greatly enhance the value obtained from education and training. For example, a considerable amount of effort might go into providing education and training to change risk behaviors such as lifting incorrectly, riding a bicycle without a helmet, or driving without a seat belt. Although some people will be convinced to change their behavior, most would be more convinced to change if there are associated rules, regulations, or policies. The policy could take the form of required back safety training every six months or fines for not using safety equipment.

Policy implications can be determined "by asking the question: what could or should be done about this issue" (Public Health Nursing Section, 2001, p. 315) that could not be done with the resources or authority available to the project team. Policy recommendations need to be reasonable and strongly supported by the findings of the project.

Attachments section

The attachments to the project report are all the items that would allow work on the project to continue or others to use the process elsewhere. Although the project report provides a good overview, the products and the details of the process can be the most useful parts of the portfolio. Items such as the questions used in progressive inquiry, questionnaires, or focused discussions would save groups new to the situation considerable time and effort. Training manuals, pamphlets, pre- and posttests, and sources for information are invaluable to people. In the binder for the project, create different sections, such as assessment measures, graphs from assessment, evaluation forms, tabulations of results, and slides from the presentation. The project report and attachments can facilitate steady improvement in the health of communities because practitioners are sharing information and are not continuously "recreating the wheel."

SUPERMARKET BACK HEALTH SCENARIO (continued)

After the excitement of the presentation, the four team members found it difficult to pull their thoughts together to complete the final report. Maria and Jose had been working on the report and had completed the assessment section and most of the plan. They wanted some help on how to describe the products. In their original plan the products were to include the back injury prevention video, a workshop on back injury, training of Health and Safety Committee members to provide the workshop, and the store contest. Everyone agreed that they had produced these products, but that more description was needed to indicate that the training and materials were relevant and were produced collaboratively. Together they came up with a few appropriate terms.

The next section that Marie and Jose had just started was collaborative action. They knew that listing all the activities from the Gantt chart (Application 7-1) would take up too much space, and besides, some of the activities had changed. When they looked at the Gantt chart again, they realized that they could group the activities by time. They filled in the number of participants from the tables they had constructed.

The key findings were something that they had already discussed at considerable length when they were preparing for the presentation. They felt it was important to mention in the process evaluation that the workshop was modified based on feedback from participants in the pilot programs and that the contest did not involve a competition between departments, but involved the development of a slogan.

In the impact evaluation, they included the results for the accomplishment, environmental, and ability objectives. Another addition was that the workshop conducted by the trained Health and Safety Committee members had the same results as the earlier workshops. At first they were not certain about where to include the information about the three hazardous areas in the store. They decided that it belonged in the conclusions section under limitations because it limited the results that they were able to achieve. The other limitations were time and the unusually high activity in the store during the evaluation.

Another limitation that they considered was initial reluctance of the store manager to participate. When they discussed his attitude with their instructor, she asked them how they would word the limitation and what purpose it would serve. They really did not have an answer for the questions. They realized that the store manager became more helpful when he saw that they stuck to the hour and a half for the workshops.

They felt that sustainability had been an integral part of their project from the beginning because of the involvement of the Health and Safety Committee members, especially Letecia. Sustainability was confirmed by the workshop conducted by the store trainers and by the announcement by the district manager.

They did not have a lot more to discuss about the recommendations. Three of the recommendations had been discussed and confirmed at the presentation, and the fourth, to maintain the workshops, had never really been in question. However, as they were writing them down they realized that they were making recommendations for changes in the policy of the grocery store chain. They felt a bit audacious at first, but reassured themselves that they had the data to support what they were recommending.

Which attachments to use was also an easy decision. Along with the reference list, the presentation slides, and the instructor's manual for the workshop, they decided to itemize other elements of the workshop such as the pre- and posttests, the handouts, and the tabulation of the evaluation data.

When they had completed reviewing the project report, they sat back with sighs of relief. They thought that it would have taken them a lot longer than it did. In most cases they already had the information and had just needed to decide where to put it. They were pleased to think that their project portfolio would probably be used in the other supermarkets in the district, and that other project teams could build on their work. Their project report is found in Application 8-1.

COLLEGE STUDENTS' SMOKING KNOWLEDGE SCENARIO (continued)

When the team working on college students' smoking completed their evaluation of the pilot display, they decided to start putting their results directly into the project report. They knew that the report would be far too long initially, but at least they would have all the information in the right place. When they went to *complete the report, they did not feel that it would be too difficult because they were just reorganizing and condensing the needed information.*

As they were deciding what should be included in the attachments to the project report, they remembered some of the comments from the presentation. They decided to include an explanation of the Transtheoretical Model and the table they had developed to display the findings from the systematic reviews (Table 7-5). They also included the slides from their presentation and tabulations of responses from smokers.

When the team thought about the information that would be in the project portfolio presented to the health clinic and to their instructor, they felt that the Lung Association and Public Health would also appreciate a copy. They wanted other people to learn from what they did.

The final task that they had for their community placement was a presentation to their classmates and invited guests. They did not have much more to do to prepare for that presentation because they only had to add the results from their presentation in the health clinic. To keep the presentation interesting and interactive, they decided that they would form their classmates into small groups and have them work on the questions they had posed to the community practitioners. Other teams were planning to focus on one aspect of their project, such as difficulties that they overcame or humorous incidents. For these presentations to classmates, use of a variety of formats was encouraged. The team presented in one room with 14 other teams while other classmates presented in other rooms. Each team had 20 to 30 minutes, depending on the size of the team. At the end of the presentations, everyone was overwhelmed by the work that had been done and would continue to be done on the projects. The students suggested, and the invited guests agreed, that the faculty should collect all the two-page reports for the class into a single document and distribute it to the community agencies. They wanted the information out in the community where it could be used.

DISCUSSION QUESTIONS

1. What is the value of having a two-page project report using a consistent format?
2. What would be an efficient way to work between the workplan and project report near the end of the project?
3. Who do you think could use the project portfolios in the future?

Teamwork to the end

The three challenges to the team at the end of the project are coordinating and allocating all the tasks, maintaining communication, and completing a team evaluation. Ending well means ensuring that there are no loose ends, every task is completed, and every person has been properly treated and respected.

Coordination and allocation of tasks

Coordination of activities as the project is ending is particularly important because of the variety of tasks that need to be done in a short period of time. The most effective use of time is to begin or continue planning for the presentation and report during the completion of the evaluation. This means concurrent activity with team members working alone or in small groups. When the tasks range from determining invitation lists to analyzing evaluation data, coordination can be daunting.

Similar to this stage during assessment, the team leadership function may have become shared among the team members. Although that shows maturity in the development of the team, one person, or at the most two if the team has expanded to include collaborators, need to track the tasks that must be done to meet deadlines.

The team leader should develop a task list together with the team members about three to four weeks before the end of the project. At each subsequent meeting, the task list should be used to document progress in completing the tasks. If tasks are not being completed on time, reassess the priority in completing all the remaining tasks. There simply may be too many tasks for the time available. Determine whether the tasks are a necessity or a nicety. If the task is a necessity, it could be scaled down to be manageable in the time remaining.

Early preparation and thinking about the presentation are particularly important and need to be assigned to people who have an understanding of the issues. Experienced presenters advise that you spend 80% of your preparation time on delivery and 20% on content (Bender, 2000). The presentation at this time can have quite an impact on how the project information is used in the future. Therefore, the team needs to make a considerable effort to determine what message they want to impart at the presentation. Often the presentation audience will include people who have not been directly involved in the project but who can affect the future use of the products. The team needs to consider the implications of this situation and consult with the instructor, agency representative, and relevant managers.

Coordination can be difficult at the end because team members may be feeling both sad about the end of the teamwork and rushed for time. The team leader and instructor need to work closely with individual team members to help them make fair and rational decisions to respect both the work done on the project and the people doing the work.

Communication

Communication of team decisions, especially if the team is working in small groups, becomes particularly important because of complicated arrangements. For example, the team leader may be informed that certain people need to be invited to the final presentation. That change can affect who else can be invited or the focus of the presentation and needs to be quickly communicated to team members.

Because the time available is short and last minute changes may be necessary, communication by email or phone may be far more frequent than during earlier parts of the project. Team members may need to be reminded to be more diligent in check-ing for messages. More people may also need to be included in the email distribution list.

Team evaluation

Along with the tasks, take time to reflect individually and as a team on what you have accomplished and learned. Look back to what you felt as you started this project, and ask yourself some questions: Did you learn what you wanted to learn? Did you learn what you expected to learn? Did you learn more than you expected to learn? What individual and group skills can you now add to your resume? How did your team make a difference in the community? As a team, review the high points and the low points as well as the stage of development that you are at now (Chapter 2). Also refer to the team agreement to evaluate the team and document the results in the workplan.

Ending can be a time of celebration as well as a time of mourning. Some team members may start feeling sad as soon as most of the tasks are done; others may have a delayed reaction. To assist people in recognizing what they have done and preparing them to move on, take time to recognize the contribution that each team member has made. One team member may have found a talent for identifying key messages, another for developing a role play, or another for preparing an electronic presentation. When those hidden or taken-for-granted talents are recognized, people can gain confidence to move on to new challenges.

The end of any accomplishment deserves to be celebrated. Plan a party, plan a trip, or plan on writing an article or giving a presentation on what your team has accomplished in collaboration with the community group. Community health groups and community health nursing need to hear about those accomplishments if we are to make a difference in the health of the population.

Summary

Ending well means that the team is satisfied by their accomplishments, the collaborators have gained from the experience, useful resources have been produced, and most people who have been involved have positive feelings about the experience. Although some team members may have regretful feelings because there may not have been the time or resources to accomplish all that was planned, positive movement in the right direction means that the project made a difference. Ending well also means that there will be some continuation of use of the products and the relationships that have been formed. Both will eventually contribute to improved health of the population.

PRACTICE AND APPLICATION

1. For the college students' smoking knowledge project, prepare an outline with timelines and responsibilities for their presentation.

2. For the college students' smoking knowledge project and material developed in Exercise 2 of Chapter 7, complete the collaborative action and findings sections of the project report.

3. Your team has completed collecting evaluation data on the use of three different methods of providing information on nutritional food to people who have difficulty speaking and reading English. Describe how your final presentation would vary if given to
   a) A community group who have difficulty speaking and reading English
   b) Lay workers who work with the community group
   c) Health professionals who work with the community group
   d) The board of directors of a large healthcare organization providing services to the community group

4. Your team is just about to start collecting evaluation data on three objectives for your project. Prepare a table with four columns. In the first column, list every task that must be accomplished by the end of the project. In the second, indicate when the task must be completed. In the third column, indicate the people or person responsible for each task. In the fourth column, indicate what could delay or prevent completion of the task.

REFERENCES

Bender, P. (2000). Secrets of power presentations. Toronto: The Achievement Group.

Health Communication Unit, University of Toronto. (2000). Strengthening presentation skills. Toronto: Author.

Karas, B., & Conrad, K. (1996). Back injury prevention interventions in the workplace: An integrative review. American Association of Occupational Health Nurses Journal, 44, 189-96.

KU Work Group, E. (2000). Community Tool Box: Part B, chapter 4, section 5: Making community presentations. Lawrence, KS: University of Kansas. Retrieved July 15, 2000, from the World Wide Web http://ctb.lsi.ukans.edu/tools/en/sub_section_main_1029.htm.

Occupational Safety and Health Administration. (1999). *Ergonomics Program.-64:65768-66078.* Washington, DC: U. S. Department of Labour.

Public Health Nursing Section. (2001). *Public health interventions-Applications for Public Health Nursing Practice.* St. Paul: Minnesota Department of Health.

van Tulder, M., Jellema, P., van Poppel, M., Nachemson, A., & Bouter, L. (2002). Lumbar supports for prevention and treatment of low back pain (Cochrane Review). In: *The Cochrane Library,* 1, 2003. Chichester, UK: John Wiley & Sons.

APPLICATION 8-1

PRESENTATION

East Coast College, School of Nursing

Community Health Project in Collaboration with Eastern Supermarket
WE WATCH OUR BACKS!

December 1, 2004

Team members: Maria Lopez, Stephanie White, Denny Hoi, Jose Rupierez
Instructor: Janet MacWilliam
Agency representative: Letecia Marcos
Agency manager: Joseph Offenbach

Importance of issue/problem Occupational Safety and Health Administration (1999) indicates that musculo-skeletal disorders [MSD] comprise one third of all lost work days and low back pain is the most prevalent and costly form of MSD. People doing manual handling jobs, which includes grocery store stocking, are at risk for MSD.

Agency mandate: (Human Resources) Provide a safe and healthy work environment.
Agency priority or issue: Work-related injuries and days off work of staff
Community of interest: Staff working at Eastern Supermarket

ASSESSMENT

Assessment goal: Determine issues contributing to work injuries from management and workers
Methods: Review statistics on injuries and days off work, key informant interviews with Health and Safety Committee members.
Validated key results/findings with supporting evidence:
Present health situation
Barriers to health: back injuries as result of work situation

Evidence: injury statistics for previous three years showing back pain as the most common cause for days off work, stockers have the most days off work from back pain, no back injury prevention training available to staff working evenings and nights

Strengths: Health and Safety Committee's interest in providing training and supports to reduce back injuries. Management interested reducing cost related to back injury

Preferred health situation: healthy backs

Issues for action: lack of back injury prevention training for stockers

Priority action statement: Stockers have potential for improved back health related to accessible back injury prevention training

PLAN

Project Goal: Stockers have improved back health

Products: Locate back injury prevention video appropriate for supermarket staff, workshop on back injury and workshop materials tailored to meet needs of supermarket staff, 3 Health and Safety Committee members demonstrate ability to provide workshop, and slogan for back safety determined through a contest among supermarket staff.

Strategy, theory, evidence base: Educational activities and framework on health communication. Evidence from Cochran Library that education for back injury prevention and exercise flexibility training programmes decreased back injuries (Karas & Conrad, 1996); no consistent evidence for the use of lumbar supports (van Tulder, Jellema, van Poppel, Nachemson & Bouter, 2002).

Accomplishment objective: 40% of stockers demonstrate safe lifting techniques and flexibility exercises by the third week of November.

Ability objective: 50% of participants in back injury prevention training for stockers demonstrate safe lifting techniques and flexibility exercises at end of training.

Environmental objective: 75% of Health and Safety Committee members trained to provide back injury prevention training to all shifts on a regular basis.

COLLABORATIVE ACTION
Administrative activities and participants:

Preparation, Sept. 21–Oct. 7: Conduct literature search for evidence base, observe and document lifting and carrying behaviors, acquire room and equipment for workshops and final presentation.

Develop workshop resources, Sept. 28–Oct. 14: locate training video, develop, test and rehearse material for workshop and evaluation forms.

Pilot test, Oct. 21: Two pilot workshops with total of 12 participants

Action, Oct. 28: Revisions to workshop

   Nov. 1: 2 workshops for 13 and training of 3 trainers

   Nov. 7: 1 workshop for 6 given by trainers

Evaluation: week of Nov. 7: observation of stockers for use of lifting techniques and flexibility exercises by 7 people for one hour each night

KEY FINDINGS

Process: Video of 25 min, had appropriate techniques, exercises, did not show use of lumbar belt, and was approved by participants in workshop; workshop modified to suit needs of workers, competition between departments not mounted, slogan for back health selected from 15 submissions.

Impact: Only 42% of participants in workshop demonstrated safe lifting techniques and flexibility exercises. No stockers used lumbar belts after training compared to two prior to training. Only 20% of stockers used correct lifting technique during observation and none were observed doing flexibility exercises. Three members of four members the Health and Safety Committee received training on the workshop and conducted one workshop session that received similar evaluations as other workshops.

Limitations: Three areas of the store which did not allow for the use of safe lifting techniques were identified through observation and feedback from workers. Limited time and high activity in store reduced results.

Sustainability: Three staff members are trained to provide workshop and have provided one workshop. Management is supportive in making changes to environment and hiring staff to promote back health.

Recommendations: 1) Workshops are given to all staff on a regular basis and become part of an orientation package, 2) workers are given incentives to watch each others' lifting techniques and take flexibility breaks, 3) 3 areas of the store need to be modified to provide a safer work environment, 4) Distribute posters throughout the store demonstrating techniques pertinent to that area.

Attachments: (the following would be attached but have not been attached here) Reference list, instructors manual for workshop including pre and post tests and handouts, slides from presentation, tabulation of evaluation data.

Collaborative Assessment and Action: Across Settings, Populations and Issues

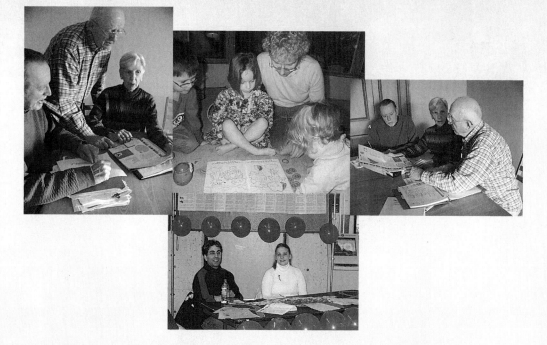

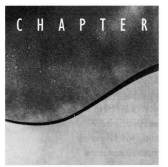

CHAPTER 9

Family Home Visiting Projects

ELIZABETH DIEM

FAMILY HEALTH PROMOTION IN THE HOME

A home health nursing organization received a small fund from the head office to develop a procedure to incorporate health promotion and illness prevention in the home visit. The home healthcare nurses in the region had asked the head office for a procedure that was brief and would be relatively easy to adapt to different situations. The procedure was to be developed and pilot tested within the local organization, and then the head office would organize a pilot test for the region.

The management of the nursing organization felt that the grant provided an opportunity to add a peer support component to their orientation program. Four new graduate nurses had recently been hired and were completing their initial orientation, which included home visits with experienced home healthcare nurses. The new graduates had varied clinical experience: Natalia had completed an extended practicum in community health nursing; Jennifer had received considerable experience in maternal–child family nursing in various settings; Denise had experience in working with the elderly in institutions during her education and in the summers; and Ron had worked as a home healthcare aide. The team first needed to determine the parameters of the project and establish relationships. This step is similar to step 1 (establish relationships within the project and community) of the collaborative assessment workplan given in Chapter 3. The group had three months to complete the pilot testing of the procedure and three hours a week together to work on the project. Emilie, the manager assigned to work with them, would meet with them every week for the first four weeks and every second week thereafter. They decided on an early morning meeting time to ensure that no one's attendance at the meeting would be delayed by extended home visits.

OBJECTIVES **After reading this chapter and answering the questions throughout the chapter, you should be able to**

1. Compare the community health nursing process used with groups and communities with that used with families in the community.
2. Identify the main components of family nursing in the home.
3. Determine an approach to develop a collaborative relationship with families.
4. Organize home visits that are safe and resource efficient, and consider other service providers.
5. Identify issues and procedures that are applicable to a number of families or home nursing situations.
6. Manage teamwork during home visits.

KEYWORDS   case manager or care coordinator ■ commendations ■ contextual approach ■ family ■ family circle ■ family interaction diagram ■ family nursing ■ home healthcare worker ■ referral ■ service providers ■ social support

Family home visiting projects

Projects based on visiting families in their homes follow the same steps of the community health nursing process as do projects for groups and communities. Some adaptations of the substeps are necessary to accommodate the home situation, however, especially during assessment. Tables 9-1 and 9-2 detail the adaptations to the community health nursing process collaborative assessment and action for families in the home.

TABLE 9-1   Comparison of Collaborative Assessment with Groups or Communities to Families at Home

GROUPS AND COMMUNITIES	ADAPTATIONS FOR FAMILIES AT HOME
1. Establish relationships within project and community.	Determine responsibilities, assessment goals, and meeting times with project organizers and team. Review mandate, policy, and procedures of organization.
2. Assess secondary data.	Conduct literature review on issues related to populations served at home, such as families with newborns, families living with chronic illness, or frail elderly. Review census tract data and maps to determine areas with a high number of elderly and low income families.
3. Initiate assessment of community.	Interview key informants such as other nurses and service providers to identify issues, challenges, and strengths; conduct windshield surveys of designated areas; determine community resources available to families receiving home nursing visits.
4. Conduct specific assessment.	Determine the number and characteristics of families that will be involved, time period, approach that will be used to engage families, and observations that will be made. Use and revise questions and observations to collect data from families meeting characteristics during allocated time period.
5. Determine action statements.	Similar process using both family barriers to health and strengths to identify collaborative issues for action and then action statements for "Families living with _____ (e.g., infants, adolescents, frail elderly) with _____ (health challenge)" Provide a report in a format that is useful to the organization.
6. Evaluate team work.	Same process as with groups and communities.

TABLE 9-2	**Adapting Collaborative Action Process with Groups or Communities to Families at Home**

GROUPS AND COMMUNITIES	ADAPTATIONS FOR FAMILIES AT HOME
1. Plan.	Determine priority action statement through discussions with families in the home and communication with relevant community health staff. Similar to communities and groups, which is to identify goal from action statement, strategies, theories, research, final products and activities, objectives, and evaluation measures.
2. Take action.	Similar to communities and groups, which is to take action on the collaborative plan, which includes evaluation.
3. Determine results/impact.	Similar to communities and groups, which is to analyze the results of the process and impact evaluation measures. Provide report in format that is useful to families and organization.
4. Evaluate team work.	Same process as with groups and communities.

Family nursing

Illness and health are a family affair. Family nursing crosses most domains of nursing practice and is an integral part of community health nursing. **Family** is defined as "two or more persons who are joined together by bonds of sharing and emotional closeness and who identify themselves as being part of a family" (Friedman, Bowden, & Jones, 2003, p. 10). This very broad definition of the family allows people to define who is important to them and who they want to involve in their healthcare. The family can include a mother, father, children, and any other close or distant family member, or a friend who might be living with them; a single mother, her children, and a female friend; same-sex partners and their children; two homeless men who are friends; or two single women from another country who are sharing accommodations while they attend school. Although the initial reason for the home visit may be the health of one individual, the community health nurse considers at least one other person in the nursing care and in increasing the integration of the family with the community.

Family nursing has been based on three types of theory: family social science theories, family therapy theories, and nursing models and theories (Hanson & Kaakinen, 2001). Of these, theories from the social sciences, which include structural-functional theory, systems theory, interactional theories, stress theory, developmental theories, and change theory, are the most developed and are being adapted to clinical practice (Hanson & Kaakinen, 2001). Three integrated family nursing models are consistently mentioned in the nursing literature: Family Assessment Intervention Model and Family Systems Stressor Strength

Inventory (FS³I) (Hanson, 2001), Calgary Family Assessment Model and Calgary Family Intervention Model (Wright & Leahey, 2000), and The Friedman Family Assessment Model (Friedman et al, 2003).

An alternative approach to family nursing is based on viewing the family context rather than considering the family as a system or unit of interacting parts (Hartrick & Lindsey, 1995). This approach to family nursing means that the nurse works with the family to increase the family's capacity to deal with health and healing. The four interactive activities of the **contextual approach** to family nursing are 1) listening openly to understand the meaning that the family has attributed to health and healing experiences, 2) engaging in therapeutic communication, 3) recognizing and reflecting on patterns, and 4) providing opportunities for the family to imagine possibilities to enhance their relationships and promote health and healing (Hartrick & Lindsey, 1995; Hartrick, Lindsey, & Hills, 1994). This approach to family nursing promotes change at the structural level rather than simply providing health information (Hartrick, 1997). In contrast to the contextual approach, the provision of information places the health practitioner in the role of expert and the family as dependent on expert information.

The theories and integrated nursing models provide different perspectives and approaches for nurses working with families. Some aspects of the Calgary Family models and the contextual approach to family nursing are used throughout this chapter.

As with assessments of individuals, groups, and communities, the family assessment is used to plan collaborative action with the family. Community health nurses are particularly interested in the family's social support system, which is included in the external and context portions of Wright and Leahey's (2000) family structure. The contextual approach to family nursing also places strong emphasis on the relational experiences of the family (Hartrick & Lindsey, 1995).

Social support is "interactions with family members, friends, peers, and healthcare providers that communicate information, esteem, aid and emotional help" (Stewart, 2000, p. 85). Families usually expect different types of support from different people. For example, Stewart (2000) stated that many families perceive that their families provide instrumental or practical support, healthcare professionals provide informational support such as education and referral resources in the community, spouses or partners provide emotional support such as encouragement and reassurance, and peers or friends provide affirmational or feedback support. Community health nurses need to learn about the family so they can assist them in connecting with people to meet each type of social support.

The type and depth of family assessment that the community health nurse conducts depends on the family situation and the expected length of time for which nursing care will be provided. Community health nurses may see mothers with infants when they are first discharged from the hospital, families with a disabled member, families dealing with an acute or chronic illness in the community, or families at risk for illness or injury. When the contact is to screen for risk, such as identifying mothers having difficulty caring for an infant, short and specific assessment tools for the mother and infant may be required. In other situations, extensive assessment tools may be required by agencies or funding bodies. Before these tools are used, the nurse is expected to spend some time conversing with the family members to gain some understanding of their experiences and explain the tool before launching into the assessment. Part of the role of the nurse is to assess the value of assessment tools in the provision of nursing care. If the tool requires an excessive amount of time with little contribution to nursing care, an appropriate action would be to advocate elimination of the tool.

Many of the families who are visited by nurses are struggling to survive as well as care for a family member who is ill. These families may have just arrived in the country, may not speak the language, may be poor, or may in other ways be dealing with difficulties not experienced by the nurse. When working with these families, community health nurses are expected to learn about their cultural practices, especially as they relate to children. They are also expected to consistently engage in reflection, as described in Chapter 2, or a self-discovery process (Hartrick & Lindsey, 1995). Although an interpreter from the cultural community could assist with obtaining the family history, building an ongoing relationship requires that the family and nurse converse directly. Suggestions for using plain language are given in Appendix B.

Family nursing in the home

Nursing families in the home is the traditional base for nursing practice. In recent years, nursing care in the home has increased as hospital stays decrease and preventive care in the home is found to be cost effective for some population groups.

Community health nurses use the home visit as the main strategy to reach families who have members who are ill, at risk, or vulnerable. Home visits provide a viable option to institutional care for those needing medical and nursing care. Home visits can also assist in identifying, monitoring, and providing education and supportive services for people at risk for illness. Groups who might benefit from a home visit include families who have physical needs or conditions, emotional needs, family role changes, health education needs, psychosocial needs, and other conditions such as those at risk for abuse, developmental delay, and poor medical outcomes (Clark, 2003).

A home visit may occur once, periodically, or regularly over a long period. A single home visit may be made to screen for risk. Periodic home visits are a useful way to monitor families at risk, especially if they are unable or unwilling to use central services. Ongoing visits often are the most effective way to support families under stress and assist them in connecting to others in the community.

Home visiting process

Each home visit begins with the receipt of a referral for a new family client or the record of a family that has already been admitted to a program and ends with completion of activities related to the visit, documentation, and evaluation. For families receiving more than one visit, the end of one visit begins the planning for the next, and the cycle does not end until discharge. Each home visit includes three phases: preparation, conducting the visit, and postvisit evaluation. The phases and activities are detailed in Application 9-1.

In comparison to other places where the community health nurse provides services, the people in the home may not be aware that they have been referred for a home visit. A **referral** is a request for services for clients that can be made by another person, such as a health professional, teacher, family member, or neighbor, or one can be automatically generated as part of a program. Often women who have had their first baby are referred for a home visit as part of a maternal–infant program. An elderly man or woman living alone may be referred for a home visit if the neighbors become concerned. This situation means that the community health nurse must pay particular attention to providing explanations at the initial phone call and provide the opportunity for the person to accept or reject the visit. During the visit, the community health nurse will again explain the purpose of the home visit and the role of the nurse in the home.

Home visits are distinguished from other sites used in the provision of community health nursing care by the intimacy and privacy of the situation. Because the home is under the control of the people living there, the community health nurse is a guest in the home. This can bring up issues such as who determines the agenda and how to distinguish between a professional and social visit.

The privacy of the home visit also means that the nurse is much more vulnerable to unsafe situations in both the neighborhood and the home itself. Application 9-2 provides safety guidelines for nurses during home visits. These guidelines will have some relevance for all home visits, but are particularly necessary in areas that are associated with crime and drug use, in homes in which drinking or drug use is a problem, or in homes in which members of the household are dealing with mental or emotional difficulties. These safety guidelines are to be considered in conjunction with the phases and activities of home visiting detailed in Application 9-1. For nurses new to home visiting, a discussion of the guidelines with experienced home healthcare nurses would be particularly beneficial.

Advantages and disadvantages of home visits

Several authors have pointed out that home visits have both advantages and disadvantages for families, community health nurses, and the healthcare system (Clark, 2003; Hitchcock, 2003; Loveland-Cherry, 2000; Smith, 2000). The advantages for families are accessibility and a sense of control. Community health nurses doing home visits have the opportunity to focus on the family; develop a relationship; observe the physical, social, and emotional environment surrounding the client/family; and work with the family to identify their strengths and address their specific needs and potential health problems. Home visits are more cost effective than institutional care for parents and their children and for elderly people and their caregivers (Elkan et al., 2000), and also help prevent fragmented care for specified groups such as infants who are vulnerable because of poverty, social risk, or prematurity (Kearney, York, & Deatrick, 2000).

Home visits also have disadvantages for clients and community health nurses. Families may prefer more formal surroundings or be overburdened by providing care in the home (Hitchcock, 2003; Smith, 2000). For community health nurses, home visits are more time consuming (Hitchcock, 2003; Loveland-Cherry, 2000), can create difficulty in maintaining professional distance (Clark, 2003), have safety concerns related to the home and neighborhood, and have more interruptions and distractions. Community health nurses can find home visits stressful because initially there is no immediate access to equipment or consultations with others is available (Hitchcock, 2003), clients are diverse and have a multiplicity of problems (Clark, 2003), and situations are constantly changing, which is stressful for nurses who need to be in control (Hitchcock, 2003).

The advantages and disadvantages to clients, community health nurses, and the healthcare system emphasize the need to capitalize on the advantages and minimize the disadvantages of home visits. Because the cost of home visits is a major factor, community health nurses work collaboratively with families and other service providers to prepare the family to assume responsibility for handling their own healthcare needs.

Acting to overcome disadvantages

Two types of actions can address most of the disadvantages of home visits for community health nurses and promote health and injury prevention in the home. The first is supporting nurses while they learn to develop collaborative relationships with families and service providers in the community. Developing health-promoting practices with families requires time and considerable reflection. Health-promoting practices include changing from an emphasis on disease or behavior modification to a focus on helping the family deal with the socioenvironmental aspects of health (Hartrick, 1998). Practitioners new to the home environment also need to be aware that long-term involvement with a family in the home can lead to a loss of professional distance (Clark, 2003). Signs of overinvolvement rather than a professional relationship include providing services that could be done by a family member or a friend, such as picking up items at a store, or feeling that you are the only professional who can provide the appropriate care to that family.

The second action is providing guidelines for effective and safe nursing care in the home. As mentioned earlier, guidelines for safety considerations are given in Application 9-2. These measures are particularly important for nurses doing home visits because they usually work independently from each other. Support from peers and guidelines for community health nurses will encourage the maximum health benefit for families receiving nursing home visits.

FAMILY HEALTH PROMOTION IN THE HOME SCENARIO (continued)

After their week of orientation and home visits, the four nurses met to discuss what they had learned so far and to begin planning for the project. Ron opened with: "Wow, those home visits were really an eye opener for me! As a home care worker I'm used to going into homes, but I didn't have so much to think about!"

"Well, I have never really been in other people's homes as a nurse," stated Jennifer. "I felt like a guest, not a nurse, and found it difficult to think of these people as patients."

"That's what got me," claimed Natalia. "They had definite views about what they expected from the nurse I was with. She wasn't the only one with expertise on what was needed! It took a bit of time to get used to the idea, but when I did, I realized that that is how it should be. It is their life after all!"

"I went on an evening visit with the nurse to a client in a rundown area of town," said Denise. "I was feeling uncomfortable. I had never been there before even in daytime. The nurse explained all the precautions that she took and I wrote them down. I wouldn't have thought of them myself."

After discussion about the differences between visiting families with infants and the elderly, Emilie, the manager working with them on the project, asked them what they had learned about doing home visits. Ron said that there was a lot to think about when planning their own home visits. Jennifer added that she had been on home visits with two home healthcare nurses and was amazed at the differences in the way they prepared and conducted their home visits. Denise said that she was feeling worried about doing visits on her own and had looked at several texts on community health nursing. She found that all of them had considerable information on doing a home visit, and she had started to make a checklist. Ron volunteered to work with her in drafting a checklist that they would share with the others.

Emilie then asked about what they noticed about health promotion or illness prevention during the visits. Jennifer mentioned that both of the nurses that she was with provided information on other resources that were available in the community. Ron said that he was surprised that the nurse he was with routinely asked the elderly clients about getting their influenza immunization because flu season was approaching.

Natalia spoke up at that point and explained how she had been comparing the team project that she had done during her nursing program with visiting families in their homes. In the team nursing school project, the team had worked with a group of single mothers in an educational program to determine their priority issue and the action they wanted to take. Her team collected their data by first deciding on the two questions that they would use that day, and then each of them asked the women the questions during their normal conversations (progressive inquiry, Chapter 4). At the end of the day, the team members compared their results and decided on the questions for the next time. She wondered if they could use the same kind of process during home visits.

A general discussion followed as they questioned Natalia. Emilie then asked them who was going to be team leader and what they were going to do for next week. Everyone turned to Natalia. She agreed to lead at first until everyone felt more comfortable, and then someone else could take over. She would draft a plan and send it to everyone by the next meeting. She asked everyone to observe or ask other home care nurses about including health promotion and illness prevention in their visits. Denise volunteered to do a literature search to identify issues related to young children and the elderly.

DISCUSSION QUESTIONS

1. How were the team members preparing themselves to do visits with families in the home?
2. What do you feel would be the greatest difference in working with families in the home compared with working with communities or groups?
3. How do you think that health promotion and illness prevention information could be included in every home visit?

Guidelines for collaborative relationships with families in the home

Home visiting provides the opportunity to build a health-promoting relationship with families, especially when nursing care extends over a period of time. This relationship is fostered by privacy, a sense of intimacy, a relaxed environment, and continuity of care in the home environment. A synthesis of qualitative studies indicated that building and preserving relationships with clients in the home is at the core of home nursing (McNaughton, 2000).

Guidelines for establishing professional, collaborative relationships with families are adapted from Wright and Leahey's (2000) brief family interview guide and the contextual or phenomenological approach to family nursing. This latter approach concentrates on meaningful conversations that lead to understanding and enhancement of the lives of families rather than dealing strictly with a health problem (Hartrick, 1997). The components of the collaborative guidelines are 1) orientating conversations, 2) mapping relationships, 3) participating in therapeutic conversations, and 4) imagining possibilities.

Orienting conversations

Conversations in the brief family interview are purposeful and time-limited and acknowledge and affirm people (Wright & Leahey, 2000). The purpose of the initial conversations in the contextual approach is to orient yourself to the family's experiences (Hartrick & Lindsey, 1995). This is "listening to learn," not to determine problems but to understand the family's view of the world. This means that the nurse asks an open-ended question, such as "What has it been like for you living in this situation?" and allows people the time to think and respond. The nurse responds in a way to indicate an initial understanding of the person or family's experience.

As well as the nurse becoming oriented to the family, the family needs to become oriented to the nurse. Initial discussions need to involve practical issues such as timing and expectations for each visit. If possible, the nurse should try to accommodate the preferred visiting time identified by the family, which will hopefully reduce the number of interruptions such as phone calls or visitors.

Establishing a collaborative relationship requires trust and understanding. When first meeting people, introduce yourself and provide your title, such as "I am Gill Roland, a nursing student working with public health," establish eye contact, provide the reason for contacting them, and invite their participation in the care (Wright & Leahey, 2000). As you meet other family members or friends, continue to introduce yourself, and explain your role. If appropriate, invite their participation. For example: "Hi Jean, my name is Gill Roland, a student nurse working with public health. I've been working with your mother and younger sister to figure out an easier way to feed your sister. Do you want to watch? Maybe you'll have some ideas."

Another aspect of a collaborative relationship is fulfilling promises and being honest (Wright & Leahey, 2000). If you say that you will do some task, ensure that you will remember to do it within the time period. If you are not able to perform the task or forgot, be honest. Honesty means telling people what you can provide and what you cannot. This needs to be done in a manner that is noncritical and clearly provides limits. For example, if you are asked for a ride, say, "The organization has quite strict rules. I am not able to take anyone anywhere in my car" rather than "I cannot take you to the store because I do not have time right now." The latter response suggests that at other times you would be willing to take the person in the car.

Another aspect of the collaborative relationship is establishing boundaries. For example, refreshments or gifts may be considered appropriate by the family, and the nurse could be considered unsociable if the offers are not accepted. A middle ground could be to accept the offer of refreshments at the end of the visit if time allows rather than the beginning (Wright & Leahey, 2000). This shows willingness to accept hospitality while indicating some boundaries on the interaction. Gifts, especially expensive gifts, are not acceptable in a professional relationship. The spirit of giving needs to be recognized, and possibly a smaller token such as food can be substituted. When family members talk about what you have done for them, emphasize how they have helped you gain a greater knowledge about working with families.

Mapping family relationships

Mapping of family members and relationships within the family and with the community is necessary if you are working with a family for more than three interactions (Wright & Leahey, 2000). Although similar information may have been originally collected in an admission form, the use of the family mapping diagrams provides a visual depiction of the family and greatly facilitates a collaborative effort. If the situation is appropriate and there is no map of the family, you are encouraged to initiate one on your first encounter with a family, especially if you will be seeing them again. If there is a map available, review it and possibly update it with the family.

Two types of family mapping diagrams are usually used: the genogram and the ecomap. The genogram depicts the family tree. It includes three generations: the parents, siblings, and offspring. The ecomap is a visual representation of the family in relation to the community and indicates the nature and quality of relationships (Hanson, 2001). The symbols and instructions for genograms and ecomaps are provided in most community health and family health texts. Genograms and ecomaps may help the community health nurse sort out difficult or complicated relationships.

An alternative, simplified system is proposed that uses two diagrams that are completed in phases either during one visit or over several visits, depending on the family situation. The first diagram is called the **family circle** and the other the **family interaction diagram**. Together they help to provide a picture of the family connections for both the family and the nurse. The family circle, described in the following section on phase 1, provides qualitative data, and the interaction diagram indicates the people who are physically and emotionally available to the family. Involving the family in developing the diagrams of the family is a strategy that quickly engages family members and sends a clear message that you are interested in them as a family (Wright & Leahey, 2000).

The completion of these diagrams with families who do not speak the same language as the nurse will be difficult, but is worth pursuing. Possibly another family member, a friend, or an interpreter can assist in obtaining the information for the mapping. Often, if the family understands the symbols used in the map, the symbols can be pointed to during discussions to be sure that the relationships are understood.

Phase 1. Mapping relationships: Family and friends

The family circle quickly identifies the people in the family and the people important to the family (Thrower & Walton, 1982) and can be included in every first encounter you make with a family. The family circle would probably take the family only two to three minutes to complete.

Introduce the idea by drawing a large circle to represent the family as it is now and by saying: "As a health professional, I am interested in you, your family, and the people who are important to you." Invite all available family members to take part in completing the circle. Ask the family members to draw in smaller circles for women or squares for men to represent themselves and the people important to them—family and others. The size of each circle or square indicates the person's significance or influence. Ask them to include the person's age and name in the middle of the square or circle. People can be inside or outside the large circle, touching or far apart. Encourage them to include people who they would call upon if they needed help. There are no right or wrong circles.

The result is a family circle that is a schematic diagram of a family system completed by family members (Thrower & Walton, 1982). Date the family circle and additions or revisions. The diagram can then be used as a point of discussion about family connections and the support provided by different people.

If the family will be seen for more than two visits, ask them to draw a circle around the people who live with them. The symbols for the people in the household are then placed in the inner circle of the family interactions diagram in Figure 9-1. The various circles in the family interaction diagram are explained in Figure 9-1.

Phase 2. Mapping weekly interactions

The next phase in mapping the family connections is to include the people in the family circle who interact with the ill family member or caregiver each week. The people are

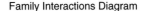

Family Interactions Diagram

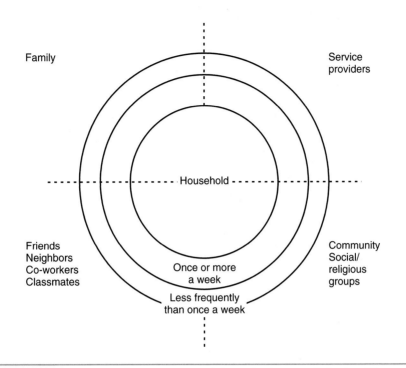

FIGURE 9-1. The family interactions diagram consists of three circular areas indicating different frequencies of interaction among people and the categories of people involved in the interactions.

The diagram is an adaptation of an ecomap developed for use with elderly persons by Moyer, Jamault, Roberge, & Murphy (1998). People in the inner circle live in the same household and interact daily. People in the outer two circles interact less frequently and are divided into four categories. **Inner circle:** The people who are in the household are shown in the inner circle. A square is used for a male; a circle is used for a female. Age and name are included. If a person from the household has died, this is shown with an X through the appropriate gender symbol, and a date of death is included. Pets may be included in this circle. **Middle circle:** This circle includes people with at least weekly contact with the person requiring care or the primary caregiver. The same symbols apply. Four categories are used to indicate the source of support: family, friends and neighbors, informal clubs and groups, and service providers from the community. These four categories are shown as four quadrants. The quadrants are not meant to be absolute, but do give an indication of the sources of support. Connections to the person requiring care or to the caregiver are provided by different types of lines. An unbroken line means a face-to-face interaction. A line made with dashes means the contact is not usually face-to-face. When contact is usually made by telephone, email, or letter, a T, E, or L, respectively, is used with the dashed line. An arrow in one direction or another means that the visitor always comes to the home or the person always makes the visit. Arrows in both directions indicate that there is visiting both ways. A line with crossed lines is an indicator of negative emotions attached to the relationship. **Outer circle:** The four categories in this area include people who interact with the family household less than once a week. The system of recording the social connections is the same as that used in the middle circle.

included in the family interaction diagram in the middle circle and in one of the four categories. Not all these people may have been included in the family circle. Because of the broad definition of family, the distinctions between family and friends may be blurred. **Service providers** are people who receive pay to provide services and include nurses, social workers, physicians, ministers, and house cleaners.

After completing the inner and middle circles, the nurse and family will be able to clearly see the number of people who interact with the family often and the importance of those people to the family. Some categories, such as community organizations, may not be involved at all and could be a potential source of support for the family. The family interaction diagram allows the family and nurse to objectively see what connections the family has and, if needed, what sources of support could be expanded.

Phase 3. Mapping less frequent interactions

The diagram is completed by including the people who interact with the family less often than weekly. Checking with the family will reveal whether the interaction diagram is complete. When the family interaction diagram is first completed, the start and completion dates should be indicated. As changes occur, such as a death, birth, or someone leaving home, the changes can be added in another color to keep the diagram up-to-date. New connections, such as joining a self-help group, also need to be added. As new health practitioners encounter the family, the diagrams can be used to orient them to the family situation. Examples of completed family interaction circles and diagrams are given in Figures 9-2 and 9-3.

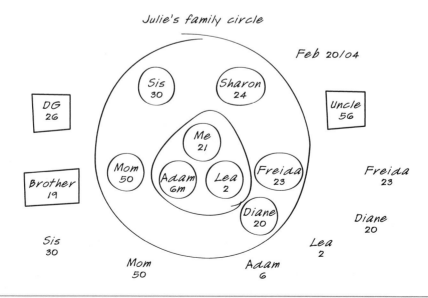

FIGURE 9-2. Example of a family circle and a family interaction diagram.

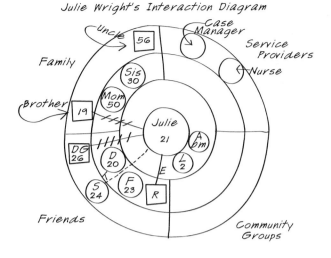

FIGURE 9-3. Example of completed interaction diagram.

Participating in therapeutic conversations

The nurse engages the family in therapeutic conversation to help each other understand and express the meaning of common and unique experiences (Hartrick & Lindsey, 1995). The conversation, although purposeful, is more free flowing than an interview, to allow new ideas to emerge. This means that when questions are posed, answers are not cut off prematurely by opinions or conclusions (Hartrick & Lindsey, 1995). For example, in a family living with a confused elderly grandparent, the nurse would seek each family member's experience and perspective on living with someone who is confused. As a general guide, some possible questions (adapted from Hartrick & Lindsey, 1995; Wright & Leahey, 2000) follow:

What is it like to live with someone who has _____ (name condition)?
What makes it easier or more difficult?
What has the family done that has made it easier for you?
What has worked for your family in the past? What has not worked?

In the home, a major issue is the burden on caregivers. Often caregivers can be putting forth a tremendous effort to the detriment of their own health. When caregivers have the opportunity to converse about the effect the illness has on their lives, they are better able to sustain and conserve family relationships (Tapp, 2001). Various questions related to caregiver burden need to be included with every visit.

According to Hartrick and Lindsey (1995), the nurse opens up possibilities in these conversations by providing information from different sources, linking the family with other community resources, or using other means such as art or literature to stimulate discussion. They stated that the purpose is to clarify what has been taken for granted and to discover new patterns to promote family health and healing.

During the conversations the nurse reflects **commendations** on their functioning back to the family. Wright and Leahey (2000) state that commending for family and individual strengths is an important role of the nurse. They describe commendations as observations or reports of strengths, resources, or competencies that have occurred over time and suggest that at least one or two should be offered in each 15-minute interview. Commending is providing affirmational support. Qualitative studies, particularly with families of children with a chronic illness, emphasize the importance of acknowledging effort, recognizing the burden of responsibility, and providing an orientation to strength and hope (Hodgkinson & Lester, 2002; Robinson, 1998).

Examples of commendations are: "I see that everyone in your family has a part to play in the care of grandmother. You all work together." "Children at four can be a handful. But I notice that when the baby starts crying, Jake starts gently rocking the crib. It's great that you have found something that makes him feel that he can help." In contrast to commendations, compliments are usually based on something that is displayed once and is more likely an attribute rather than a sustained behavior. Wright and Leahey (2000) state that families experiencing ongoing illness, disability, or trauma suffer from "commendation-deficit disorder" (p. 282), and nurses can never offer too many sincere commendations.

Families experience forces that draw them into attachment as well as making them resist attachment. The nurse and family need to identify and reflect on the family patterns and themes that include both autonomy and relatedness (Hartrick & Lindsey, 1995).

Imagining possibilities

In the contextual approach to family nursing, once families have a sense of their themes and patterns, they need time and space to think about these experiences without judgment and expectation (Hartrick & Lindsey, 1995). The nurse can offer various options to encourage further exploration by the family. Hartrick and Lindsey suggest that the family can be asked to think of a question to stimulate discussion or to determine concrete actions that can be taken. Some possibilities of the latter could be a family conference with all service providers coming into the home or the format for a contract that the family can develop on their own.

FAMILY HEALTH PROMOTION IN THE HOME SCENARIO (continued)

By the fourth week of the project, the team had decided that the specific assessment methods would be the guidelines for collaborative family relationships, and they had started to use them the previous week. As a modification in the procedure, they decided to ask if there was any specific health information that they could bring with them when they made the phone call to set up the appointment. The team offered specific information in three areas: 1) injury prevention, 2) immunization, and 3) access to healthcare after reviewing the leading health indicators from Healthy People 2010 (U.S. Department of Health and Human Services, 2000) to determine information that would apply to all age-groups served by home care. They collected fact sheets on injury prevention and immunization for different age-groups and each carried a book listing community resources. They were excited about using their nursing skills in the home and had stories to tell.

"I've got to tell you about this one older fellow," Ron began. "I hadn't visited him before, but he has been on the program for ages because of diabetes and leg ulcers that don't heal. When I phoned him

to make the appointment, I asked if there was some information that I could bring for him and gave him some suggestions such as social events for seniors and mall walking programs. He seemed surprised by the question, but said no. When I arrived at his door in the seniors' apartment building, the door was ajar. I gave a firm knock on the door, gave my name and where I was from. When I heard a response, I went in to find him in the living room with his leg up on a footstool all ready for the dressing to be done. I introduced myself again and explained that since he was ready, I would do the dressing first, and then I would like a few minutes to talk to him about the people in his life. He seemed surprised, but nodded. I should mention that ashtrays filled with cigarette butts were all over the place and he kept smoking the whole time I was there.

"When I introduced the family circle, he drew a circle for himself, a fairly big circle for a man who lived down the hall, and a small circle for an older sister who lived in another city. We talked about different things that interested him to identify if he could be connected to a community group. As I went to leave, he told me that no one had ever asked him about his family and friends before. I felt quite pleased with the visit and the interaction.

"I decided to start using the brief family interview with a single mother who has two children, one six months and one two years," said Jennifer. "When I phoned to make the appointment and asked her if she wanted any information, she said she wanted to know about what food she should be feeding the baby. We didn't have any information in the office, but I was able to find it on a good Web site and printed it off for her. When I arrived at her place the next day, she was in a state of panic. Her landlord had told her that she had to move because of a loud party that went on half the night. Her brother had come to her place with a bunch of friends and had just taken over. She felt helpless and had left the apartment with her children to stay with a friend. I asked her for the name of her social worker at the children's service organization. She couldn't remember her name. I called the organization, found out the social worker's name, and then passed the phone to the mother. By then she was able to explain the situation and set up an appointment with the case manager. I commended her on being able to summarize the situation for the social worker. She seemed surprised that I mentioned it."

Jennifer continued by saying, "Since she was now more settled and it seemed appropriate, I asked her if she would complete the family circle. She had a sister who lived fairly nearby and who she felt would help her deal with the brother. The sister was represented by quite a big circle within the family circle diagram. The friend she stayed with also had a large circle. Her mother who also lived nearby and helped her at times with the children was given a medium-sized circle. A couple of other single mothers who she met regularly in the mall had small circles. (Julie's family circle is shown in Figure 9-2.) Her brother and ex-boyfriend were outside the circle, but an uncle helped her at times. I commented that she had really used her resources well to protect herself and her children the previous evening. She seemed to enjoy talking about her family and friends, so we went on and completed the family interaction diagram (Figure 9-3). We didn't get to talk about feeding the baby, but the baby was bright and smiling, and I left the mother the information to read. We agreed to discuss it on the next visit. It certainly made me aware of how we have to be prepared for anything!"

"Denise and I have been talking, and we have been having the same results as you two in following the guidelines," said Natalia. "However, I have been feeling uncomfortable about the question on the information when the call is made to set up the visit. I told her about this article I read by Gwen Hartrick (1998) on developing health-promoting practices. I started to realize that by asking them what they needed, I was in the problem-solving, servicing mode rather than thinking about the skills and knowledge that they have. I would rather think of the family's resources as being half full rather than half empty."

Jennifer responded, "I don't see it that way. It gives us a chance to provide something in an efficient way."

"Now that you mention it," stated Ron, "it does seem a bit forced. Many people don't have any idea or their concerns have changed when I get there. If I've spent time finding information, I want to be able to talk about it. I would rather feel free to talk to them about their experiences rather than feeling that I have to carry out an agenda that I have created."

"Well, the rest of you seem to want to give it up," reflected Jennifer. "When I think about being with that single mother, information on nutrition was not what she needed at that time. And yes, I admit I was thinking *about it even when she was telling me about the crisis she was in. I, too, want to spend time discussing what they want to discuss. But didn't Emilie especially like that aspect of what we were doing?"*

Emilie spoke up at that point. "Yes, I felt that taking a few minutes in the initial phone call to check to see if people needed information was an efficient way to provide health promotion. I am now starting to realize that the way you are talking about health promotion is far more than providing information. If you are not comfortable continuing with that aspect of the procedure, you do not need to. However, I will need to spend some time explaining this to other managers and the head office."

Natalia nodded to her and continued, "Okay, we have agreed to cut that out of our procedure. Now, moving to the rest of the guidelines, I feel that I naturally use the components of the brief family interview format, except for using the diagrams and commendations. I cannot imagine any nurse that wouldn't introduce themselves or ask about family."

At that point, Emilie explained that funding for home care had been steadily reduced over the previous few years, and nurses just had less time and sicker people to deal with on each visit. Some nurses cope by just focusing on getting the task done. They feel that if they stopped to talk, it would take too much time and delay the next visit. The team members commented that they had observed the task-driven behavior and had been told by some home healthcare nurses not to get caught up in family affairs. The team members started to wonder if they would be expecting too much to have the nurses use the family mapping. At least cutting out the initial questions would reduce some time. They decided to document the approximate time it took them to do the mapping. They felt quite strongly that the other parts of the brief family interview would be an expected part of nursing practice.

At their meeting on the sixth week of the project, they had a considerable amount of information from more than 200 visits to 100 families in the two preceding weeks. Each person had calculated the amount of time it took them to develop the family interaction diagram on the first and second visit. There was considerable variation in the amount of time taken. For some people, the complete diagram could be done in 15 minutes at the first visit. For others it took longer and more visits. Older people tended to take longer because they described each person.

Before they moved into a more detailed discussion, Natalie asked them to think about what they felt encouraged the relationship with the family.

"Now that you ask," mused Ron, "I was wondering why I was feeling more responsive in some situations than in others. I have had more visits this last week and have felt too rushed to really have a good conversation with some of the families or to work on the diagrams. I realize now that it has been those families where I have been feeling less satisfied with the care I have provided and probably also because I was rushed."

"I find that it has been the diagrams and the commendations that seem to make a difference for me," said Natalia. "Completing the diagrams allows them time to talk about themselves and the help that they have available to them. I don't have any trouble recognizing their ability to cope, but I wouldn't have thought of that as part of nursing practice before I read about collaborative guidelines."

"Yes, I agree," added Denise. "I'm used to talking to older people, but never before made a point of commending them."

"What concerns me," said Jennifer, "are the women out there who are caring for a sick or disabled child, mother, father, or husband without any help from anyone including their family. I don't think I could manage like they do!"

"When I looked at some of the diagrams, they were almost empty!" said Denise. "I can tell how lonely and stressed they feel, not by what they say in front of their spouse, but what they say in the 'door-knob' conversations as I'm leaving!"

"It's not just the elderly," exclaimed Jennifer. "Poor mothers with young children feel abandoned. Mothers with older children and a sick or disabled child feel that they must do all the care and look after everyone else, too. They ask how others manage, as if feeling stressed about caregiving means that there is something wrong with them!"

"We have to do something!" declared Ron. "We can do all the commending we want, but that won't help them. Well, it helps them, but it would sure be better if we could look at lightening the load they bear."

"It doesn't do any good for us to keep doing things for them," countered Natalia. "We need to consider how we can help them get more help from others. Isn't there some saying about not just giving people food, but working with them so they can grow their own food?"

"When I commend them on how they have worked out a difficult problem, such as getting everyone in the family to help, they have some pride in what they have done, but feel that they could really learn from others in a similar situation," countered Jennifer.

"Well, I have found that by looking at the diagram together and discussing how they are managing, they start talking about what they do well and where they can use some extra help," stated Denise.

"That's it!" declared Natalia. "It's all about working with them so that they can see their potential and take over control of their family's health. If we keep doing things for them, we don't allow them that opportunity. We are into service delivery and keeping them dependent on us!"

In further discussions about the assessment data they had collected, they realized that statements about risk did not really belong. They had substantial evidence from families that they wanted to improve the sharing of caregiving roles within the family and wanted to share their experiences with other families.

DISCUSSION QUESTIONS

1. In Ron's description of his visit with the elderly man, he did not say that he asked about the man's smoking. Do you think he should have said something?
2. What commendations did Jennifer include in her interactions with the upset mother?
3. What do you believe is involved in a health-promoting practice?
4. Why was the use of the collaborative family guidelines going to be more difficult for Emilie to support than providing information?

Collaboration with service providers

Working effectively in the home with families also requires collaboration with other disciplines, paraprofessionals, and lay workers. The family's interaction diagram will help to identify the service providers who are involved with the family on a regular basis. For clients receiving home care services, the other services involved are usually indicated in the client's record.

Nursing students and beginning practitioners would begin to develop a collaborative practice by first forming a collaborative relationship with families and identifying and learning about the service providers in the practice area. A basic understanding of the scope of practice of the different professionals can be obtained from journals, texts, Web sites (see Web Site Resources), discussions, and home visits with other professionals. The contribution of paraprofessional home healthcare workers can be determined from discussions with experienced colleagues, job descriptions, and talking with workers in the home.

Professionals who could be involved with families receiving care in the home are social workers, physical therapists, occupational therapists, psychologists, general or family practice physicians, and medical specialists. Interdisciplinary practice involves professionals working together in a coordinated way compared with multidisciplinary practice in which aspects of practice are provided independently by people from different professions (Ervin, 2002). Collaboration with other professions is important to ensure that common goals for the family are being sought.

The most prevalent paraprofessional in the home is the unregulated care provider. This job label changes from one location to the next and includes home healthcare worker, home healthcare aid, or service support worker. The educational preparation of **home healthcare workers** also varies in different areas, but mainly involves learning basic personal care skills, communication skills, and home management skills including meal preparation, doing laundry, and housecleaning. Home healthcare workers are usually in a home for at least an hour to provide a specified task such as assistance with a bath or for longer periods to complete several tasks, engage in social interaction, or provide respite for the caregiver. For some families and isolated individuals, the home healthcare worker is considered part of the family. Home healthcare workers can provide valuable information on how the family functions when the nurse is not present. Collaboration with the worker will ensure that the family is being supported in a consistent manner and is not receiving mixed messages. Other workers and technologists with specific training such as respiratory technologists and child development workers can also be involved in specific home care situations and can contribute to the home healthcare team.

In home healthcare, the coordination of services often is assigned to one person who is called a **case manager** or **care coordinator.** The case manager is usually a community health nurse or a social worker and has responsibilities that include designating the type, frequency, and duration of services that are provided to families in the home. The case manager may work for the same organization that employs the community health nurse or may be employed by a government organization that assigns contracts for home nursing visits. The case manager for a family receiving home care would be a key informant in planning nursing care, particularly care involving other service providers.

In addition to knowledge about the different service providers, a collaborative practice requires skill in interpersonal relations and communication (Ervin, 2002). These are the same skills needed to effectively function on a team, whether the team is composed of people from the same or different professions. The development of team skills is explained and applied in Chapter 2. In home care, communication is particularly important because the team may need to function with few, if any, face-to-face meetings.

Opportunities to collaborate with other service providers can emerge from dealing with difficulties faced by a single family or a problem faced by many families. When working with a family of a premature infant, a community health nurse would be collaborating with the parents and could be collaborating with a child development worker and a social worker. For a family member who is disabled and therefore restricted in performing major life activities such as walking, talking, breathing, seeing, or working, a different collaboration team would be involved. An example of interdisciplinary practice to reduce falls by elderly persons is provided in Box 9-1.

Agreements or contracts with an individual family member, a family, or a home healthcare team are a valuable tool in community health nursing in the home. An explanation of the use of collaborative agreements for families with children and service providers is given in Box 9-2.

FAMILY HEALTH PROMOTION IN THE HOME SCENARIO (continued)

Emilie invited a home health nursing representative from each of the six geographical areas served by the home health nursing organization, two case managers, and the supervisor of the largest home healthcare worker organization together to discuss the findings from the assessment.

BOX 9-1	**Examples of interdisciplinary practice to reduce falls by elderly persons**

In a systematic review of interventions to reduce falls by the elderly, Gillespie et al. (2003) identified four interventions that were likely to be beneficial and could be delivered in the home:

1. A program of muscle strengthening and balancing prescribed by a trained health professional
2. A home hazard assessment and modification professionally prescribed for elderly persons with a history of falling
3. Withdrawal of psychotropic medication
4. Programs that included different disciplines and factors, health and environmental risk factor screening, and interventions

In home healthcare, screening for risk of falling would involve everyone providing care in the home to the elderly person and would consist of questions at admission to home care, reliable measurement tools, and questions and observations of clients presently in the program. Home healthcare workers would play a prominent role in identifying symptoms of falls such as abrasions and bruises observed while giving personal care.

Once an elderly person at risk of falling is identified, the home care physical therapist would prescribe the exercises, the occupational therapist would conduct the hazard assessment and supervise the modifications, and the community health nurse would review the medications with the family physician. Once the exercises and home modifications are in place, the nurse and home health worker would continue to work with the client and family to provide education and support in maintaining the fall prevention program.

If the fall prevention program is delivered through an official public health organization, the same health professionals could be involved, but the manner of screening and ongoing monitoring and support would be different. Elderly people could be recruited to the program through referrals from hospital emergency departments, physician offices, or families or by self-referral. The organization would probably work in collaboration with organizations in the community such as churches and seniors' apartment buildings and organizations. Once people at risk are identified, the four components of the program—exercises, hazard reduction, review of psychotropic medications, and coordination of activities—would be instituted in the home. The community health nurse working for the public health organization would probably continue to provide the educational portion of the fall prevention program to the client and family for a certain number of home visits.

The team explained the concerns that they had with trying to provide health information on the first visit. That stimulated lively discussion. Some of the home health nurses were excited about the focus on family capacity rather than trying to find the problem to solve; others were worried that they could be accused of not doing their job. The latter were assured that crises would be addressed. All were willing to go ahead with the pilot test focusing on family capacity for caregiving and opportunities for families to come together to provide mutual support. After that consensus was reached, they discussed the potential impact on other people.

Everyone agreed that the development of family capacity related to family caregiving was important and had definite possibilities for collaboration, particularly with home healthcare workers. A case manager explained that there would be some situations of caregiver burden that would require the involvement of a

BOX 9-2	Using agreements (contracts) in families with children

Agreements, or contracts, among families, community health nurses, and service providers are a collaborative way to set goals and work toward those goals. The simplest agreement identifies the people, what action is to be taken by whom, and the deadlines when evaluation will occur. The agreement or plan may be verbal or written. Everyone who could be involved should have a chance to review a draft of the agreement. The agreement must be easy to manage or it will not be followed. Once the use of a contract has been introduced, the family may use it in other situations.

The following is an example of how a collaborative agreement can be used. A small child in a family with four children and two parents needs specific exercises at least six times a day. The physical therapist was prepared to train the family members and monitor the child's progress. The community health nurse would work with the family to draw up an agreement for the first week. The agreement included a seven-day schedule with the exercise times indicated and a reward at the end. The two oldest children and the father took the times in the early morning, evenings, and weekends, and the mother took the two remaining times during the day. The four-year-old girl helped the mother. When they completed the exercises, they put a check beside their time. After a week, the physical therapist came in to assess the progress and was pleased with the results. She asked them to continue in the same way for another week, and then the length of the sessions or the frequency might be changed. The mother was pleased because she did not need to remind anyone. Everyone seemed to enjoy the time alone with the child. The 12-year-old boy drew up the schedule for the next week. The family celebrated by having their favorite meal together.

social worker. These could include situations in which a discussion or agreement about the sharing of tasks within a family with the community health nurse was not effective or appropriate or if more financial resources are needed. If institutional placement is being considered because the health of the client or caregiver has deteriorated, a social worker or case manager would be involved in certain jurisdictions to assist the family in making decisions and to complete the application papers. The case manager would be involved if the referral involved another home care service such as Meals on Wheels.

There was considerable discussion regarding opportunities for families to learn from each other. Everyone agreed that the opportunity should be available, but did not agree on who should provide the service and how it should be organized. They decided to create an interagency task group to study the situation.

The team members were pleased with the result of the prioritizing meeting. They had a good idea of what they needed to do because they realized that they had already been testing the intervention themselves. The team developed their goal and determined strategies and theories. They decided to focus their literature search on social support for families.

They found several systematic reviews that indicated the value of social support in the perinatal period for supporting smoking cessation during pregnancy (Lumley, Oliver, & Waters, 2003), breast-feeding mothers (Sikorski, Renfrew, Pindoria, & Wade, 2003), and mothers with postpartum depression (Ray & Hodnett, 2003). Social support was found useful for families living with chronic conditions, such as the mental health of mothers of children with chronic illnesses (Ireys, Chernoff, DeWet, & Kim, 2001) and patients with moderate chronic obstructive pulmonary disease (Smith, Appleton, Adams, Southcott, & Ruffin, 2003).

The biggest problem they faced was how to take action. The action and objectives in this case would pertain to home healthcare nurses. They wanted to test whether home healthcare nurses on their own or in collaboration with other service providers would find the collaborative guidelines useful in their interactions with families. Although they had several nurses from each of the six geographical areas who were willing to take part in the test, they wanted to make the best use of everyone's time. They did not want to jeopardize the results by asking too much and overwhelming people.

They decided that each member of the team would work with two nurses on the use of the collaborative family guidelines and diagrams. They would meet with the volunteer nurses twice: once before the test and once after to discuss the results. Each volunteer was asked to send an email at the end of the first week reporting their progress. They were to use the guidelines and diagrams with at least five families who they would see at least twice in the two-week period.

While the team members were waiting for the results, they started working on the report. The head office had asked them for a description of the procedure, the results they had obtained, and their recommendations. They described each initiative and included the initial findings from their work.

The team found the results from the guidelines surprising. Most of the nurses stated that if they used the diagrams with someone who they had been seeing for awhile they could almost fill it out themselves and it did not take much time. Some found asking questions of all family members quite time consuming but also quite interesting; others liked the use of commendations. All agreed that the diagrams would be best initiated on the admission and completed on subsequent visits unless a crisis or concern took priority. They were to be updated periodically. They felt that if caregiver burden and community connection were the only points of discussion, other experiences and issues could be missed.

The participants in the test were quite zealous in advocating for the importance of working collaboratively to connect people They gave examples from their own practice that they wanted included in the report to the head office. In one example, a home healthcare nurse was able to connect two women who were living in the same apartment building and were both caring for a husband with a stroke. In another, a discussion of the family interaction diagram with an isolated mother and the lay home worker resulted in a decision that the lay worker would accompany the mother and children to a neighborhood play group, rather than concentrate on mother-child interactions in the home.

The team was ready to put the results of the pilot test in the report. They needed to explain the initial use of a contact phone call with the question about health information and why it was dropped. They suggested as an alternative that age-appropriate fact sheets on the leading health indicators should be compiled and made available, possibly on the organization's Web site.

The initiative with the collaborative guidelines was more complicated. It was difficult to determine the amount of extra time that was involved. From the posttest discussions with the nurses, most of what was included in the interview was already being done, but not specifically in that way or by everyone. The additional time needed to start the diagrams would be available at the admission visit.

All eight nurses who took part in the pilot test of the collaborative guidelines felt that they should become part of their practice to remind everyone about the importance of the family. All had some comment about receiving either positive comments from clients or clients being more assertive. They stated that they enjoyed learning together. They were not certain that they entirely understood what health-promoting practice was yet, but felt that they were starting to question what they had been doing in the past and were moving in a different direction. They cautioned that not all nurses would feel the same way as they did, because they were different—they volunteered!

After discussing their final report with Emilie, they decided to attach an outline procedure that covered the whole home visit and included some details from their project. They had already developed and had been using a checklist that helped them organize their visits. The collaborative family guidelines would be attached to provide more explanation. They felt that by including the collaborative family guidelines, those would become a part of usual practice. Their checklist is given in Application 9-1. They recommended that nurses could be introduced to the new procedure in a large presentation, but that small learning groups using email communication would help to implement the new procedure.

As they were finishing the final details on their report, they received the first results from the task group looking into family support groups. Task force members had contacted various local organizations to determine whether support groups were available. Some were identified, but more were needed. In the process, more people were recruited to their group, and they were planning to approach city council for funding for a pilot project.

DISCUSSION QUESTIONS

1. Why would some home health nurses be concerned about not doing their job if they focused on family strengths?
2. What was the value of asking for volunteers rather than assigning nurses to take part in the pilot test?
3. Why is time a particular factor to consider in home health nursing?

Summary

Nurses working in home health care provide individual and family nursing care for family members with acute or chronic illness and those at risk for illness to build family capacity and promote health and healing. The relationship with the family needs to be nurtured and monitored. A professional relationship is collaborative and is characterized by mutual respect, an understanding of the family structure and dynamics, and a reflective process. Nurses working in the home start with the narrow end of the telescoping lens to consider how a particular family can be supported and linked with community resources. They work closely with other service providers in the community to coordinate the support provided to families. Then, as community health nurses, they consider the common needs faced by families they serve and advocate with families or on their behalf to health care agencies and governments. Family home health nurses work with families as they develop their capacity to thrive in the community.

PRACTICE AND APPLICATION

1. Compare the strategies that were used in this scenario with those described in Chapter 6.

2. Item 22 in Application 9-1 states that the nurse will identify issues from the visit that could apply to other families. What "cross-cutting" issue was identified by the team in the scenario?

3. Write an agreement to include all family members in a family of four (both adults smoke) to reduce environmental tobacco smoke in the home.

4. Using your own practice or experience, develop the following:
   a) Family circles for different families
   b) Family interaction diagrams after the first, second, and third visits
   c) Examples of how caregivers react when asked about their own health
   d) Examples of collaboration in home visits
   e) Examples of when collaboration would have reduced problems

REFERENCES

Allender, J., & Spradley, B. (2001). *Community health nursing* (5th ed.). Philadelphia: Lippincott.

Clark, M. (2003). *Community health nursing* (4th ed.). Upper Saddle River, NJ: Prentice Hall.

Elkan, R., Kendrick, D., Hewitt, M., Robinson, J., Tolley, K., Blair, M., Dewey, M., Williams, D., & Brummell, K. (2000). The effectiveness of domiciliary health visiting: A systematic review of international studies and a selective review of the British literature. *Health Technology Assessment, 4*(13), i–v, 1–339.

Ervin, N. (2002). *Advanced community health nursing practice: Population-focused care.* Upper Saddle River, NJ: Prentice Hall.

Friedman, M., Bowden, V., & Jones, E. (2003). *Family nursing: Research, theory, and practice* (5th ed.). Upper Saddle River, NJ: Prentice Hall.

Gillespie, L., Gillespie, W., Robertson, M., Lamb, S., Cumming, R., & Rowe, B. (2003). Interventions for preventing falls in elderly people. In *The Cochrane Library 2.* Chichester, UK: John Wiley & Sons.

Hanson, S. (Ed.). (2001). *Family health care nursing: Theory, practice and research* (2nd ed.). Philadelphia: Davis.

Hanson, S., & Kaakinen, J. (2001). Theoretical foundations for family nursing. In S. Hanson (Ed.), *Family health care nursing: Theory, practice and research* (2nd ed., pp. 37–59). Philadelphia: Davis.

Hartrick, G. (1997). Beyond a service model of care: Health promotion and the enhancement of family capacity. *Journal of Family Nursing, 3*(1), 57–69.

Hartrick, G. (1998). Developing health promoting practices: A transformative process. *Nursing Outlook, 46*(5), 219–225.

Hartrick, G., & Lindsey, E. (1995). The lived experience of family: A contextual approach to family nursing. *Journal of Family Nursing, 1*(2), 148–170.

Hartrick, G., Lindsey, E., & Hills, M. (1994). Family nursing assessment: Meeting the challenge of health promotion. *Journal of Advanced Nursing, 20,* 85–91.

Hitchcock, J. (2003). The home visit. In J. Hitchcock, P. Schubert, & S. Thomas (Eds.), *Community health nursing: Caring in action* (2nd ed., pp. 500–518). Clifton Park, NY: Thompson Learning.

Hodgkinson, R., & Lester, H. (2002). Stresses and coping strategies of mothers living with a child with cystic fibrosis: Implications for nursing professionals. *Journal of Advanced Nursing, 39*(4), 377–383.

Ireys, H., Chernoff, R., DeWet, K., & Kim, Y. (2001). Maternal outcomes of a randomized controlled trial of a community-based support program for families of children with chronic illness. *Archives of Pediatric & Adolescent Medicine, 155*(7), 771–777.

Kearney, M., York, R., & Deatrick, J. (2000). Effects of home visits to vulnerable young families. *Journal of Nursing Scholarship, 32*(4): 369–376.

Loveland-Cherry, C. (2000). Family health risks. In M. Stanhope & J. Lancaster, *Community and public health nursing* (5th ed.). St. Louis, MO: Mosby.

Lumley, J., Oliver, S., & Waters, E. (2003). Interventions for promoting smoking cessation during pregnancy. *Cochrane Database for Systematic Reviews, 1.*

McNaughton, D. (2000). A synthesis of qualitative home visiting research. *Public Health Nursing, 17*(6), 405–414.

Moyer, A., Jamault, M., Roberge, G., & Murphy, M. (1998). Designing and testing individual and community-based interventions for the elderly in need using action research. (Publication No. M98-05). Ottawa, ON: University of Ottawa, Community Health Research Unit.

Ray, K., & Hodnett, E. (2003). Caregiver support for postpartum depression. *Cochrane Database of Systematic Reviews, 1.*

Robinson, C. (1998). Women, families, chronic illness, and nursing interventions: From burden to burden. *Journal of Family Nursing, 4*(3): 271–290.

Sikorski, J., Renfrew, M., Pindoria, S., & Wade, A. (2003). Support for breastfeeding mothers. *Cochrane Database of Systematic Reviews, 1.*

Smith, B., Appleton, S., Adams, R., Southcott, A., & Ruffin, R. (2003). Home care by outreach nursing for chronic obstructive pulmonary disease. *Cochrane Database of Systematic Reviews, 1.*

Smith, C. (2000). The home visit: Opening doors for family health. In C. Smith & F. Maurer, *Community health nursing theory and practice* (2nd ed., pp. 211–236). Philadelphia: Saunders.

Stewart, M. (2000). Social support, coping and self-care as public participation mechanisms. In M. Stewart (Ed.), *Community health nursing* (2nd ed., pp. 83–104). Toronto, ON: Saunders.

Tapp, D. (2001). Conserving the vitality of suffering: Addressing family constraints to illness conversations. *Nursing Inquiry, 8*(4), 254–263.

Thrower, S., & Walton, R. (1982). The family circle concept for integrating family systems concepts in family medicine. *Journal of Family Practice, 15*(3), 451–457.

U.S. Department of Health and Human Services. (November 2000). *Healthy people 2010: Understanding and improving health* (2nd ed.). Washington, DC: U.S. Government Printing Office. Available at: http://www.healthypeople.gov.

Wright, L., & Leahey, M. (2000). *Nurses and families: A guide to family assessment* (3rd ed.). Philadelphia: Davis.

WEB SITE RESOURCES

Home health nursing

These are just some examples; many more exist.
Visiting Nurse Associations of America: http://www.vnaa.org
Victorian Order of Nurses: http://www.von.ca
St. Elizabeth Visiting Nurses' Association: http://www.sen.on.ca/programs.htm

Professionals providing home care services

Case Management Society of America: http://www.cmsa.org
Ontario Case Managers Association: http://www.ocma.on.ca
American Network of Home Health Care Social Workers: http://www.homehealthsocialwork.org
Canadian Association of Social Workers: http://www.casw-acts.ca
National Association of Social Workers: http://www.naswdc.org
American Physical Therapy Association: http://www.apta.org
Canadian Physiotherapy Association: http://www.physiotherapy.ca
The American Occupational Therapy Association, Inc.: http://www.aota.org
Canadian Association of Occupational Therapists: http://www.caot.ca

APPLICATION 9-1

FAMILY HEALTH PROMOTION: HOME VISITING CHECKLIST

For each item on the checklist, indicate the following rating:

0 = Does not apply
1 = Unsatisfactory
2 = Satisfactory

HOME VISIT CHECKLIST

Rating	Preparation for Visit
_____	1. Studies referral, record, or other information on family.
_____	2. Contacts family to a. Set up appropriate time for home visit. b. Obtain address and directions to home c. Ask if there are any particular issues or concerns in the neighborhood that the nurse should know about.
_____	3. Plans a route to the home that is the most resource efficient.

CONDUCTS HOME VISIT

_____	4. Travels with safety and easily locates the home.
_____	5. Makes arrival known through knock or doorbell and gives name and organization name.
_____	6. Introduces self with full name to each person present, and establishes and maintains eye contact* throughout visit.
_____	7. Allows a few moments of socialization before beginning visit. If offer of refreshment made, request that it be shared at end of visit.
_____	8. Clearly states that the expected purpose of the visit is to discuss the family's experiences in dealing with a family health issue to orient everyone.
_____	9. Asks family if there is a pressing concern that they would like to deal with first, and if so, follows their lead.
_____	10. If this is the first visit, discusses expectations and management of future visits.
_____	11. Introduces the family circle and asks which people are living in the house and the people that family members see each week (first visit). Complete family interaction diagram for two to four weeks and the following two to three weeks. Update interaction diagram (as changes are mentioned).
_____	12. Encourages discussion about connections with family, friends, and community that have worked in the past.
_____	13. Proposes and discusses options about increasing family connections to community if necessary.
_____	14. Explains any procedure before, during, and after care.
_____	15. Asks about the caregiving requirements, such as who provides care, when care is required, how the family or primary caregiver has managed in the past, and any changes that have increased caregiving requirements.
_____	16. Proposes and discusses options about increasing support for caregiving, if necessary.
_____	17. Commends family unit and family members individually at least twice for progress or accomplishment; e.g., "Your family really works together." "Anna, I see how you help your mother." <div align="right">(continued)</div>

Rating	Preparation for Visit
_____	18. Ends the home visit by summarizing the main points.
_____	19. Discusses possible plan for next visit with family.
	Postvisit Evaluation
_____	20. Reviews information for visit to plan next visit.
_____	21. Documents home visit in a timely manner.
_____	22. Notes family needs or interests that are consistent with those of other families and passes these on at team meetings.
_____	23. Completes a self-evaluation of home visit.

Source: Adapted from Allender & Spradley (2001) and Wright & Leahey (2000).
*Eye contact: If family member is not comfortable with eye contact, direct your gaze at a nearby object.

APPLICATION 9-2

SAFETY GUIDELINES FOR HOME VISITS

Preparation

1. Connect with family:
   - Call ahead and arrange visit time with family.
   - Ask family for location and directions and about any precautions that you should take.
2. Locate home and check safety:
   - Locate address on map and carry map.
   - Confer with others about safety of neighborhood.
     —If location is associated with gangs, crime, or drugs, arrange for visit during morning or with an escort.
     —If people in household have threatened nurses in the past, arrange joint visits or visit when potentially dangerous people will not be present.
3. Ensure that organization has accurate information about you:
   - Provide organization with daily visit schedule including phone numbers.
   - Provide organization with vehicle description and license number.
4. Transportation:
   - If using public transportation, determine closest bus stop and bus schedule.
   - If using vehicle, ensure that it has sufficient fuel.

5. Appearance:
   - Appear as a professional by wearing modest clothing or a uniform and a name tag.
   - Do not carry a purse or wear expensive jewelry; leave valuables at home.
6. Safety equipment:
   - Cell phone with emergency number on speed dial
   - Whistle
   - Money for phone calls or taxi
7. Personal confidence:
   - Determine organization policy and procedure about potentially dangerous situations.
   - Discuss and possibly role play different safety situations with colleagues.
   - Learn personal defense techniques.

Conducting the visit

8. Arrival:
   - Park vehicle as close to home as possible.
   - Ensure that you have the correct address.
   - Avoid isolated and dark areas or where people are loitering, especially in evening or night.
   - Walk directly to home.
   - Keep one arm free.
   - Knock on door even when door is open.
   - State your name and the name of your organization.
   - Do not enter until you are certain that the person that you are to see is present. Show official identification if this is an agency expectation.
   - Do not enter unless you feel comfortable.
9. During visit:
   - Greet each person present and establish eye contact.
   - Leave if you feel threatened or if the environment does not allow you to establish a relationship.
10. After visit:
    - Report to organization at end of clinical day.
    - Record and discuss with supervisor any threatening or difficult behavior during home visit.

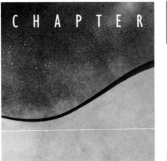

CHAPTER 10

Community Capacity Building

ELIZABETH DIEM

SCENARIO *DETERMINING RURAL PRIORITIES*

Susan has been working as a public health nurse in a rural farming county for three years. Recently she was approached by the Farming Women of Northeast County (fictional name). The women's group belongs to the Associated Country Women of the World, which works to improve the standard of living of women and families worldwide. A year ago, the women's group and one of the six local churches decided to apply for a government grant to develop a resource center in a former gas station located near the intersection of the two major county roads. They are successful in obtaining funding and were now providing social activities and lunches for seniors twice a week. They are very concerned about the cutbacks in government funding for medical and social services and are considering an expansion of the services offered at the resource center.

Susan felt that the possible expansion of services would be a good opportunity for nursing students to learn about working with the community groups in the rural area. The students would need to have a vehicle and be available to attend meetings on different days. Four students, Gabriela, Rosa, Greta, and Colleen, willingly volunteered. Two of the students had a car, and Rosa had grown up in the area. The students had different schedules, and with the two cars at least two people would be able to attend meetings at different times.

OBJECTIVES After reading this chapter and answering the questions throughout the chapter, you should be able to

1. Compare the process used in community capacity building with the community health nursing process.
2. Identify the characteristics of rural communities and rural nursing.
4. Identify qualities needed by organizers working to build community capacity.
4. Establish relationships with various community organizations.
5. Use presentations and meetings effectively.
6. Work according to the community's direction and timeframe

KEYWORDS assumptions about adult learners ▪ community capacity building ▪ dialogue ▪ rural nursing ▪ social capital

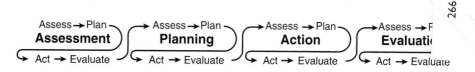

FIGURE 10-1. Cycles within components of the community health nursing process.

Community capacity building projects

Most communities have people, groups, and organizations that have come together over the years to make changes, such as building a library or a park or starting an annual community event. **Social capital** refers to the ability of communities to successfully come together to identify problems and needs and determine and achieve goals to improve community living (Mattessich & Monsey, 1997). **Community capacity building** is working with the people in the community to recognize and effectively use the resources or social capital that they have (Mattessich & Monsey, 1997). This type of work has been called community development, organizational development, and citizen engagement (Ontario Prevention Clearing House, 2002).

Projects based on community capacity building follow the same steps of the community health nursing process as the projects used for community groups in Chapters 3 through 8. They would probably focus more on one aspect of the process, however, such as assessment or planning. Because community capacity building is an ongoing process and is expected to include groups from different segments of the community, it would not be feasible to complete a full cycle of assessment, planning, action, and evaluation in less than two or three years. With this longer timeframe, each component will have an internal cycle to assess, plan, act, and evaluate. This is depicted in Figure 10-1.

In community capacity building, the emphasis is on the process used to bring together community members from across geographical areas or different interest groups to solve common problems. The type of problem is less important than the development of community skills, knowledge, and capacity. For example, the community may be interested in reducing speeding on local roads, rather than public health issues of smoking reduction or increasing exercise and immunization.

Collaboration in the community health nursing process is considered a fairly equal partnership between the team and the community. In contrast, in community capacity building, the community is the leader. The difference in the relationship is shown in Tables 10-1 and 10-2.

Community capacity building

Community capacity building is used in this chapter as an orientation to the ways in which people who identify as members of a shared community engage in the process of community change (Minkler & Wallerstein, 1997). Community capacity building starts where the people are (Nyswander, 1956) and increases when community members work together effectively to 1) "develop and sustain relationships," 2) "solve problems and

TABLE 10-1 *Comparing Collaborative Assessment with Groups or Communities for Community Capacity Building*

GROUPS AND COMMUNITIES	ADAPTATIONS FOR COMMUNITY CAPACITY BUILDING
1. Establish relationships within project and community.	Establish relationships with those immediately involved. Define an assessment goal that is feasible within the time available. The goal can range from determining who needs to be involved in the assessment to actually conducting the assessment.
2. Assess secondary data.	Review history of area. Review issues or organizations that have come together over issues in the past at a broader level (e.g., regionally, nationally).
3. Initiate assessment of community.	Similar to communities and groups, but with emphasis on determining the geographical dimensions of the community, organizations and community groups, history of working together, and emergence of issues.
4. Conduct specific assessment.	Join/augment plan that community has started or build plan from their interests and issues, conduct assessment, and expand membership.
5. Determine action statements.	Similar process as with communities or groups, but with emphasis on working with community; provide report in format that is useful to community groups.
6. Evaluate team work.	Include collaborators from community in team evaluation.

TABLE 10-2 *Comparing Collaborative Action with Groups or Communities to Community Capacity Building*

GROUPS AND COMMUNITIES	ADAPTATIONS FOR COMMUNITY CAPACITY BUILDING
1. Plan.	Similar to communities and groups, but with emphasis on joining/augmenting community initiative, expanding membership, and providing planning skills as needed. May occur concurrently with planning for assessment.
2. Take action on planned activities.	Similar to communities and groups, but with emphasis on building skills and knowledge with community members and increasing community ownership. May occur concurrently with conducting assessment.
3. Determine results/impact.	Community members would report what they have accomplished and learned.
4. Evaluate team work.	Include collaborators from community in team evaluation.

make group decisions," and 3) "collaborate effectively to identify goals and get work done" (Mattessich & Monsey, 1997, p. 61).

Community capacity building is a refinement of previous terms such as community organizing and community development, which have been used for many years and have different meanings for different people (Mattessich & Monsey, 1997; Mittelmark, 1999). Community capacity building, in comparison to community organizing or development, emphasizes a strengths-based approach that is of and by the community (Minkler & Wallerstein, 1997). It includes the identification, strengthening, and linking of resources, such as local service groups and motivated community groups (Ontario Healthy Communities Coalition, 2002) and the extension of those resources to others in the community. The generation of a civic spirit is an important aspect of community capacity building.

Community capacity building is an important strategy used by community health nurses; however, it is a very lengthy and time-consuming process. As the Public Health Nursing Section (2001) pointed out, it is best used in combination with other interventions.

Theoretical basis of community capacity building

Community capacity building is based on the premise that "change is more likely to be successful and permanent when the people it affects are involved in initiating and promoting it" (Thompson & Kinne, 1999, p. 30). Thompson and Kinne state that this premise evolved from two principles: participation and ownership. They state that the principle of participation means that the people who are the most affected by the problem need to be engaged in defining the problem, planning, taking steps to resolve the problem, and setting up structures to maintain the desired change. Ownership means that local people feel responsible for and continue to maintain the change after the initial organizing efforts are over (Thompson & Kinne, 1999). A strong relationship exists between the two principles: as participation increases, feelings of responsibility or ownership increase.

Minkler and Wallerstein (1997) identify participation and relevance as the two principles that evolved from social learning theory and adult education. Relevance would underlie both peoples' willingness to participate and their feelings of ownership. If the issues that are raised are not relevant to them, they will neither participate nor take ownership. Ensuring that issues remain relevant will increase active participation and feelings of ownership.

In community capacity building, participation, for at least some people living in the community, is at the level of working in partnership or having control. Participation means that the community is engaged in creating a healthy community and better quality of life (National Association of County and City Health Officials, 2000). A good way to determine different levels of participation is by using Arnstein's (1969) ladder of participation, given in the middle column of Table 10-3.

DETERMINING RURAL PRIORITIES SCENARIO *(continued)*

The four students met with Hilda, the president of the Farming Women's group, and Susan, the public health nurse, on the first clinical day. The next meeting of the Farming Women was in two weeks, and the two women wanted the students to know something about the county before the meeting. Hilda explained

TABLE 10-3	Levels of Citizen Participation	
CATEGORY	**LADDER**	**AMOUNT OF CITIZEN CONTROL**
Degrees of citizen power	Citizen control	People control all decision making.
	Delegated powers	People have some areas for which they control the decisions.
	Partnership	Decision making is collaborative.
Degrees of tokenism	Placation	A minor change is made in plans in response to feedback from people.
	Consultation	People are asked which of a few options they would like.
	Informing	People are told what is going to happen.
Nonparticipation	Therapy	Professional directs changes.
	Manipulation	People are exploited.

Source: Adapted from Arnstein (1969); Goeppinger & Hammond (2000).

that the Farming Women's group had worked on different issues over the years and wanted to keep working with the community. She felt that it would be useful for the students to talk to a couple of the pioneer members of the club. Those members would provide a historical perspective on the women's group and the county. Susan added the name of the editor of the county newspaper, Joe Johannson. She explained that Joe had been running the newspaper for more than 30 years and really knew who to see and talk to in the community.

Susan asked Hilda if the women's group had decided what they wanted to accomplish at the resource center. Hilda said that they were not certain. They had recently been informed that the foot care service that had been provided by a visiting home health nurse was going to be discontinued in 3 months. The group had conducted an informal survey of their members and found that 30 to 50 people in the county could be affected. She added that she did not know if that issue was the most important one for the people living in the county.

Susan asked the students if they had some information from the course that they were taking. Gabriela explained what they had been learning about doing a community assessment to identify priorities. She said that some or a combination of methods such as community meetings, focus groups, or a survey could be used. Susan added that a community meeting could be a way to include other groups. Hilda asked if the students would present a summary of the methods at the upcoming meeting. They agreed.

In the car on the way back to the university, the students were wondering about the direction of their project.

Greta asked, "I don't know why we need to do this presentation. I'm sure that Susan knows this stuff."

Colleen complained, "Why do we have to go and see these people? I think we should just get on with planning something for the people who need foot care."

"Well," responded Gabriela, "I've been thinking about why Susan asked us about assessment methods. Maybe she wants the information to come from us. It also gives the women an opportunity to see what we can do."

"Yes, I think so," responded Rosa. "I'm looking forward to talking to the pioneer women. I wonder what it was like here when they were our age?"

"I suppose we might as well get on with it," stated Colleen.

"I'll take notes. We might as well use our driving time to come up with the questions we'll ask," added Gabriela.

DISCUSSION QUESTIONS

1. Why was it important for the team to meet the pioneer women and the editor of the newspaper?
2. How easy or difficult would it be for the team to present the information on assessment methods rather than material that they had collected themselves?

Rural communities and rural nursing

Rural communities develop their own culture based on their history, geography, and major occupation. This culture affects the health status of rural residents and the role of the community health nurse working in rural areas.

History and culture of rural communities

Rural communities have usually been formed by self-reliant and independent people determined to eke out a living from the land (Keating, 1991; Leipert & Reutter, 1998). Their pioneering spirit allowed them to harvest natural resources such as crops, domestic animals, fish, minerals, or trees to support the economic growth of the country. This spirit is also associated with right-wing politics, traditional family values (Keating, 1991; Leipert & Reutter, 1998), and less experience in dealing with differences and change compared to people living in more urban areas.

The culture of rural communities can mean that male preferences dominate in both the community and the delivery of healthcare (Leipert, 1999; Leipert & Reutter, 1998). Other groups in the community, notably women who are elderly, lesbian, disabled, or First Nations people, suffer from lack of appropriate health and social programs (Leipert, 1999; Leipert & Reutter, 1998). Often a major part of the nursing role in rural areas is to work with women to develop programs that are appropriate for them and their families.

Rural geography

The term *rural* is not used consistently. In Canada, the recommended definition from Statistics Canada is that *rural* is the population living in towns and municipalities outside the commuting zone of an urban center of 10,000 or more (du Plessis et al., 2002). Greater degrees of isolation exist for communities in the three northern territories and the northern parts of the larger provinces. These northern isolated communities are characterized by severe climatic conditions and either great distances between areas of habitation, lack of road access, or road access only at certain times of the year (Leipert & Reutter, 1998).

For the United States, Bushy (2003) felt that a continuum of rural–urban residency that takes into account residency and population density is the best approach. The continuum ranges from farm residency or frontier areas with less than six persons per square mile to metropolitan residency in cities with more than 1 million people.

The land of a state or province is divided into various areas with defined boundaries. The most common in approximate order of increasing geographic size is municipality or township, county, and state or province. The usual description of a county is that it is a geographical unit of administration intermediate between the larger state or province and the smaller township or municipality. The jurisdiction of each unit will be similar within the same state or province but is likely to vary between states and provinces and countries.

A part of the early assessment when one works in a county would be to determine the boundaries of the county, the names of the county administrators, the location of their office, and their responsibilities. As these boundaries become known, further assessment would involve determining whether the people living in the county identify with being a resident and are concerned about county matters. For example, there may be many people living in the county who have little interaction with others. They would meet one aspect of being a community by sharing the same location, but lack the relational ties that bring people together to work on common issues.

Occupations in rural and northern communities

Occupations in rural areas are based on natural resources and therefore are vulnerable to changes in the economic and environmental climate. The rural industries are farming, fishing, logging, and mining (Rennie, Baird-Crooks, Remus, & Engle, 2000).

Farming has traditionally been the main occupation in rural communities. Although farming families share the independent and entrepreneurial spirit of business owners, the type of farming, such as wheat, cattle, or mixed farming, will have a great influence on the attitudes and practices of members of the particular rural community. For example, the timeframes of dairy, cattle, and wheat farmers will vary greatly on a daily, weekly, and seasonal basis. In working with a farming community, the nurse needs to determine times when people will probably be available that would not interfere with farming tasks such as milking or harvesting.

The other rural industries involve fishing, logging, and mining (Rennie et al., 2000). When one industry is the main employer in an area, the hiring, firing, and other policies of the industry dominate the economy. The community health nurse could be in a position to advocate on behalf of the community for a change in company policy to improve the health of the community.

Occupational choices, particularly for women, are limited in rural and northern communities (Leipert, 1999; Leipert & Reutter, 1998). Often this means that women are unemployed or underemployed. In addition, women and families have fewer resources to compensate for their isolation, such as public transportation or a vehicle to allow them to meet with others.

Health status of rural populations

Geographical isolation, resource-based occupations, and fewer healthcare resources and personnel all probably contribute to a poor health status for people living in rural areas. For example, people living in the rural areas of Canada have lower life expectancy rates and lower disability-free life expectancy than people in urban areas (Shields & Tremblay, 2002). Reasons for the differences have not been determined through research. Lack of research is particularly an issue for rural women's health and the health of First Nations people (Leipert, 1999; Leipert & Reutter, 1998; Young, 2003).

The health status of U.S. residents in the most rural areas has the following characteristics compared with those of residents living in the fringe counties of large metropolitan areas: highest death rates for children and young adults, highest unintentional and motor vehicle traffic-related injuries, highest death rates among adults for ischemic heart disease and suicide, highest level of smoking among adolescents, highest physical activity during leisure time among men, highest obesity among adults, and highest percentage of adults with activity limitations caused by chronic health conditions (Centers for Disease Control and Prevention, 2001).

Rural nursing

The characteristics of rural communities influence the way nurses practice in those communities. Several authors have identified the characteristics of **rural nursing** practice (Bushy, 2000, 2003; Dunkin, 2000; Leipert, 1999; Leipert & Reutter, 1998; Rennie et al., 2000). In Table 10-4, the factors have been sorted into positive and negative columns, indicating the challenge of the practice.

Community health nurses working in rural areas have a particular opportunity as well as a challenge to build on the capacity of community groups. As identified in Table 10-4, community health nurses who are new to a rural area will have a challenge to gain the trust and acceptance of community members. Scarce resources also mean lack of services for disadvantaged groups such as women, the elderly, and minority groups. Community health

TABLE 10-4 *Positive and Negative Factors in Rural Nursing Practice*	
POSITIVE FACTORS	**NEGATIVE FACTORS**
Generalist skills used in a variety and diversity of experiences with clients of all ages having a full range of conditions/diagnoses	Sparse professional and community resources Difficulty maintaining specialist skills
Opportunity to use full scope of practice and be creative, flexible, and independent	Challenge for those wanting structure and control
Status in community, professional role model, overlap with other disciplines	Undue expectations, professional/personal isolation
Continuity of care for clients in community, hospital, and during discharge through formal and informal interactions with co-workers and clients	Lack of anonymity
Opportunity for community involvement and informal health education	Gaining acceptance and trust is a challenge to overcome outsider/insider or old-timer/newcomer phenomenon (Bushy, 2000; Leipert & Reutter, 1998).

nurses will need skills and knowledge to encourage the organization of these community groups.

Examples of community capacity building initiatives with women used by public health nurses in northern British Columbia are an informal women's coffee group and a women's wellness day (Leipert, 1999). In a northern Ontario mining town, the author and a colleague worked with women in the community to determine a community project. The event they decided on included discussion groups on menopause and parenting adolescents, child care, displays of household and kitchen merchandise, and a fashion show of casual clothes. The women continued the event on their own.

This chapter will help nurses working in rural areas to understand the importance of trusting relationships with people in the community and begin building on community capacity. These relationships are foundational to bring about the health benefits that the community desires.

DETERMINING RURAL PRIORITIES SCENARIO (continued)

After the student team was starting to get some sense of the county, Susan sat down with them to discuss her role as a rural nurse. She explained that although she had been working as a Public Health nurse in the county for three years, some people are just starting to accept her. She felt that one thing that has helped is that she also lives in the county. She still feels that she is a newcomer, and most people think of her that way also.

Gabriela exclaimed: "I can't believe it! A newcomer still after three years. In most places with a great turnover of staff you would be the most senior person there."

"I can understand it," said Rosa. "Most of the people who live in the county, like my family, count generations, not years!"

Susan added, "Well, you can't blame them in one way. There has been a great turnover of nurses coming here. Before I came, nobody seemed to stay more than six months."

Susan went on to say that even if she is still viewed as a newcomer, people are starting to accept her. People who she has met in her practice are starting to approach her for health information as she goes about her daily business at the bank or grocery store or when she is picking up her children at school. She explained that other colleagues on the rural team who commute to their area from the city are having more difficulty forming relationships with people.

She explained that she makes a point of listening and making certain that she understands what is wanted before responding. At first she had difficulty realizing how much of the residents' lives and priorities revolved around farming. Another lesson is that she needs to consider how she is viewed in the community. For example, one of the first contacts she had was with the Farming Women. They had come to her with a concern about a weed that was being used by the teenagers to get high. A youth in a nearby county had become seriously ill from it. Susan was able to bring in experts to talk to parents, teachers, and the students. Through their efforts the practice seems to have been stopped. During that situation, Susan met Joe, the editor of the newspaper. He explained that the work she did with the Farming Women was valued, but she must also work with other community groups so that she would be considered fair. She has started to work with businesses in the county to distribute information on farm safety.

In addition to working with community organizations, Susan explained that she has responsibility for other required public health programs such as testing of well water and immunizations. Sometimes she feels a bit overwhelmed because she is viewed as the public health practitioner in the county and has an interdisciplinary practice with physicians, social workers, and home health nurses, as well as an intersectoral practice with teachers, municipal leaders, businesses, and community organizations. She told then that some public health or outpost nurses working in more remote areas can be involved in providing clinical services as well as health promotion and illness prevention.

The students were at first overwhelmed; then they all started exclaiming over the many things she had to do.

Susan stopped them by saying, "Yes, I have a lot to do, but I can decide how and when I do it. I enjoy the freedom and flexibility. I call myself a generalist in rural health. Not every nurse would be happy with this practice, but I am. I enjoy the challenge."

DISCUSSION QUESTIONS

1. How is Susan dealing with being a newcomer?
2. How would Susan's role differ if she was practicing in a more isolated area?

Community capacity building practice

In community capacity building practice, community health practitioners, often called organizers, work with and between people, groups, and organizations to identify and use the resources they have for the betterment of the community. They build capacity by providing particular types of services, programs, and goods that help community members feel like a community and address their health issues (Ontario Prevention Clearing House, 2002).

For some community health practitioners, such as social workers or community developers or organizers, their complete practice is composed of community capacity building. Often for community health nurses working for a Public Health agency or other community health agency, community capacity building will be only a part of the practice. The other parts could be health teaching, immunizing, or running medical clinics. These multiple roles of the community health nurse can be confusing for community members who are unfamiliar with the social determinants of health. People may ask, "Where is the health in what you are doing?" For example, nurses could be working with community groups on controlling street traffic, obtaining legal assistance, or building a playground. Superficially, these activities do not appear to be directly related to health, although they do relate to the determinants of health. Community health nurses need to take time to explain how community capacity building can be as important to the health of the community as other Public Health or medical services.

Although most community health nurses are building community capacity part time, they can include the concepts in all their relationships within the community. This requires an emphasis on the social dimensions of the community. For community members, the social dimension of community is often more important than geographical boundaries (Billings, 2000; Lindsey, Stajduhar & McGuinness, 2000). The social dimension means that community is a relational experience that includes belonging, sharing, caring, and being important to one another (Lindsey et al., 2000). This means that community is an emotional involvement similar to saying, "We are family."

Experienced practitioners and researchers consistently identify similar factors that contribute to successful work with communities. These consistent factors have been identified at the national (Wolff & Kaye, 1995) and international levels (SIL International, 1997) and by experienced public health nurses (Public Health Nursing Section, 2001). Mattessich and Monsey (1997) conducted a systematic review of the literature on community building to identify the key factors that resulted in the success of community building initiatives. The factors from both experienced practitioners and the review of community capacity building apply to five areas: characteristics of organizers, characteristics of the community, relationship process, and task functions.

Characteristics of organizers

Although community capacity building usually occurs without any dedicated involvement of a professional organizer, organizers with knowledge, skills, and abilities associated with community capacity building are able to assist communities in using their resources to the best advantage. Organizers are people from inside or outside the community who design, implement, and manage the community capacity building effort (Mattessich & Monsey, 1997). The definition of who is an insider and who is an outsider has considerable variation. In some rural communities, for example, a person can still be considered a newcomer after being a resident for more than 10 but less than 20 years (Bushy, 2000).

When organizers have more of the following three characteristics, likelihood of success in community capacity building is increased (Mattessich & Monsey, 1997):

- Understanding the community
- Sincerity of commitment and relationship of trust
- Level of organizing experience, including the ability to be flexible and adaptable

Understanding the community

Successful organizers need to understand the community's culture, social structure, demographics, political structures, and issues (Mattessich & Monsey, 1997). The types of knowledge needed emphasize the multidimensional nature of communities (Walter, 1997) and the need for organizers to be out in the community interacting with a variety of people on a regular basis. For example, organizers would know who is friendly with whom, who likes to get things done, and who likes to support others. Organizers need to know the history of the community, especially how decisions are made. Although organizers may not know the history personally, they take the time to talk to the people who do know and who are respected in the community. Through talking, listening, and observing over a period of time, organizers will be able to identify the issues that are important to the community. For community health nurses, listening and observing would be included in their conversations with people in the course of their activities.

Sincerity of commitment and relationship of trust

The characteristics of organizers' commitment to the community and trust by the community are closely related. A sincere commitment to the community is conveyed when organizers demonstrate an interest in the long-term development of the community, a sustained attachment to community members, honesty, and actions that serve the community and not an outside group (Mattessich & Monsey, 1997). For example, organizers could emphasize that people within the community should be employed to do a task or give a presentation rather than bringing in people from the outside.

Community members learn to trust organizers when they share the same vision and when the organizers attend to their interests, do not favor one group over another, use words that have the same meaning for everyone, and follow through with commitments (Mattessich & Monsey, 1997). The development of both the organizers' commitment and the community's trust of the organizers takes time and requires ongoing interactions. When organizers are working as a team, often each member will form stronger relationships with different groups in the community and thus the team can develop a more comprehensive view of the community. For community health nurses, commitment and trust come from demonstrations of their desire to promote the health of all members of the community.

Level of organizing experience, including the ability to be flexible and adaptable

The extent of the organizers' experience in working with communities and the ability to be flexible contribute to successful community building (Mattessich & Monsey, 1997). Experienced organizers are better able to estimate the amount of work that is required, motivate people, and plan and be productive, while still being flexible and adaptable (Mattessich & Monsey, 1997). Additional characteristics are the ability to share responsibility, good communication skills, a sense of humor, patience, the ability to view the "community as client," and utilization of the wisdom learned from previous organizing efforts (Public Health Nursing Section, 2001). Experience provides organizers with the opportunity to view the situation and determine the action that will be most suitable at that time, according to the readiness of the community. Experience is greatly augmented by engaging in self-reflection and team reflection and evaluation (Chapter 2), especially when one is working with vulnerable and disenfranchised groups.

From experience, organizers need to learn which type of approach works best at different stages. In a review of programs using empowering group strategies with low-income families, Diem (1996/1997) stated that organizers could err in two opposing directions. They could be just receptive and supportive or they could be directive. A more successful approach begins with just being supportive and evolves into a more challenging or questioning approach to encourage people to take action. Throughout all stages, organizers need to provide a forum in which people can discuss the issues important to them.

According to Freire's (1972) three-stage listening–dialogue–action approach, listening means being receptive and supportive. **Dialogue** is the skillful interaction between people that develops shared understanding as a basis for trust, ownership, true agreement, and creative problem solving (National Association of County and Health Officials, 2000). During dialogue, a leader moves from a totally receptive listening role to a position that starts challenging the people to look critically at their beliefs in what has been called a problem-posing approach (Wallerstein & Bernstein, 1988). Being challenging does not mean that the organizers impose ideas on a group, such as wanting to address poverty rather than a more manageable project. It does mean asking questions, and introducing other ideas, issues, perspectives, or underlying problems. It also means that the organizers offer hope and a vision that will inspire the community. The challenge includes encouraging and supporting community residents to take action on the issues that they have identified.

Although the relationship-building process starts earlier, it does not stop during the task activities. An experienced organizer recognizes that the relationship process nourishes people for the tasks, and the completion of tasks provides the food for the relationship. An organizer interested in community capacity building begins leading from the middle of the group to hear what is being said and to support group leaders and gradually withdraws to the rear as the group takes over.

DETERMINING RURAL PRIORITIES SCENARIO (continued)

In preparation for the Farming Women's meeting, the team looked over the information they had on assessment methods. They prepared a draft and asked Susan for feedback. She suggested that they identify one or two advantages of each method and talk over their ideas with Hilda. Hilda said that it would be a good idea to include an example to indicate situations for which each method would be particularly useful. In addition to interviewing key informants, they had been collecting county sociodemographic information.

More than 20 women were present at the meeting, which was considered a good turnout for the beginning of the harvest season. Rosa and Greta presented the information on the assessment methods early in the meeting. They gave examples of the best use of each method and how more than one method could be used together or in sequence. Several specific questions were asked at the end of the presentation. Then one woman asked why they would bother to do an assessment at all. Rosa explained that a community assessment could identify the issues of people throughout the county and could also be a way of including other people if that is what they wanted. Hilda suggested that they consider the assessment information along with the information on foot care services.

The expected discontinuation of foot care services in the home was next on the agenda. The president announced the issue and provided the results of the informal survey, which identified that 30 to 50 seniors could lose the service in three months. She asked for members' views on the issue. Two people immediately sprang up and told how their relatives were really upset about losing the foot care service. They wanted the association to look into options to address the problem. After they finished, an older woman took the floor and talked about different issues that were facing seniors in the rural area. She said that she had visited the national Web site of the association and found that other groups around the country had conducted formal surveys on the needs of seniors. Others added comments about how their informal survey may have counted the same people more than once and how they were being questioned by different community members about what was going on at the resource center.

One woman summed up what was being said by stating, "I feel uncomfortable about going ahead on our own at this point. A year ago, only one church wanted to work with us. Now others see the possibilities of providing better health services through the resource center. The people in my church ask me why they cannot take part in what is happening at the resource center. I have also been called by someone from the seniors group. I don't know what to say to them. We have always prided ourselves in working with the community!"

These comments stimulated considerable discussion. When they were considering various options such as continuing with the foot care issue or considering other issues, they asked Susan what she thought. She suggested that they consider the following questions: Can they take on more than one issue? Do they want to work with other groups in the community? Are they certain that foot care is the most important issue? They decided that they could not take on more than one issue, that they did want to work with others, and that only a few felt that foot care was the most important issue.

After more discussion, the group agreed to hold a community meeting in about four weeks to get all the issues "on the table" and to begin to identify the most prominent healthcare issue. An ad hoc committee was formed of the students and women from different areas of the county to organize the meeting.

DISCUSSION QUESTIONS

1. How did the questions Susan posed to the women's group indicate that she knew issues that were important to them and how they made decisions?

2. What would have been the likely response if Susan had given them advice instead of posing the questions?

Characteristics of the community

The basic ingredient of working in and with the community is being able to determine to what degree the community is likely to take successful action. Mattessich and Monsey (1997) conducted a systematic review of the literature on community building and identified the social and psychological attributes of the residents that were associated with successful community building. When the community showed more of the following factors, the chance of success was greater:

  ■ Community awareness of an issue
  ■ Motivation from within the community
  ■ Small geographical area
  ■ Experience from previous community building

When communities are assessed for these characteristics and are found to be lacking in one or more, this does not mean that community capacity building should not proceed. It just means that some preliminary work on the missing factors would probably increase the potential for successful community building.

Community awareness of an issue

Successful efforts are more likely to happen if the community is aware that a problem or issue exists and it has significance for most community members (Mattessich & Monsey, 1997). The same types of problems motivate people nationally and internationally. These include the need for housing, community safety, threats to natural resources, health concerns or fears of disease, and concerns about the future of children (Mattessich & Monsey, 1997).

To assess whether community awareness is present, organizers would listen to hear whether people in one area express the same types of concerns and whether the concerns are relevant in other areas. Community health nurses would do this as they go about their work in the community and would note what concerns people raise in conversation and check to see whether the concerns have broader interest by asking others. For example, in the scenario there is some concern raised about the availability of healthcare in the county.

Many of the assessment methods described in Chapter 4, such as key informant interviews, mapping the area, meetings, and questionnaires, can be extended to identify community-wide issues. A concerns survey involving as many people as possible in the community is valuable, not only in identifying common issues, but also in including the community members and providing credibility for their issues.

The University of Kansas's Community Tool Box (KU Work Group, 2000a) suggests that the items in a survey be limited to 30, with an additional 8 to 10 questions for demographics. This limit is suggested because it would take the average person 15 minutes to complete a survey of this length. Their Web site provides examples of properly worded items and demographic questions. When you work with a community, it is preferable to include demographic questions that will assist with planning programs. These types of questions need to be checked with community members to determine whether they are acceptable. Usually people are receptive to providing information on their age, sex, number and ages of children, language(s) spoken, level of education, and the location of their residence.

Motivation from within the community

Successful efforts are more likely to occur if the community decides on their own to take action and determines the ideas and goals (Mattessich & Monsey, 1997). The motivation can be assessed when the issue is raised to determine whether community members are ready to take action. For example, in the scenario, the chairperson of the women's group is concerned about the healthcare services in the community.

Small geographical area

A small geographical area allows people to interact and organize activities that contribute to successful community building (Mattessich & Monsey, 1997). One way to assess the dimensions of a community is to determine how far people presently travel to attend regular meetings of community organizations or groups. When people have further to travel, the chances of getting together are also less because of time, weather, and the pressure of more immediate concerns. In the scenario, there was both a county women's group and a resource center, indicating that people identified themselves as being residents of the county.

Experience from previous community building

Communities that have learned from a previous community capacity building experience have an advantage over communities that have not had the experience or have not learned from the experience. From previous experience, communities are expected to have learned to be flexible and adaptable; have social cohesion; be able to discuss, reach consensus, and cooperate; have identifiable leadership; and have some success with community capacity building (Mattesich & Monsey, 1997).

Successful community capacity building depends on people who are ready to look at different options and choose those that have the best chance to work, rather than simply reusing methods that have been used in the past or sticking to methods that are not working (National Association of County and City Health Officials, 2000; Mattessich & Monsey, 1997). Although rules or guidelines may have been necessary in the past, they may also become a hindrance. For example, the organizers of an annual event may find that each year fewer and fewer teenagers are participating in the event. The rules of the organization are that each organizer must be a business member of the community. To include teenagers, they must consider how they can change the rules so teens can assist in organizing the events.

Social cohesion, which is the strength of the relationships among community residents, is associated with community problem solving, good communication, and a large number of associations within the community (Mattessich & Monsey, 1997). Usually social cohesion is associated with a stable population. If the population is not stable, the institutions that provide services to the transient population are often encouraged to work together; an example would be a coalition for the homeless.

Although the number and names of organizations can be determined from a telephone directory or a community resource list, a list will not necessarily provide information on how well associations work with each other. Another consideration is whether all people in the community are represented by an effective organization. Both aspects can be determined by observing who is involved in community events and asking whether and how well the concerns of community members are represented.

Successful efforts are more likely to occur if community members have been able in the past to openly discuss their problems and needs or have come together previously to help each other or work on events (Mattessich & Monsey, 1997). An important aspect of this characteristic is to determine whether the community has had the opportunity to practice dialogue, develop trust, and develop skills in decision making (National Association of County and City Health Officials, 2000; Mattessich & Monsey, 1997). If the community has not had an opportunity to come together, this can be a crucial contribution of organizers. For example, a community health nurse might be told by different parents of children in the same grade or different grades of a school about verbal abuse by teachers. The nurse can organize a meeting in a neutral location where the parents can compare the information they have and consider different courses of action.

Successful community capacity building requires people who are used to leading and who others will listen to and follow (Mattessich & Monsey, 1997). Although there may be community leaders, they may have so many commitments that they cannot take on additional ones, or they may be functioning as leaders in less prominent situations such as organizing a baseball league or regularly organizing church events. Busy prominent leaders can acknowledge the importance of an issue or mentor potential leaders. Leaders with less experience can gain more confidence by first working on small tasks and working with a team.

If communities have no previous experience in community work, or the experience was negative, different approaches are needed. If the community has had no experience, they need to start with small steps. For example, if the tenants in a rundown building have not worked together previously, they should not be encouraged to confront the landlord immediately, but could instead organize an event to discuss the issue with more people in the building and to hear from people who have experience in dealing with landlords. If the community has had a negative experience, the community could be asked to review the experience to identify the factors that contributed to the failure. The community would probably be unwilling to embark on a new initiative unless they feel it has a very good chance to succeed and the negative factors associated with the previous initiative have been minimized. For example, a neighborhood would be very reluctant to become involved in any government-funded projects if they had previously received government funding to build a playground, only to have the money or materials reduced by half after they had started.

DETERMINING RURAL PRIORITIES SCENARIO (continued)

When the team met with Joe, the editor of the newspaper, he seemed unwilling to talk very much until Rosa mentioned her family. He then brightened up and told them how Rosa's uncle had been a part of the county's fight to stop the establishment of a waste disposal site four years ago. A large waste disposal firm had approached county officials and sold them on the idea because of the jobs the site would provide. When the residents heard about it, they demanded a meeting. The firm came to the meeting with a lot of fancy slides to show them how much money and jobs would come to the county. Questions about traffic, seepage into the water table, or pollution from the smokestack were not answered. The firm realized that the meeting did not go well, so they came back to the community with three options involving different locations for the waste disposal site. Most residents were not happy with any of the locations. The firm then tried to tell them that they would use higher-than-required standards for the smokestacks and for lining the pits. By this time the community was really angry and forced the officials to reject the application. He said that many groups from the community came together to fight the firm: the service clubs including the Farming Women, all the churches, and some of the businesses.

When he mentioned the Farming Women, he said that they were another issue. The students asked him what he meant. He said that he had nothing against them, but some people in the community questioned why only the Farming Women and one church from the six in the area were managing the county resource center.

After meeting with the pioneer women, the students had quite a different perspective. They learned that the Farming Women and the church were the only two groups that were willing to work together on the proposal for the resource center. Because they felt that others were not interested, they had formed a board from their members and a few businesspeople and professionals. The older women talked proudly about issues that had been dealt with over the years and the challenges they had faced because they were a women's group. On the drive home in the second week, ideas were spinning in the students' heads. "Well, I don't know what to make of it," said Gabriela. "Why aren't they happy with what the women's group is doing?"

"It's difficult to explain," responded Rosa. "What I remember about the waste disposal site was that everyone joined in. In contrast, it seems that the county resource center is viewed as being exclusive to the women's group and the one church."

"I get the feeling that we are going to have to use all the assessment skills we're learning as well as conflict management," stated Greta.

"I'll second that," confirmed Rosa. "I hadn't really thought that community health nursing was political!"

DISCUSSION QUESTIONS

1. For each of the eight levels in Arnstein's ladder (Table 10-3), provide an example from the scenario.
2. Discuss possible sources of resentment in the community about the management of the resource center.

Relationship process

Community capacity building is unique in identifying the central role of relationship building and the fact that building a relationship precedes any action. The relationship must also include as many people in the community as possible. The following identify the characteristics of a successful relationship process:

- Start where the people are (Nyswander, 1956).
- Develop relationships based on understanding, sincerity, and trust (Mattessich & Monsey, 1997; SIL International, 1997; Wolff & Kaye, 1995).
- Provide fulfilling roles for community members (Wolff & Kaye, 1995).
- Involve as many people as possible from the start, and keep recruiting, including establishing links with local leadership, community organizations, and government (Mattessich & Monsey, 1997; SIL International, 1997).
- Provide a good system of communication (Mattessich & Monsey, 1997).
- Create opportunities to recognize community members, and show respect for their contributions on an ongoing basis (Wolff & Kaye, 1995).

The only difference between the type of relationship needed to work successfully with community groups, as listed here, and working in a small group, as discussed in Chapter 2, is the number of people involved. The relationship process is similar to addressing team morale.

Start where the people are: Listen to learn

The important message in the relationship process is to spend time talking to people so that you know about them and the things that matter to them. "Start where the people are" (Nyswander, 1956) means listening to their existing interests to determine the things that are important in their lives, their perceived needs (SIL, 1997), and the skills they have to offer. The same kind of listening to learn needs to occur over and over again as you meet with different groups in the community at different times and in different places.

Difficulties can arise when organizers have become quite familiar with the issues of one group and assume that the same issues apply to others. The best approach is to listen to learn when meeting new people and until similar issues start emerging. As you learn about the community's issues and why members feel the way they do, you will find yourself committed to the community's future, and they will learn to trust you.

Develop relationships and provide fulfilling roles

Relationships draw people to groups and keep them involved. The most effective way to recruit individuals is to ask them to join the group and identify what they could contribute. When I was recruiting women for a support group for mothers of adolescent girls, one mother felt that she would have nothing to contribute. I pointed out to her that she had a wealth of information from raising five daughters. Often women do not appreciate the skills they have learned in caring for a family because their contributions have not been recognized.

People may join a project initially because they can provide the perspective of a particular group of people in the community. As they become more comfortable on the team, they will probably find that they have hidden talents to contribute to the success of the project. These talents can include artistic or writing abilities, knowing people in the community who have resources, finding people who are isolated, or helping new members feel welcome.

Widespread and ongoing participation

From the beginning, always consider how to expand participation. You may feel more comfortable initially settling down to plan only with people you know. However, the danger is that what you plan will belong to the planners and not to the community (SIL International, 1997). Relationships also need to be extended to others: those external to the community, such as government agencies; others from the community who have not yet been involved; and those in need who do not usually participate in community activities.

Widespread participation must be representative of most segments of the community and be continuous (Mattessich & Monsey, 1997). Representative participation has the following advantages: 1) provides the talents of a wider and more diverse group of people, 2) provides more political acceptability of any endeavors that result from the participation, and 3) increases the chances of connections to people outside the area who can contribute to the community effort (Mattessich & Monsey, 1997).

Although people may be attracted initially to a community effort, their circumstances and priorities can change. To keep up the motivation and effort, recruitment and training must be ongoing (Mattessich & Monsey, 1997). Although bringing in and orienting new participants may make you feel like the project is being slowed, the overall effect is that the project will continue to grow, expand, and adapt.

Participation can be expanded by holding community meetings. Two types of community meetings, described as specific assessment methods in Chapter 4, provide the means to open up the process to others. A community forum or town hall meeting allows people to air their concerns and can be the beginning of an initiative. An invitational group meeting brings people together to obtain their views, support, and involvement in an issue. Meetings provide the opportunity to identify and include community opinion leaders and representatives of most segments of the community who could greatly assist the initiative if involved or, conversely, could damage the initiative if not involved.

Representatives of organizations that are important to the community initiative need to be included in planning meetings in terms of date, time, location, and agenda items. For example, if the meeting is planned when one organization has planned another event, the openness of the process may be challenged. Other important issues are determining who will facilitate the meeting and who will present information. Often the meeting chairperson sets the tone for the meeting, not by what is said but by how fair or considerate the person is viewed to be by the community.

Effective dialogue during meetings greatly contributes to engaging the community. Box 10-1 provides tips for including dialogue in meetings.

Presentations at meetings can also encourage dialogue if they are used as a way to open up discussion rather that to provide pat answers. In a consultative presentation, some information is provided along with a process to engage participants. The content of a community presentation needs to be carefully considered because adequate time must be allowed for discussion. This type of presentation is quite different than presentations in a course for which you are graded on your skill in presenting content or in a business setting in which the bottom line is increased sales.

In the University of Kansas's Community Tool Box, the following reasons are given for presentations: to increase community awareness; to increase understanding of you, your group, and your issues; to increase support for you and your group; and to encourage involvement and action regarding your cause (KU Work Group, 2000b). The details of preparing and delivering a consultative presentation are given in Appendix A.

Communication

An important way to keep people involved is to keep them informed. This requires a dependable communication system. Usually individual organizations have their own communication system, such as a telephone fan-out, regular meetings, or a newsletter; but as more people or organizations are recruited, the communication system needs to be expanded to include the new recruits. Communication encourages community members' awareness, motivation, involvement, ideas, problem solving, and ability to mobilize (Mattessich & Monsey, 1997).

Recognition and respect

Similar to group work, people feel that they belong in a group when they are recognized, are shown respect, and have developed relationships. Recognition is important on both a

| BOX 10-1 | Including dialogue in meetings |

1. Arrange room so people can see each other (circle or horseshoe) (National Association of County and City Health Officials, 2000).
2. Begin each meeting with a check-in and end with a wrap-up to provide each member a 5 minute (or less) opportunity to give his or her views (Wheeler & Chinn, 1984). The check-in and wrap-up should be conducted like a brainstorming, without interruption. Initiate each "round robin" with a question such as "What do you want to get out of this meeting?" or "What do you like about our community?" for the check-in and "What did you learn?" and/or "What can be improved about how the meeting was conducted?" for the wrap-up.
3. Once dialogue starts, ask each speaker to summarize the points of the previous speaker before adding new points. This contributes to clarity of meaning and validation (National Association of County and City Health Officials, 2000).
4. Allow time for increased understanding of both particular and broader perspectives by seeking views from everyone and posing questions to stimulate a broader view of the situation.
5. Summarize the dialogue by going around the circle and have someone record the main points (National Association of County and City Health Officials, 2000).

one-on-one level by thanking a person for what he or she has done and publicly at a meeting, event, or in written material. Ensure that any contribution of community members is recognized whenever possible. People respect you when you listen to them and take their wishes and concerns into account when planning meetings, events, and project goals.

DETERMINING RURAL PRIORITIES SCENARIO (continued)

When the student team and women started planning the date and location of the community meeting, Greta suggested that maybe they should start with a list of the people and organizations they felt should be invited. Then they quickly determined that they should hold the meeting at a central meeting place, such as the central high school or township office, in the early evening. They knew that they would not get the farmers to come earlier in the day when they were harvesting and had the milking to do. One of the women agreed to phone the high school and township office to determine when room would be available.

In short order, the group had quickly determined who to contact and what specific information they would ask. As decisions were being made, Rosa and Greta sketched out a form they could each use to collect the data. Each person copied the form and added the names of those they were to contact. The woman determining the availability of a meeting room promised to phone each person with the possible locations and dates to include in the questions.

On the way home from the meeting, the students were excited about being included and feeling that they had something to contribute.

"That stuff we learned in class was okay," stated Gabriela, "but after working directly with the women, I realize why Susan and Hilda wanted us to keep it simple and provide examples. I don't think the women would understand the different assessment methods otherwise. I know I felt confused the first time we learned about it."

"They really are trying now to include others from the community," said Rosa. "They are really good at organizing among themselves. Look at all the money they've raised. They just hadn't thought that others were concerned about healthcare and now wanted to be part of the resource center."

At the meeting of the committee the following week, the women reported that it was easy to contact the people about their preferences because most were at the fall fair held on the weekend. Through informal discussions at the fair, the most acceptable location and date were determined. People usually seemed pleased about being asked to attend and provide their input. Names of new members who had not been on the original list were mentioned, and those people were also contacted. Most people were able to attend on the chosen date, and if they weren't, they felt that others who were available would represent their interests. A complete list of names with phone numbers was compiled.

Now they were down to planning the meeting. Several names had been suggested for chairing the meeting, but often these people were associated with a particular organization. Susan, the Public Health nurse, was selected because her name came up the most often. People mentioned her because they felt that she could keep a meeting on track and was fairly "neutral." Joe Johannson and one of the pioneer women would be invited to give a short historical review on what the county had leaned from the fight with the waste disposal site and forming the resource center. The students offered to prepare a short presentation on the sociodemographics of the elderly persons living in the county and would also present the various ways that could be used to assess the community. Four groups with differing views wanted to present and would be given time to do so. The time for the meeting was carefully blocked out to allow time for discussion after each presentation.

On the way back to town, the students considered ways to present their material.

"I think the best thing is to use a map of the county," stated Colleen. "People like to see maps of where they live."

"Great idea!" declared Gabriela. "I'm sure we can download a map with the county lines from the county Web site. We can use numbers or shading with the map to show where more elderly people live."

"Okay, now what about the assessment methods?" asked Rosa. "I think we should concentrate this time on how a survey could be developed and used."

"Well, I heard one of the Public Health nurses who works on the rural team with Susan mention that they did a survey with the elderly in that county last year," stated Greta. "I could call her. I'm sure she'll give us a copy so we'll have somewhere to start."

DISCUSSION QUESTIONS

1. What characteristics, skills, and knowledge are displayed by the students?
2. What characteristics, skills, and knowledge are displayed by the women?
3. Compare the meeting that is being planned with the first meeting held by the waste disposal firm.

Task functions

Once people in the community have started to indicate that they trust the organizers, various tasks that they can work on together will be considered. Although the types of tasks will vary, the most successful have the following characteristics:

- Make decisions together on the goals, priorities and directions for the project (National Association of County and City Health Officials, 2000; Mattessich & Monsey, 1997; Wolff & Kaye, 1995).
- Work on process and task concurrently (Mattessich & Monsey, 1997).
- Start with projects that are simple and winnable and address community-identified issues (Mattessich & Monsey, 1997; Public Health Nursing Section, 2001; SIL International, 1997; Wolff & Kaye, 1995).
- Introduce new ideas about tasks that relate to the community's issues only after the relationship has been built (SIL International, 1997).

■ Systematically gather information and conduct analysis (Mattessich & Monsey, 1997).
■ Train trainers to train others in an accessible location and using methods familiar to community members (Mattessich & Monsey, 1997; SIL International, 1997).

Determine goals and objectives together

Once people have come together over issues in their community, one of the first tasks is to determine goals, priorities, and directions. These are not the specific goals and objectives that are determined after an assessment (Chapter 6); these are the goals and objectives used to identify the original direction for their effort. Sometimes groups first decide on the goals or direction; at other times they determine the name of their group first. In either case, the goals and direction should be reflected in the name.

Determining a name and an identity is an important exercise for a group. Mattessich and Monsey (1997) offer the following questions to assist in the naming process:

■ What do we want to accomplish?
■ What geographical area do we cover?
■ How do we want people in the community to think of us?

An additional question could be the following:

■ Do we consider only a particular age-group or everyone?

Take, for example, the previously mentioned event for women living in a northern mining town, that group spent a considerable amount of time coming up with the name of a community event that would be fun and interesting to women and families without being labeled a "women's" event. Eventually they arrived at the name "Healthy Living Festival."

Although determining the name may seem like a minor decision, how the decision is made and the name itself help to clarify the goals and priorities of the group and provide a spirit of collaboration. To determine initial priorities, (National Association of County and City Health Officials, 2000; Mattessich & Monsey, 1997) the most successful groups take time to ask each person to state his or her needs and then to decide as a group which needs are the most important.

Work on process and task concurrently

Similar to building small teams, the relationship process or building morale must continue as tasks are undertaken. As mentioned in the characteristics of successful organizers, the relationship process and the completion of tasks support each other. Without both, participation will decrease.

To ensure that the relationship process continues, organizers need to suggest that celebrations are scheduled along with tasks, that people are recognized for their contributions, and that social events are held. These social events need to be organized according to the "4F" principle: fun, free, food, and friend (bring a) (University of Manitoba, 2002). Also, organizers need to ask people on a regular basis whether they are learning what they want to learn and to provide other opportunities if they are ready for a change.

Winnable projects

The first initiatives need to be considered both manageable and therefore winnable to increase the community members' confidence in their ability to effect further change (Eisen, 1994). They also need to be clearly relevant to community members rather than problems envisioned by health professionals (Eisen, 1994; Stevens & Hall, 1992). Usually people will consider a project simple or winnable if they have done something like it, possibly on a smaller scale. For example, a new group that covers a large geographical area may decide to raise funds by holding a bazaar or raffle, which has worked in a small community within the area. They could also gain confidence by learning what others have done outside the community. People who have never worked together before could start by organizing a meeting or a picnic. As people become more experienced in working together and have more confidence in their abilities, they can take on more complex tasks.

To keep tasks simple, complex issues often need to be broken down into more manageable steps by experienced organizers. For example, a small group of parents may want to improve the nutritional value of the food available at the school, or seniors may want a more accessible source for purchasing medications. Organizers can lead them through a problem-solving session to identify preliminary steps that will provide both progress and confidence.

Tasks in projects that are successful must also be relevant to what the community considers as issues. Although smoking rates, teenage pregnancy, or underage drinking rates in the community may be high, the community may be more concerned about the lack of jobs or vandalism. When community members work on issues that will benefit them, they are likely to be more motivated and ready to gain the knowledge, skills, and abilities necessary to consider other initiatives that may not be as pressing.

Prepare people for new ideas

The process of building relationships can seem quite prolonged, especially when organizers have deadlines and want to show some tangible results for their work. Pushing issues or ideas can backfire if relationships have not been sufficiently developed. The best option is to prepare people for new ideas by asking questions, proposing options, or waiting to introduce new ideas until people start asking questions or asking for suggestions. The two situations given in Box 10-2 give you some idea of the importance of timing and preparation.

In situation A, the students are not prepared and the requests would seem bizarre. Situation B provides an introduction and context to understand and consider the requests. The students would probably be willing to try something new in situation B.

Community members who have less experience working in groups or planning projects are going to be even more reluctant to follow the lead of someone who they do not know. For example, if people have not had advanced education or experience working in a large business or government, planning a project might seem quite different to them than planning a family reunion or working on a committee. When they have learned to trust a person in small matters, they will be more ready to listen to the person's ideas (SIL International, 1997), especially if the needed knowledge and skills are related to something that interests them. Often women need to be encouraged to realize that their skills in running a household and managing a family are useful in other situations.

| BOX 10-2 | **Imagine your reaction** |

In the following two situations, imagine how you would react:

Situation A
A woman walks into the classroom when everyone is waiting for the instructor. The woman talks very quickly and mentions something about the instructor, but people are not certain what she said. She asks the class to do something that is quite different from whatever has been done before, such as drawing a graphic for a poster or writing a song.

Situation B
The class instructor has told you that you will be having a guest lecturer who has trained healthcare workers in developing countries. On the day of the class, the woman is introduced and tells you a bit about working in undeveloped countries. She says one of the important lessons that she has learned is that messages need to be simple and supported by pictures or songs. For example, she said that the healthcare workers made up a song about oral hydration for diarrhea that they could teach to the women in the village (Werner & Bower, 1982). The women loved the song, and the number of babies dying from dehydration was greatly reduced. She asks you if you want to create a picture or compose a song to promote breast feeding.

Systematic approach

A systematic approach to collecting and analyzing information is crucial to ensure that the community issues and strengths are clearly identified for the benefit of both the community as a whole and potential funders outside the community. The actual process of determining what information to collect and how to collect it is also a meaningful way to involve community members, develop relationships, and increase everyone's knowledge about the community (Mattessich & Monsey, 1997). The community assessment and analysis that are described in Chapters 3, 4, and 5 can be offered as an approach to community groups who want to systematically gather information. Community mapping and surveys are useful ways to include a variety of people once the direction for the project has been determined.

Train-the-trainer

Train-the-trainer involves training a certain number of people in a community group so they can train others within the community. This approach is considered an effective and efficient method of extending skills and knowledge because the trainers have a continuing presence and work within the culture of the community. The train-the-trainer approach is based on the premise that if you give a woman a fish, you are helping her and her family for a short time; if you teach her to fish, she is able to help herself and family for a lifetime; if she teaches others, many are helped (SIL International, 1997).

Preferably people who receive the training should be either present or emerging leaders in the community (SIL International, 1997). To ensure that people who receive training have some credibility in the community, the community needs to have the opportunity to determine who receives the training. The selection process can be used to increase interest in the project and the training. Similar to recruiting new members, recruitment and training of leaders is crucial to the sustainability of the project.

To train others, the person needs knowledge about teaching adults as well as knowledge about specific content. Train-the-trainer approaches are based on Knowles's (1980, 1989) **assumptions about adult learners.** Those assumptions are that adults

- Need to know why they need to learn.
- Have a self-concept that is capable of self-direction.
- Base learning on previous experience.
- Are ready to learn.
- Are motivated when learning is based on solving present problems and achieving life goals.

Knowles's assumptions are met when people learn to do something that they see will be a benefit to themselves and others.

A train-the-trainer approach is similar to group members learning to apply their particular skills and knowledge to the project and then teaching other members to take over the task. When greater numbers of people are involved, the teaching usually becomes more formalized into workshops or training sessions with printed educational material. Train-the-trainer is an educational activity that is planned in Chapter 6, implemented in Chapter 7, and evaluated in Chapter 8. When used in community capacity building, train-the-trainer approaches would involve the trainees in all aspects of the training including planning. The workshops described in the grocery store scenarios for Chapters 7 and 8 are compatible with community capacity building.

In community capacity building, training is more successful when it occurs close to home and when familiar methods are used (SIL International, 1997). When it is close to home, more people are able to take part, and they can assist each other in maintaining their learning. Adult learners learn best when they can build on the experience they have. New methods would need to be related to something they already do. Another approach is to explain what you want adults to learn and then ask them to brainstorm different ways that they feel would make it easier for them to learn.

An organization that initiates a train-the-trainer program has a responsibility to maintain and support ongoing training. Without support, trainers can lose their motivation and lack appropriate information. Supported trainers, on the other hand, will continue to expand their skills and recruit others.

DETERMINING RURAL PRIORITIES SCENARIO (continued)

The students were feeling anxious when they arrived for the community meeting. They had heard the meeting had generated considerable interest in the community and people wanted to be sure that they were heard.

More than 30 people were already in the room when they arrived; they were crowded together in small groups talking among themselves. Susan started the meeting right at 7 p.m. because she knew that most people would expect to leave by 9 p.m. at the latest. She welcomed everyone and explained the timing for the meeting. She stressed that everyone who wanted to would have a chance to speak, but that each speaker would be limited to five minutes. Notes would be taken on the flip charts at the front of the room. At 8 p.m. she would form small groups to discuss the issues. The issues would be reviewed at 8:30 p.m.

The two historical speakers went first, and the lessons learned from those experiences were noted on the flipcharts. The elderly woman who described the beginning of the resource center was challenged by a farmer who asked why only the Farming Women and one church were involved. The woman explained that they were the only two organizations that came forward when the government offered funds for a resource center two years ago. He then asked why more people weren't involved now. Several people from the audience started to speak. Susan requested that only one person at a time speak. She asked the farmer if he agreed with the points made on the flip chart about the resource center. He said he did.

The students were next on the agenda and presented a map showing where seniors were located throughout the county. The audience was interested in learning about the differences between areas. The students then presented their description of different methods that could be used to determine the issues in the county. When they mentioned surveys, one participant said that surveys had to be done by scientists if they were going to be believed. Greta explained that the residents of the next county had conducted a survey a year ago and were able to get funding for rural transportation. The response was that the next county was smaller than theirs.

Joe Johannson, the editor, spoke up at that point and asked if people were concerned about the lack of services for the elderly. Most hands in the room were raised. He then said that he knew that if they were concerned about something they would be able to work something out to address it because they had done it before.

The meeting moved on to presentations by different community groups. One group raised the concern about the distance people had to go when they needed long-term institutional care. The nearest facility was a two-hour drive away. Because of the distance, families were wearing themselves out trying to keep ailing elderly family members at home. Many in the audience agreed with the comments. Others raised issues about the isolation of young mothers and the lack of recreational facilities. A few raised issues that involved only themselves or a neighbor. Their points were recorded.

By 7:50 p.m. no major issues remained. Susan asked the audience to count off from one to seven and then asked people with the same number to form a group. When they were rearranged into groups, she asked them first to group the issues by location or issue and then to identify issues that stood out more than others. After working together for 30 minutes, the groups were ready to present their findings. All the groups agreed that the issues related to seniors were from people throughout the county. As the groups presented the issues that stood out, Susan circled them on the flip charts: loss of home foot care services, the lack of accessible institutional care, the limited services provided at the resource center, the control of the resource center, and other issues related to seniors such as the cost of medications. Other issues discussed related to mothers with young children and teenagers.

Susan asked if questions about the control of the resource center could be dealt with separately. Hilda, the president of the Farming Women agreed, and said that she would bring up the issue of control at the next board meeting. She invited people to give her their names if they were interested in the outcome.

At that point, a pastor stood up and said that his group had been looking over the issues related to seniors and said that there were too many items. He did not know how to decide which ones should be the priority. A woman from another group stood up and said if the next county could do a survey, they could do one too to find out what was the most important to the seniors. A general murmur of approval rose from the participants. She wanted to know how they would start.

Susan said that the first thing would be to set up a county task force. She brought out the map of the county prepared by the students and asked for nominations for representatives for each area. She quickly had 12 names. Joe Johannson volunteered to have the receptionist at the newspaper office function as the communication center. Other people suggested that volunteers could work with the receptionist to sort through messages and to telephone people. People who wanted to be informed of future meetings were asked to sign up on a list before they left.

Although it was nearly 9 p.m., Susan had one more question to ask. She wanted to know whether the participants felt that the group they were forming would be dealing only with the elderly or would other groups in the county be considered? She asked them to indicate by a show of hands whether the initiative would be for the benefit of the elderly in the county or for all residents of the county? The overwhelming number supported a county effort for all residents. Many stated that they were starting with a survey of the elderly because they had the most need at the moment. They would probably follow that survey with a more *general one. One person suggested that they call themselves the "Northeast County Health Council." Susan concluded the meeting by noting the progress that had been made and the people who had contributed and stated that the next meeting could deal with determining a name and selecting a chairperson.*

After the meeting, Mr. Gerard, a member from the seniors' council, approached the students and asked if they wanted to come to speak to the council the next week. He said that the council met only once a month, and he wanted them to know what was happening. The students were happy to accept the offer because they felt that it would get them started on the survey.

In the car on the way home, they went over what had happened at the community meeting.

"Wow," said Colleen. "Susan was amazing! I can't imagine being able to handle those angry people so easily."

"Yes," added Gabriela. "I guess it's experience. She told me that she had previously worked as a street nurse and had to deal with a lot of angry people, including politicians."

"Now we need to think about our presentation to the seniors council," stated Greta. "It will be great to get started doing something."

"I think we have been doing a lot of good work so far," countered Gabriela. "But I'm ready to start on the survey too."

DISCUSSION QUESTIONS

1. What features of the community meeting encouraged participation?
2. Why were the groups formed by counting off people?
3. Would the participants of the meeting feel that their views would be heard?
4. What preparations for the meeting with the seniors' council did the student team ignore?

Desired outcomes of community capacity building

The desired outcomes in capacity building are that people and groups have gained experience and confidence in working together to improve the community. These skills, knowledge, and abilities mean that more people in the community are capable of bringing about beneficial change by raising issues, bringing people together, training others, and making connections outside the community that are beneficial to the community. The following are the characteristics of desired outcomes:

- Many people in the community benefit from the capacity building, and the benefits are visible (Mattessich & Monsey, 1997).
- Community members receive training in community capacity building skills and can train others (Mattessich & Monsey, 1997; SIL International, 2002; Wolff & Kaye, 1995).
- Relationships are built with local leaders, community organizations, and government that are interdependent rather than dependent or totally independent (Mattessich & Monsey, 1997; SIL International, 1997).

These characteristics result from the relationship process and the completion of tasks that have built on the characteristics of communities and organizers. Community capacity building emphasizes the mutual reinforcement of both physical or economic benefits and the social capital that has accrued during the process.

Projects within community capacity building are only a small part of the action. Although projects would probably contribute to the development of skills, knowledge, and abilities of only a fairly small number of people, this adds to community capacity. If a series of projects with the community consistently address the four components necessary to achieve the desired outcomes, community capacity will steadily increase.

DETERMINING RURAL PRIORITIES SCENARIO (continued)

When the students presented at the seniors' council, they expected to quickly have people involved in providing feedback on their draft survey. They soon found that they were too abrupt. The participants were confused about who the students were and who they were working for. Arlene, a senior who had attended the community meeting, stood up and explained what had occurred at that meeting. She also explained that the nursing students were working with the Public Health nurse to identify health issues in the county. She asked the students if they had copies of the county map they had made. They did and distributed them to those present. They discussed the map and possible different needs of seniors living in different areas. Arlene invited the students to stay to attend the meeting of the services committee to discuss more details about the survey.

After the meeting, the students discussed what had happened.

"I was really floored when you were asked who we worked for," stated Colleen.

"I was too," declared Rosa. "Especially when the second question was asked about filling out the form. I realized that they had no idea what we were talking about or why we were there. Thank goodness Arlene rescued us."

"Yes, we blew it," stated Gabriela. "We were in too much of a rush to get started. We assumed too much."

"Well, they liked the map," stated Greta.

"Yes, they did," confirmed Rosa. "And they liked us. They invited us back to work on the questions. That was a good idea, Gabriela, to ask each person on the service committee what problems were faced by the elderly."

"I remembered what Susan did," stated Gabriela. "I knew that since they were on the seniors' council that they would know what the issues are. When we go back we can show them how those issues compare with the questions on the sample surveys that we have."

In the remaining weeks, the students continued to meet with the service committee of the seniors' council to develop the questionnaire for the survey. The seniors decided that elderly people would not complete anything that took them longer than 15 minutes or was more than 2 pages long. They also decided that it would be easier for them to read if the font size was larger. When a draft was prepared, it was reviewed and approved by the task force. The students' time was running out, but they wanted to conduct a small pilot test with the questionnaire.

The six people on the service committee were feeling reluctant at first about trying out the questionnaire. The students asked them if it would help if they did a role play, and the seniors agreed. The seniors tried using it on each other and could call on the students if they had any questions. They gained confidence from that and suggested that they try it out at an early Christmas bazaar the next week. Two of the students were available for the bazaar and were on call if any questions came up. Soon the seniors were competing with each other to see how many questions they could do. They found that one question was a bit confusing and needed to be changed.

On the students' last day, they and the people from the seniors' service committee gave a presentation to a combined meeting of the seniors' council and the task force. The students talked about how much they had learned in working with people in the community. They realized that if they had not developed the questionnaire with the help of the seniors' service committee, the questionnaire would have been too long and complicated, it would not have asked questions pertinent to the county, and no one would have been comfortable using it.

When the service committee presented the questionnaire, Arlene stated that if the students had not worked with them, their group would not have learned about how to put together a questionnaire or how to *interview someone to complete a questionnaire. Their group was now planning to train others in all areas of the county on how to use the questionnaire. They told Susan that if other nursing students would be coming to continue with the work, the students had to be as knowledgeable, accommodating, and friendly as Rosa, Gabriela, Greta, and Colleen. Susan said that she hoped so, too.*

Susan thanked the nursing students on behalf of the community. She stated that with their assistance the community had learned about doing community-wide assessments, a county map showing statistics, and a questionnaire developed with seniors; the community had also learned how to produce those things themselves. She said that to her, the important thing that the students had demonstrated was that they had become skilled at learning from what they heard, saw, and did.

DISCUSSION QUESTIONS

1. In what ways did the students learn to adjust their approach with the people on the seniors' council?
2. Discuss the work with the service committee of the seniors council in terms of the train the trainer approach.
3. Were the desired outcomes discussed earlier attained in the scenario?

Summary

For successful community capacity building, the characteristics of organizers and the community, the relationship process, completion of tasks, and desired outcomes must be considered. Community health nurses new to community capacity building need to assess their own skills and knowledge and those of the community. Once they have some understanding of both, they need to begin developing relationships with an ever-expanding network of people. As the community health nurse joins groups or brings people together, more community members will form or strengthen relationships among themselves. These relationships and a commitment to bettering the community are the basis of community capacity building.

The characteristics of successful task functions identify the ways that organizers and community members can work together for mutual benefit. In most cases, the organizers are providing some structure and process that can be subsumed and adapted by community leaders.

Community health nurses using community capacity building as a component of their practice often need to defend what they do. Superficially, community development activities may not appear to be directly related to health, although they do relate to the determinants of health. Nursing involvement in these activities is usually initiated because communities have an established relationship with community health nurses and trust that the nurse will work on their behalf. The arguments for nursing involvement in community capacity building relate to expected and desired outcomes. Communities that are involved in capacity building are expected to be improving their health because they know how to use the knowledge, skills, and abilities of their people to benefit everyone.

PRACTICE AND APPLICATION

1. Identify how community capacity building in an urban setting compares with that in a rural area.

2. In the four presentations given by the students in the scenario, identify which ones seemed to be appropriate according to the criteria given in Appendix A.

3. Take one of the following issues and identify how community capacity building would differ from a health education approach:
   a) Teenage pregnancy
   b) Women's or men's health
   c) Parenting practices

4. Describe a community group you are familiar with and explain which circumstances faced by the group could be best dealt with by using community capacity building.

5. Take one of the issues or circumstances described in 4 and identify what actions you would take to address the successful characteristics of an organizer, community, relationship, and task.

REFERENCES

Arnstein, S. (1969). A ladder of citizen participation. *Journal of the American Institute of Planners, 35*, 216–224.

Billings, J. (2000). Community development: A critical review of approaches to evaluation. *Journal of Advanced Nursing, 31*, 472–480.

Bushy, A. (Ed.). (2000). *Orientation to nursing in the rural community*. Thousand Oaks, CA: Sage.

Bushy, A. (2003). Community and public health nursing in rural and urban environments. In M. Stanhope & J. Lancaster (Eds.), *Community and public health nursing* (6th ed., pp. 374–395). St. Louis, MO: Mosby.

Centers for Disease Control and Prevention. (2001). *United States, 2001—Urban and rural chartbook*. Retrieved December 4, 2003, from http://www.cdc.gov/nchs/data/hus/hus01.pdf.

Diem, E. (1996/1997). Empowerment for mothers of early adolescent girls in low SES neighbourhoods. *Dissertation Abstracts International, 58*(1), 134B (UMI No. AAC97-19343).

Dunkin, J. (2000). A framework for rural health nursing interventions. In A. Bushy (Ed.), *Orientation to nursing in the rural community* (pp. 61–69). Thousand Oaks, CA: Sage.

du Plessis, V., Beshiri, R., Bollman, R., & Clemenson, H. (2002). *Definitions of "rural."* Retrieved December 4, 2003, from http://www.statcan.ca/english/research/21-601-MIE/2002061/21-601-MIE2002061.pdf.

Eisen, A. (1994). Survey of neighborhood-based, comprehensive community empowerment initiatives. *Health Education Quarterly, 21*, 235–252.

Freire, P. (1972). *Pedagogy of the oppressed.* New York: Herder and Herder.

Goeppinger, J. & Hammond, R. (2000). The renaissance of primary care: An opportunity for nursing. In J. Hickey, R. Ouimette, & S. Venegoni (Eds.) *Advanced practice nursing: Changing roles and clinical applications* (2nd ed., pp. 175–189). Philadelphia, PA: Lippincott.

Keating, N. (1991). *Aging in rural Canada.* Vancouver, BC: Butterworths Canada.

Knowles, M. (1980). *The modern practice of adult education: From pedagogy to andragogy.* Chicago: Association Press/Follett.

Knowles, M. (1989). *The making of an adult educator: An autobiographical journey.* San Francisco: Jossey-Bass.

KU Work Group. (2000a). *Conducting concerns surveys* (Community Tool Box: Chapter 3, Section 10). Lawrence, KS: University of Kansas. Retrieved May 29, 2002, from http://ctb.lsi.ukans.edu/tools/EN/sub_section_main_1045.htm.

KU Work Group. (2000b). *Making community presentations* (Community Tool Box: Chapter 4, Section 5). Lawrence, KS: University of Kansas. Retrieved July 15, 2000, from http://ctb.lsi.ukans.edu/tools/en/sub_section_main_1029.htm.

Leipert, B. (1999). Women's health and the practice of public health nurses in northern British Columbia. *Public Health Nursing, 16*(4), 280–289.

Leipert, B., & Reutter, L. (1998). Women's health and community health nursing practice in geographically isolated settings: A Canadian perspective. *Health Care for Women International, 19*(6), 575–588.

Lindsey, L., Stajduhar, K., & McGuinness, L. (2000). Examining the process of community development. *Journal of Advanced Nursing, 33*, 828–835.

Mattessich, P., & Monsey, B. (1997). *Community building: What makes it work*. Saint Paul, MN: Amherst H. Wilder Foundation.

Minkler, M. & Wallerstein, N. (1997). Improving health through community organization and community building. In M. Minkler, (Ed.), *Community organizing & community building for health* (pp. 30–52). New Brunswick, NJ: Rutgers University Press.

Mittelmark, M. (1999). Health promotion at the community wide level: Lessons from diverse communities. In N. Bracht (Ed.), *Health promotion at the community level* (2nd ed., pp. 3–27). Thousand Oaks, CA: Sage.

National Association of County and City Health Officials. (2000). *Mobilizing for action through planning and partnerships*. Retrieved May 30, 2003, from http://mapp.naccho.org/MappModel.asp.

Nyswander, D. (1956). Education for health: Some principles and their applications. *Health Education Monographs, 14*, 65–70.

Ontario Prevention Clearing House. (2002). *Capacity building for health promotion: More than bricks or mortar*. Retrieved May 19, 2003, from http://www.opc.on.ca.

Public Health Nursing Section. (2001). *Public health interventions—Applications for Public Health nursing practice*. St. Paul: Minnesota Department of Health.

Rennie, D., Baird-Crooks, K., Remus, G., & Engle, J. (2000). Rural nursing in Canada. In A. Bushy (Ed.), *Orientation to nursing in the rural community* (pp. 217–228). Thousand Oaks, CA: Sage.

Shields, M., & Tremblay, S. (2002). The health of Canada's communities. Supplement to *Health Reports, Statistics Canada, 13*, 1–25.

SIL International (formerly known as the Summer Institute of Linguistics). (1997). *Ten principles*. Retrieved May 19, 2003, from http://www.sil.org/anthro/communitywork.htm#principles.

Stevens, P., & Hall, J. (1992). Applying critical theories to nursing in communities. *Public Health Nursing, 9*, 2–9.

Thompson, B., & Kinne, S. (1999). Social change theory: Application to community health. In N. Bracht (Ed.), *Health promotion at the community level* (2nd ed., pp. 29–46). Thousand Oaks, CA: Sage.

University of Manitoba, Summer Institute on Population Health Promotion. (2002). *Best practices for community organizing and interviewing*. Retrieved May 29, 2003, from http://www.umanitoba.ca/faculties/social_work/summer_institute/index.htm.

Wallerstein, N., & Bernstein, E. (1988). Empowerment education: Freire's ideas adapted to health education. *Health Education Quarterly, 15*, 379–394.

Walter, C. (1997). Community building practice: A conceptual framework. In M. Minkler (Ed.), *Community organizing and community building for health*. New Brunswick, NJ: Rutgers University Press.

Werner, D., & Bower, B. (1982). *Helping health workers learn*. Berkeley, CA: Hesperian Foundation.

Wolff, T., & Kaye, G. (1995). *From the ground up: A workbook on coalition building and community development*. Amherst, MA: AHEC/Community Partners.

Young, T. K. (2003). Review of research on aboriginal populations in Canada: Relevance to their health needs. *British Medical Journal, 327*(7412), 419–422.

WEB SITE RESOURCES

Adult learning principles

The use of "adult learning principles" in a keyword search will provide a variety of examples and applications of adult learning principles.

Community organizing/development/capacity building

Academy for Educational Development: http://www.aed.org. AED is an independent, nonprofit organization committed to solving critical social problems in the United States and throughout the world through education, social marketing, research, training, policy analysis, and innovative program design and management. Major areas of focus include health, education, youth development, and the environment.

Asset-based Community Development Institute: http://www.northwestern.edu/ipr/abcd.html. The ABCD Institute at Northwestern University is built upon three decades of community development reasearch by John Kretzmann and John L. McKnight. The ABCD Institute develops tools to mobilize communities and to help identify and develop community assets. The site also links to research papers and best practice information on community development.

Environmental Youth Alliance: http://www.eya.ca/yaec/for_rsrch_story_01.html. A step-by-step manual for mapping community assets designed for use by youth.

Mobilizing for Action through Planning and Partnerships (MAPP): http://mapp.naccho.org/ MappModel.asp. MAPP is a strategic approach to community health improvement. The MAPP tool was developed by the National Association of County and City Health Officials (NACCHO) in cooperation with the Public Health Practice Program Office, Centers for Disease Control and Prevention (CDC). This site provides tip sheets on various aspects of MAPP, such as a very practical tip sheet "Engaging the Community," which is found under Tools on the home page.

Ontario Prevention Clearinghouse: http://www.opc.on.ca. Definitions and resources on capacity building are available on their Web site by following these links: Our Programs, Health Promotion Resource Centre, Resources, Community Capacity.

Public Health Nursing Section, Minnesota Department of Health: http://www.health.state.mn.us/divs/ chs/phn/interventions.html. Intervention: community organizing.

The Search Institute: http://www.search-institute.org. The Search Institute conducts research and provides resources to promote healthy children, youth, and community development. The institute developed a framework of 40 developmental assets for children and young people that identifies a combination of supports and experiences children and youth need for optimal development.

The W. K. Kellogg Foundation: http://www.wkkf.org. The Foundation Web site provides links to research papers, toolkits, and other resources that can be downloaded on topics such as community development, evaluation, and policy development. The following link is to a study on the ways to engage youth in community service: http://www.wkkf.org/Pubs/CustomPubs/ SusComBasedInits/sustaining-3/Sustaining-three-2.pdf.

Rural associations and rural nursing

Aboriginal Nurses Association of Canada: http://www.anac.on.ca. The Web site of the association provides information and links on health and medical services for Aboriginal people in Canada.

The Association for Australian Rural Nurses Inc.: http://www.aarn.asn.au. The Web site of the association provides extensive information and links on rural and remote nursing in Australia.

Canadian Rural Information Service (CRIS): http://www.rural.gc.ca/cris/about_e.phtml. CRIS is a clearinghouse for information relevant to rural Canada. Their subject areas include rural renewal, community development, funding sources, and opportunities for rural youth. CRIS serves rural residents, community organizations, rural businesses, rural practitioners, and government and educational institutions.

Centre for Applied Rural Innovation: http://cari.unl.edu/ABCD/Community/Guide.pdf. "Building on Assets and Mobilizing for Collective Action: A Community Guide" presents asset-based community development and community mobilization. Includes tools and inventories that can be used to guide these processes.

Health Canada—Nursing in First Nations Communities: http://www.hc-sc.gc.ca/fnihb/ons/nursing/introduction.htm. This Web site describes the opportunities for nursing in Canadian First Nations Communities and provides links to services and programs for First Nations within Canada.

National Rural Health Association: http://www.nrharural.org. This Web site provides information on rural health issues and minority health disparities in the United States.

National Rural Women's Health Conference: http://ruralwomenshealth.psu.edu/index.html. This is an information and learning resource related to improving rural women's health.

Office of Rural Health Policy (ORHP): http://www.ruralhealth.hrsa.gov. This Web site contains programs, research, publications, links, and an information service on rural healthcare.

Rural Information Center (USDA): http://www.nal.usda.gov/ric/. A service offering information and referrals for rural communities, officials, organizations, and citizens.

Rural Nurse Organization: http://www.rno.org/index.htm. This U.S. organization has an online journal of rural nursing and healthcare.

The Rural Nursing Web Site: http://www.usask.ca/nursing/rurnur/. This Web site is maintained by the University of Saskatchewan School of Nursing. It provides a link through "other rural sites" to an ongoing study of "The Nature of Nursing Practice in Rural and Remote Canada."

U.S. Department of Agriculture, Agroeconomic and Related Health Issues: http://www.usda.gov. This U.S. government site provides extensive information and links relevant to farming and rural living.

Train-the-trainer

Numerous sites exist that explain different train-the-trainer approaches, depending on the content area. Many also contain manuals and explain adult learning principles. Add the term "-.com" to eliminate commercial sites.

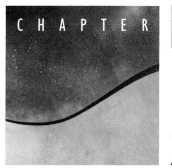

11

Building Coalitions

ALWYN MOYER

SCENARIO **PHYSICAL ACTIVITY IN SCHOOL-AGED CHILDREN AND YOUTH**

Mary completed her undergraduate degree through distance learning two months ago and has just moved to the city to take a position at the health department. She is excited and nervous about the new job, which will be the promotion of physical activity in school-aged children and youth. Mary, a keen skier, has competed in national competitions and throughout college was the assistant director of activities at a summer camp for boys and girls. She believes that her sports background and experience in working with young people helped her to get the job.

Mary is assigned to the school health program. For the first four months, she will be part of the injury prevention team, which spans the life cycle. Mary will work closely with Jean, the team leader. Jean, an experienced public health nurse, has represented the health department on an injury prevention coalition for two years. Jean tells her, "The coalition has been active for about 10 years, but there has been a big turnover in the steering group in the last year. Right now, I'm the longest serving member on the committee, and everyone comes to me with their issues." Jean will oversee Mary's orientation and prepare her to join the school-aged physical activity team, which will be formed over the summer.

Physical activity has been a component of health unit programs for many years, but a change in mandate clearly identifies physical activity promotion across the age span as a key strategy for preventing chronic disease and injury. The health department management team plans to bring together the various programs—walking programs for older adults, fall prevention, prenatal classes, and heart health—to identify the common elements and develop a comprehensive physical activity strategy. The anticipated announcement of new funding initiatives for the primary prevention of chronic disease provides an impetus to move quickly. Lately, coalitions have been a requirement for federal funding proposals. Several community partners, including the school board, have expressed interest in forming a community coalition to increase physical activity in school-aged children and youth. The health unit has a lot of experience with coalitions and is seen as a community leader because of its regional focus. In addition, a recent integration of public health with other city programs offers a chance to work more closely with the community recreation services and city planners.

"I find it difficult to get my head around the size of the programs here," said Mary. "Back in my hometown, one nurse was responsible for the prenatal program and everything to do with schools. This is so complicated." Jean helped Mary put together a workplan for the next few months and advised, "Take it a step at a time." She explained that their working together will give Mary a chance to find her way around the health department and meet future team members while preparing the ground for the school-aged

TABLE 11-1	Jean and Mary's Sample Workplan		
ACTIVITIES	**RESULTS**	**WITH WHOM**	**BY WHEN**
Interview program team leaders about physical activity component.	• Written summary of physical activity across programs • Know key players • Feel confident • Understand the programs	Team leaders: • Injury prevention • School-aged health • Seniors' programs • Prenatal program • Heart health	May 6
Learn about coalitions: Review best practices.	• Review of literature—two or three useful reference articles		May 12
Attend coalition meetings: Talk to experienced practitioners.	• Understand how coalitions work	Jean to arrange	May 17
Review evidence-based literature on benefits of physical activity in school-aged children and intervention strategies.	• Annotated bibliography, key articles, reviews • Slide presentation for community coalition	Health department researchers, epidemiologists, and community nurse specialists	June 30 (start May 17)

physical activity initiatives. "Also, you will be helping me out with the injury prevention coalition. There is no better to way to learn about coalitions than being part of one," said Jean.

Mary thanked Jean for her help in putting together the workplan—this is another skill she needs to practice (Table 11-1). "I have a lot to learn," Mary said. "We all do," said Jean. "Working in the community means lifelong learning. On the physical activity front, you've arrived at a very important time; we've been focusing on injury prevention with children for a long time. Suddenly everyone is ready to act on promoting fitness. At least we have something to build on. When you talk to the program people, get a list of their community partners. This will help to identify the common threads. By the time you finish, you'll know the health department very well and be an expert on fitness promotion with children."

OBJECTIVES   **After reading this chapter and answering the questions throughout the chapter, you should be able to**

1. Discuss the role of coalitions in health promotion initiatives.
2. Identify the skills required to accomplish the developmental tasks of a coalition.
3. Evaluate the effectiveness of a coalition meeting.
4. Share epidemiological data with a coalition to support a needs assessment.
5. Document and communicate the actions of a coalition.

KEYWORDS   **capacity building** ■ **coalition** ■ **consortium** ■ **Precede–Proceed model** ■ **socialization**

Working with a coalition

Practicing community health nursing within a primary healthcare framework requires a broad vision and long-term perspective. The focus of this chapter—working with coalitions—provides insight into the nature and timescale of community-level activities, which are becoming more and more a part of community health nursing practice (Chambers et al., 1994; Schoenfeld & MacDonald, 2002). Today's practitioners are engaged in forming **coalitions** (alliances among diverse individuals or groups to achieve a common goal), supporting the work of coalitions, and evaluating the health impact of coalitions. Given the broad scope of these undertakings, the practitioner does not work alone, but as part of a program team with management guidance and support. Nevertheless, the community health practitioner will often be the human face of the organization seen by the community. So, how do nurses acquire the knowledge and skills for this type of practice?

Bearing in mind that the life of a coalition is measured in years, not weeks, nurses may not gain experience in this aspect of community work as part of their nursing education. Typically, students spend days in a clinical setting, albeit over a three- to four-month period, and the practicum may not coincide with observable coalition activities. To complicate matters even further, coalition work extends outside the boundaries of an agency and often involves delicate negotiation between agencies and organizations—this is not a role for the novice. This chapter provides an opportunity for students and nurses to gain an understanding of aspects of working with coalitions in their formative stage.

The collaborative assessment process is adapted to the timescale and realities of working with coalitions. Forming a coalition is somewhat similar to building a team, but on a larger scale. The process of bringing together groups and agencies is more complex than bringing together individuals, and it moves more slowly. Monitoring and evaluating this foundational work is an important aspect of coalition building, as is preparing for the next stages of coalition activity, which are the community needs assessment, planning, implementation, and evaluation. Overall, the process, shown in Table 11-2 follows the community health nursing process.

Characteristics of community coalitions

A community coalition is a formal alliance among diverse organizations, agencies, and interest groups, working together to achieve a common goal (Centers for Disease Control and Prevention [CDC], 1998). Individuals also can be involved, but the coming together of organized groups is the central feature of a coalition. Typically, the relationship is goal driven, and the partnership extends over a long time. Previously, ad hoc liaisons focused on short-term interests were described as coalitions, but durability is now considered an essential characteristic (Butterfoss, Goodman, & Wandersman, 1993). The term *consortium* is sometimes used interchangeably with coalition; however, Kreuter and Lezin (1998) pointed out that a **consortium** tends to involve similar groups, such as universities or small businesses, whereas a coalition aims to engage diverse partners. Another important feature of a coalition is that members are expected to advocate on behalf of the coalition and not

TABLE 11-2	Adaptation of Collaborative Assessment Process with Groups or Communities for Building Coalitions
STEPS OF PROCESS	**ADAPTATION FOR WORKING WITH COALITIONS**
1. Establish relationships within project and community.	Review mandate, policy, and procedures of host agency and particular program(s). Determine policy and procedures of coalition or if coalition is not yet established, those that would apply.
2. Assess secondary data.	Review literature, epidemiology, and socio-demographics related to health and social concerns to be addressed by the coalition. Determine which sectors are relevant to the identified health and social concerns and explore their actual/potential involvement.
3. Initiate assessment of community.	Gain experience in coalition work: attend a coalition meeting, interview coalition members, and observe coalition activities. Identify the assessment goal in relation to the stage of coalition building (e.g., during coalition formation, assess group/agency readiness to participate) and select the information gathering approach.
4. Conduct specific assessment.	Use selected approach(es) with stakeholders: program providers, partners, service recipients, and community members. Initiate or adapt participant evaluation of meetings.
5. Determine action statements.	Determine action to move coalition to next stage. Provide report in format that is useful to agency.
6. Evaluate team work.	Monitor formation stage of coalition building using structure and process indicators.

just represent the interests of their own organization (Butterfoss et al., 1993). This is quite different from the usual practice of organizations, which tend to concentrate deliberately on their own mandate and goals. The ability of members to act in a unified way is crucial to the success of a coalition. Two examples of the scope of coalition activities are provided in Box 11-1.

Community coalitions and health promotion

A coalition is a mechanism for bringing together the diverse resources of the community for mutual advantage and to achieve synergy. Groups and organizations from different backgrounds have different ways of looking at issues and can bring a wide range of knowledge, skills, and abilities to the table. By sharing resources, the groups can achieve more together than each could do alone.

As you will recall from Chapter 3, such collaboration is consistent with the principles of primary healthcare, which recognize that the determinants of health and disease are embedded within the social, cultural, political, and economic fabric of a society (Hawe, 1994) and cannot be addressed by the health sector alone. If you think about the issues that challenge communities today—families with young children are among the fastest growing group of homeless, food banks are becoming a fixture in many cities, high rates of injury

---

BOX 11-1 **Coalition activities**

Here are two examples of the scope of coalition activities:

University and Community Partner

A university–community partnership came together to enhance the capacity of youth and families in an inner-city neighborhood by engaging them in the design and delivery of a program to promote positive youth development and/or prevent the development of problem behaviors (Ostrom, Lerner, & Freel, 1995).

Collaboration of Agency, Government, Community, and Special Populations

The Boston Healthy Start Program aimed to reduce infant mortality by 50% over five years and to improve maternal and infant health and well-being using a community-based, family-centered, and culturally competent approach. A lead agency received federal funding. As a funding requirement, the lead agency had to organize community members, providers, and groups from the affected population. This group would provide local participation, oversight, and advice for projects (Plough & Olafson, 1994).

---

among adolescents are associated with widespread substance use, and the high prevalence of chronic illness seen in an aging population—clearly they are health-related, but they are also related to the social and economic environment. To have an impact on these pervasive and complex issues, it is necessary to address the underlying conditions, which is beyond the capabilities of any one sector or organization (Butterfoss et al., 1993). Rather, the solution depends on community-wide approaches with multiple health promotion strategies that target the determinants of health at different levels of the system: individuals and families, community, and social policy. This means bringing together different sectors of the community: schools, businesses, and political groups, for example, as well as health agencies.

A second and equally important goal of a coalition is to build the capacity of a community (Hawe, Noort, King, & Jordens, 1997) so that it functions effectively and can adapt to change in a positive way; in other words, so that it is a healthy community. Drawing on earlier work by Cottrell (1976) and McKnight (1987), Robertson and Minkler (1994) defined **capacity building** as "the nurturing of and building upon the strengths, resources, and problem-solving abilities already present in individuals and communities" (p. 303). The notion of community capacity is somewhat intangible and not well understood in a theoretical way, although people have no difficulty understanding it intuitively. The sense is captured in the expression: "It takes a village to raise a child" (Wandersman et al., 1996). It is thought that coalitions have the potential to build the capacity of the community by strengthening social networks and providing an opportunity for community leadership to flourish and a forum for community problem solving. Coalitions provide a more formal structure than was described in the previous chapter, but have similar goals. When the actions of the coalition are successful and a common goal is achieved, the sense of community is likely to increase. This increased ability to solve community problems can then be applied to other issues and other situations (Moyer, Coristine, MacLean, & Meyer, 1999).

Formation and development of coalitions

Community coalitions have many possible starting points, but two approaches predominate. The first is professional-led, for which coalitions are formed in a deliberate way as a first step toward community-wide intervention to address a defined health issue. The second is volunteer or grass-roots-led, for which community interest groups come together to address an issue or concern (Butterfoss et al., 1993). As you might expect, there can also be a mix of the two approaches, and coalitions may evolve and change over time.

In recent years, professionally led coalitions have been part of the funding requirements of many large-scale health promotion initiatives that seek to reduce the mortality and morbidity from chronic disease, foster community involvement in health planning, and build community capacity (Butterfoss et al., 1993; Minkler, 1997; Mittelmark, 1996). Typically, these initiatives aim to change community norms, based on the growing understanding that the social environment greatly influences behavior. Ecological models of health (Green, Richard, & Potvin, 1996; Stokols, 1996) and social change theory (Thompson & Kinne, 1999), for example, provide theoretical frameworks for designing multiple interventions. The points of intervention are clearly delineated (with whom and where) and are underpinned with an understanding of the causal mechanisms. Consistent with a population health approach, the community-wide interventions are based on the belief that the conditions that affect health are ubiquitous and that small but pervasive changes in many people will produce significant health gains at a low cost. In addition to the low-intensity interventions targeted at the population as a whole, community-wide interventions may include more intensive interventions tailored to subpopulations at high risk (Green & Kreuter, 1999).

When coalitions emerge from the grass roots, their exact starting point may be easier to pinpoint in retrospect. For example, a particular issue might be the catalyst that brings everyone to a crucial meeting, where the decision to work together is agreed upon. Or, the process may occur gradually as, over time, community groups have occasion to work with each other and partnerships develop, and their focus broadens to incorporate different issues and perspectives.

Grass roots coalitions may be fostered deliberately by public or community health agencies with the intention of building community capacity. For example, Moyer and colleagues (1999) discuss how a project to reduce isolation in community-living older adults led to partnerships with community groups providing programs and services to older adults and eventually with community groups interested in developing friendly neighborhoods for persons of all ages. The capacity-building model derived from this project describes how professionals marry the responsibility for fulfilling organizational mandates for health promotion and disease prevention with capacity building. Key features of the model are the staged and recursive process of engaging community groups in problem solving, the partnership between professionals and diverse sectors of the community, and the empowering agenda (Moyer et al., 1999). One word of caution though: McKnight (1997) warned health professionals of the danger of extending the health system into the realm of community and supplanting the complex web of associations and informal links that underpins community life.

It is important to note at this point that although coalitions have established a loyal following and are integral to current community health practice, evidence of their success in achieving health status change has not been demonstrated convincingly (Kreuter & Lezin, 1998). As Green and Kreuter (1999) commented, the literature provides many examples of effective innovations to address specific issues, but little evidence from which to derive rules and procedures.

Building successful coalitions

Several factors have been identified as basic to the success of a coalition. Before reaching an agreement to collaborate, groups and organizations must recognize the existence of a common problem, acknowledge that they have a role in solving the problem but cannot do it alone, and see that they have enough in common with potential partners to work together toward a solution.

Negotiating the equal distribution of power and benefits to achieve a sense of "win-win" is a continuing challenge. Unless coalition members are convinced that their organization has a voice in decision making and that the benefits accruing to the organization are worth the cost of participation, they may decline to participate (CDC, 1998). The costs are mainly measured in time, effort, and money, but also can include lost opportunities. The agencies and/or their individual representatives will probably weigh these costs differently. Similarly, the benefits, described in Table 11-3 may be seen as more or less important by particular participants and agencies. Ensuring that each member is sufficiently satisfied with the arrangements to stay with the coalition is an ongoing responsibility of the coalition leaders.

Developmental tasks of a coalition

Whether formed from the bottom up or from the top down, all community coalitions have to achieve a set of developmental tasks to function effectively. These tasks include making fundamental decisions about how the coalition will be organized; recruiting, retaining, and socializing new members; and developing and carrying out a plan of action (Butterfoss et al., 1993; McLeroy, Kegler, Steckler, Burdine, & Wisotzky, 1994).

There may also be a longer-term task—institutionalization—whereby the work of the coalition is subsumed in ongoing activities of the community so that the coalition is no longer required (Wandersman et al., 1996). Little is written about this stage in the life of a coalition, however, and it is not addressed here. Before discussing the developmental tasks, it is worth noting that much advance preparation is required before the coalition emerges.

Advance preparation for coalition building

Usually, one agency or organization, working alone or through a steering group, will take the lead in bringing together a coalition. A vision has to be articulated to start the discussion and possibly a mission and goals are drafted. The early involvement of more than one agency or group is valuable because it gives broader input and starts the collaborative effort. There is consensus that coalitions with a formal structure and clearly

TABLE 11-3	*How Coalitions Benefit Organizations*
CHARACTERISTIC OF COALITION	**BENEFIT**
Shared responsibility	Organization can become involved in new and broader issues without having the sole responsibility for managing or developing those issues.
Leverage, political strength	Unified approaches demonstrate and develop widespread public support for issues, actions, or unmet needs.
Synergy	Maximizes the power of individuals and groups through joint action.
Extended reach	Multiplies services and minimizes duplication of effort and services.
Access to information and resources	Can help mobilize more talents, resources, and approaches to influence an issue than any single organization could achieve alone.
Networking opportunities	Increases potential for recruitment from diverse constituencies, such as political, business, human service, social, and religious groups, as well as less-organized grass roots groups and individuals.
Skill enhancement (CDC, 2003)	Coalition provides opportunity for individuals and organizations to develop skills.
Recognition	Coalition activities are carried out in a public forum so abilities can be recognized in the broader community.
Satisfaction	Individuals and organizations gain a sense of pride in making a contribution and helping to solve community problems.

defined policies and procedures are more likely to succeed than ad hoc arrangements. With the formal organization of the coalition will come the collaborative development of the vision, mission, goals, and action plan. The coalition also will need to decide on a governance structure, agree on rules to guide decision making, and secure the financial and human resources needed to get the work done. An explanation of the different types of structure that have been put in place to guide decision making and oversee the work of the coalition can be found in the Community Tool Box (KU Work Group, 2003a).

Strong leadership is vital to the success of a coalition. Recruiting an influential leader is one of the tasks of the lead agency or steering group. The person should command respect across the community and be able to draw into the coalition other formal and informal leaders from different parts of the community (Butterfoss et al., 1993). Examples from the literature include directors of community organizations, religious leaders, local politicians, and middle managers who can bridge the gap between employees and management (CDC, 1998; Wandersman et al., 1996). Many factors need to be taken into consideration. In addition to being acceptable to different constituencies, the leader should have energy, administrative experience, and interpersonal skills. It takes a skilled communicator to conduct public meetings, lead discussions, solve problems, and resolve conflicts. Also, as the coalition spokesperson, the leader should be able to convey clearly where the coalition is going, both to coalition members and the broader community, and possibly, through the media. Finding such a person is an exacting task, and sometimes the responsibilities are shared or a rotating leadership may be successful.

Much has been written about the advantages and disadvantages of employing paid staff to run the coalition. To some extent the use of paid staff depends on the availability of funding. On the one hand, employees are able to dedicate time to the affairs of the coalition and ensure that the activities are carried out as planned. On the other hand, the presence of paid staff may diminish the need for a high level of engagement by coalition members. In the long term, this can have a negative impact on the sustainability of the coalition activities when the project funding runs out.

The lead agency has a pivotal role in creating the conditions for success and must walk a fine line between leading and collaborating. Official community health agencies, particularly official public health organizations, often perform this role because of their mandate and regional focus. However, they have been criticized for taking too directive an approach (Parker, Margolis, Eng, & Henríquez-Roldán, 2003). Assuming the role of lead agency is not to be undertaken lightly. Mittelmark (1996) argued that an organization should take stock of its capacity before taking on the task and recognize that coalition building requires a long-term commitment and sufficient resources if it is to succeed.

Parker and colleagues (2003) designed a survey to assess the capacity of an agency and individual practitioners to work in partnership with communities. Four broad areas emerged as relevant:

- Agency's skill in working with community groups and minority populations
- Agency workers' skill in working with community groups and minority populations
- Extent and frequency of community networking
- Community participation in health department planning.

In Canada, evidence exists from other sources that public and community health are building the required capacity. Health practitioners have shifted from working solely with individuals to working with groups and communities—and at the policy level (Edwards, Murphy, Moyer, & Wright, 1995)—and there has been a commensurate increase in community health nurses' use of a broader range of health promotion strategies, such as coalition building (Chambers et al., 1994; Schoenfeld & MacDonald, 2002).

DISCUSSION QUESTIONS

1. Find an article describing a coalition. Identify the health or social issue addressed by the coalition and determine whether capacity building is an intended outcome. In a small group, compare findings and discuss the evidence supporting your decision.
2. You are the nurse member of a steering group to build a coalition to improve services for developmentally disabled adults. List the types of agencies, groups, and organizations you would try to recruit.
3. In thinking about your community, what characteristics would you look for in the leader of a coalition to improve services for developmentally disabled adults? Identify three potential sources for such a leader. Discuss whether your criteria would change if the focus were health promotion in a rural community instead of in an urban community.

PHYSICAL ACTIVITY IN SCHOOL-AGED CHILDREN AND YOUTH SCENARIO (continued)

Mary met with staff from programs involved in the injury prevention coalition. Those active in adult injury prevention provided information on their community partners and identified areas where the partners were also involved in physical activity related to school-aged children. They also supplied contact information. Mary put the information in a table (Table 11-4), summarizing the partnerships with each agency.

Mary was delighted with the quality of the information provided by staff in the injury prevention program. They identified many community contacts and offered ideas regarding physical activity and youth. She also met two future colleagues—nurses who would be transferring to the physical activity group once the school programs had ended for the year.

While conducting the interviews, Mary was able to form an opinion about the level of interest in cross-departmental collaboration and possible participation in the community-wide coalition. Through the discussions, she learned that staff were proud of their own initiatives and did not want to lose control over the way their programs were offered. Several mentioned that they feared they would have less time for existing activities. Another cause for concern was that some physical activity programs were being used to draw people into other community-building activities. Staff did not want this useful function to be displaced by a larger agenda.

Reflecting on the list, Mary and Jean recognized that some partners were probably sending different representatives to meetings with different programs. For example, a community health center might send one representative to a diabetes prevention walking program meeting, another to a seniors' fall prevention meeting, and yet another to a meeting on bicycle safety.

Thinking about the next step of bringing all the organizations to a common table, Jean determined that consolidation of resources of the community partners and the health department could be a selling point. The program manager suggested that Mary reorganize the tables to show the number and types of links with each agency or organization. This would allow them to flag the strongest partners and identify potential representatives on the coalition. Jean commented, "It's very important to have this information before you start talking to outside agencies. You feel a little foolish when you discover that your colleagues are partnering with an organization and you know nothing about it. It does not give a good impression; it makes us look disorganized, and I worry that it might also reduce my credibility." Initially taken aback, Mary then realized the importance of Jean's personal and political insights.

Jean and Mary agreed to meet later that week to identify partners. At the same time, they set a meeting date with the program manager to discuss their approach with the various groups and agencies. Jean thought the program manager would probably want to make the first contact with the senior managers of some of the larger organizations and a few groups whose relationships with the health department had not been running smoothly. Mary said she was pleased she had been able to practice her interview techniques within her own organization before meeting external partners. Jean explained, "With the injury prevention coalition, we scripted the main points of the interview and rehearsed the delivery before we started. Everyone found this useful and the interviews went smoothly." Because Jean knew the community and many of the partners, she planned to take the lead initially. Once Mary had observed one or two interviews, she would then conduct the uncomplicated interviews on her own.

The spring meeting of the Heart Health coalition provided Mary with an opportunity to gain first-hand experience of how the coalition functioned. She read the terms of reference for the committee and was introduced to the chairperson ahead of the meeting. Afterward, she asked Jean why the group was so concerned about the nonattendance of one member. Jean explained that with all the recent changes, attendance had fallen off. This particular agency had been sending a different person to each meeting and had not honored its commitment to support fundraising activities. "All the health providers have had extra responsibilities with the recent outbreak of SARS (severe acute respiratory syndrome), and local business is still suffering from the reduction in tourism after September 11th. This puts more pressure on everyone else," said Jean. "Groups and organizations have started to complain about the additional work." A

TABLE 11-4 | **Summary of Departmental Adult Injury Prevention Initiatives and Potential for Partnerships**

COMMUNITY PARTNER	INITIATIVES	POTENTIAL FOR INVOLVEMENT IN SCHOOL-AGED PHYSICAL ACTIVITY COALITION	CONTACT INFORMATION
Heart Health Coalition Heart and Stroke Foundation Diabetes Association	West End mall walking program Walk Away from Diabetes program	Walking programs may be interested in expanding to include youth.	Alex Logie, coalition chair, board member Diabetes Association, and a local politician 222-8881
YMCA/YWCA	YMCA/YWCA conduct training sessions with mall walkers	Offer many youth programs.	Janet Bryzinscki, Director of Youth Programs 222-8882
Community health centers	Sunnyside CHC and the Aboriginal Health Center are involved in Walk Away from Diabetes	Sunnyside offers bicycle safety programs; Aboriginal HC runs a youth group.	Kim Lee, Program Manager 222-8883
Family physicians network	Regular articles on injury prevention in quarterly newsletter distributed to all physicians in area	Fall prevention program distributes notepads with prescription of physical activity for older adults; could do same with school-aged group.	
City Recreation Department	Involved in Walk Away from Diabetes	Offers many youth programs in recreation centers.	Jim Brown 222-8884
Shopping mall management	Provide office space in six malls		Glenna Sandre 222-8885
Individual businesses	Support walking programs (e.g., offer discounts for coffee) Donate prizes	Car dealer sponsors after-hours youth center in West End.	
Community police, West End		Helps to run the after-hours youth center.	Sergeant Ravi Singh 222-8886

telephone call to the agency after the meeting helped to clarify the problem. It appeared that because of the lack of continuity, the agency had not been informed of its commitment. The manager was apologetic and promised to deal with the problem, saying their organization valued the work of the coalition and wanted to continue to play their part.

Recruiting, retaining, and socializing new members

The initial recruitment of coalition members may be done by the lead agency on the basis of previous collaboration and by identifying obvious partners. In addition to involving the agencies and organizations across the health sector, it is important to draw in business, education, social, and religious groups, as well as less organized grass roots groups and individuals (McLeroy et al., 1994). Particular effort should be taken to include minority groups who can make a contribution. The simplest approach is to generate a list of potential participants and, through informal discussion, determine whether the various parties are interested and have the resources to participate. This process can be time consuming, and it may require more than one contact to gain agency participation.

Community health nurses, with management support, are well qualified to assist with the formation of a coalition. Through their work, they interact daily with community members and have access to hard-to-reach groups so they understand community diversity. In addition, they are likely to have connections with a wide range of community agencies and organizations, together with well-established links with practitioners from other disciplines. This brings an intimate understanding of the community including its culture and traditions, existing and emerging health issues, and the state of existing programs, services, and resources. Furthermore, community nurses are well regarded in the community and have skills in information gathering and organizing. All of these qualities can be put to good use in talking to groups and organizations and assessing readiness to collaborate. It is worth noting, however, that early discussions may need to be conducted at the management level because of the need to commit organizational or group resources.

The challenge of bringing together diverse groups reinforces the need to understand the community context—the sociopolitical and socioeconomic conditions, community health status, and community infrastructure. The aim is to be inclusive, but this may be difficult to achieve. In a study of 15 partnerships, Wandersman and colleagues (1996) found that greater ethnic and racial diversity in a community increases the difficulty of attaining a stable coalition. They attributed this to high levels of distrust and competition between groups, as well as linguistic barriers. Social class differences can also be divisive, as can age differences and political and religious orientations. Making sure that the coalition is truly representative of the community is an ongoing task.

It is useful to identify potential stumbling blocks during the advance preparation and strategize about how to avoid them if at all possible. It is probably better to anticipate some opposition or dissenting opinions from the outset and try to achieve a compromise early on rather than setting the stage for later confrontation. For example, a coalition advocating for antismoking policies in public places is likely to be strongly opposed by restaurant and bar owners. Failing to include potential dissenters in a coalition can set back progress by many months and cause significant community ill-feeling before differences are resolved. With early involvement in the coalition, potential stumbling blocks can be anticipated and addressed along with more general issues.

Retention of new members

Having successfully recruited members, the coalition now needs to maintain support. Good interpersonal relationships are fundamental to success. Typically, coalition members will bring a range of opinions on priorities and processes, and areas of disagreement can be anticipated from time to time, both on a personal level and at an agency level. These will not necessarily threaten the partnership, as long as there are more areas of agreement than areas of disagreement, but they will require continuing attention and, sometimes, delicate negotiation.

The following principles identified by Kaye (1997), are recommended as a guide:

- *Recognition:* People want to be recognized for their contributions.
- *Respect:* People want their values, culture, ideas, and time to be respected and considered in the organization's activities.
- *Role:* People want a clearly defined role in the coalition that makes them feel valuable and in which they can make a contribution.
- *Relationships:* People want the opportunity to establish and build networks both professionally and personally for greater influence and support.
- *Reward:* People expect the rewards of participating in a collaborative partnership to outweigh the costs and to benefit from the relationships established.
- *Results:* People respond to visible results that are clearly linked to outcomes that are important to them and that they can clearly link to their participation in the coalition.

Socialization of new members

Socialization is an ongoing task for coalitions. Agencies and organizations are likely to be involved with a coalition over several years, but the representative can change as people leave or take on new roles and responsibilities. In addition, the coalition may determine it lacks certain skills or abilities and seek to recruit new members. To maintain a sense of common purpose, it is important for the coalition to plan the **socialization** of new members; that is, how they will be helped to fit into existing relationships and patterns of working and make a contribution. In addition to formally acknowledging new members and introducing them to others, orientation might include the provision of background material on the work of the coalition and a meeting to discuss roles and issues. There are likely to be many sources of written information; for example, the work of the coalition is usually captured in the minutes of meetings. Other sources of information are operational documents such as terms of reference, mission statements, goals, logic model workplans, funding proposals, and reports. Attention to the socialization of new members will help to ensure the necessary ongoing commitment and enthusiasm required to sustain coalition activities.

Being able to work with and support coalitions is a key role for community health workers. The skills required to do this are essentially the same as those outlined in Chapter 2 on teamwork. The major difference is that the skills are being applied in larger and more diverse multidisciplinary teams and that the team members come from many different workplaces.

Timelines

Bringing groups together and agreeing on how to work together takes considerable time and effort. Kreuter and Lezin (1998) report that experts in the field agree that realistic expectations for the first year of a coalition are as follows:

- Get organized.
- Establish a clear vision and mission—a common purpose.
- Clarify mode of operations.
- Formalize process and procedures, and, as necessary, establish subcommittees to address agreed-on objectives.
- Establish trust.
- Develop an unambiguous plan of action.
- Ascertain the group skills required to effectively manage the coalition.

DISCUSSION QUESTIONS

1. You have been active in your community scout/guide group for several years and have been proposed as your organization's representative on a physical activity coalition. Identify three advantages for you and three for your organization in taking on this challenge.
2. As chair of a rural coalition on injury prevention of 20 health providers and community members, you have a loaded agenda with several important budget items to discuss. A representative from the Young Farmers Association has just joined the coalition and is attending her first meeting, as is a family physician. Your co-chair suggests that you leave the introductions until next time. Discuss your options.
3. Identify three strategies a coalition chairperson might use to encourage regular attendance.

PHYSICAL ACTIVITY IN SCHOOL-AGED CHILDREN AND YOUTH SCENARIO (continued)

The injury prevention coalition has agreed to sponsor a special meeting to bring together community groups with an interest in increasing physical activity in school-aged children and youth. For some time the coalition has wanted to address the needs of this population better and feels the meeting could be of mutual benefit. The possibility of extending the scope of the injury prevention coalition has been proposed but will be debated at a later date.

Mary has been invited to present statistics on a local survey of physical activity in children and youth at the special meeting. A professor doing research in exercise physiology will provide an overview of the evidence of the benefits of exercise for children, and a school principal will talk about physical activity in the school curriculum. Presenters have been asked to keep their presentations to 10 minutes. The purpose of the presentations is to educate members and help them to explore the issues and determine common interests.

Mary feels a little intimidated, but the assignment is timely because it fits with one of the tasks on her workplan. Also, she has found on more than one occasion that her knowledge and expertise in physical activity is being tested in subtle ways. She has had many questions about the type and amount of physical activity children need as part of a healthy lifestyle. Reviewing the literature will help to reacquaint her with the latest work and reassure her that she has mastery of the subject matter. It will also help her to be a resource in preparing a draft action plan for the expected request for proposals from the federal government.

Preparing for the special meeting, Jean said, "Coalition meeting dates are set in September for the whole year and listed at the end of each set of minutes. Normally the agenda is distributed one week ahead of the meeting, but for a special meeting such as this we have to give more lead time." Jean commented that some agency representatives have only limited authority to speak for their organization. "We try to make sure that participants know ahead of time when important decisions will be made. It allows the representative to seek guidance ahead of time or to arrange for a more senior member of staff to participate."

"Another thing we learned from experience," Jean continued, "is that our process has to be transparent. We used to meet ahead of time to try to move the meetings along more quickly, but this was seen as being too controlling. Now we allow time for full discussion of issues and make sure the members have an opportunity to express their point of view and vote on the issues. We have also started to evaluate each meeting using a brief checklist—people don't have to give their name (Application 11-1). This gives everyone a chance to express their opinions and say what they want to say about the meeting, right there. It also helps prevent the concerns from being aired outside the meeting, which gives the coalition a bad name in the community. It's working well."

Developing and implementing a plan of action

Determining the mission and goals is a crucial step in the life of a coalition. Even with sufficient common interest to bring the coalition together, partners may have widely different priorities. The goal should be broad enough for everyone and yet sufficiently specific to guide planning. For example, the goal of the Harlem Hospital Injury Prevention Program (HHIPP) was to reduce childhood injury and death rates in central Harlem (baseline rate before the intervention was 1,141/100,000, compared to the U.S. rate of 656/100,000) (Kreuter & Lezin, 1998).

The next step is to undertake a planning process designed to bring about community change. Coalitions are a key element of planning models for centrally initiated, community-based health promotion (Mittelmark, 1996). Bracht, Kingsbury, and Rissel (1999) described a five-stage planning model that has been used successfully. The five stages are 1) community analysis, 2) design initiation, 3) implementation, 4) maintenance and consolidation, and 5) dissemination and assessment. These stages are similar to the steps of the community health nursing process. Because this chapter is focusing on the formation of coalitions, only community analysis and design initiation are discussed in the following section.

Community analysis and design initiation

Numerous authors have testified to the importance of starting where the community is (Labonte & Robertson, 1996; Minkler, 1990; Nyswander, 1956) and merging community concerns with public health issues. The community analysis requires a mapping of community strengths and resources in relation to the issue at hand and puts together what is known about the health issue. Gathering this information serves to raise awareness and focus the issue. (Readers may want to refer to Chapter 3.)

The **Precede–Proceed Model of Health Promotion** (Green & Kreuter, 1999) is widely used to guide issue identification and the design of interventions. The model uses a step-by-step investigative process to develop an understanding of the issue in stages (Figure 11-1). The investigator works back from the needs or quality of life concerns identified by the community to uncover the underlying health issues and their determinants. Drawing on theories and epidemiological studies, the multiple lifestyle, environmental, and causal mechanisms that contribute are identified. Each factor is then examined in terms of its

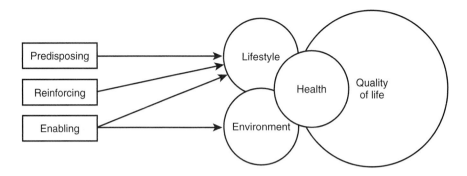

FIGURE 11-1. The Precede-Proceed Model of Health Promotion (Green & Kreuter, 2004. Reproduced with permission of The McGraw-Hill Companies. A complete diagram of the Health Program Planning and Evaluation Model can be found at http://www.lgreen.net/precede.htm).

TABLE 11-5	*Health Issues and Determinants*
CONTRIBUTING MECHANISMS	**ANTECEDENTS**
Predisposing factors	Knowledge, attitudes, values, beliefs, and perceptions that facilitate or hinder motivation for change
Reinforcing factors	Rewards and different types of feedback, either positive or negative, that encourage or discourage the desired behavior, once it has been adopted
Enabling factors	Barriers or facilitators of behavior change created by social forces (e.g., limited access to healthcare facilities; inadequate resources, income, or health insurance; and restrictive laws, regulations, policies) (Green & Kreuter, 1999)

predisposing, enabling, and reinforcing antecedents (Precede: Predisposing, Reinforcing and Enabling Constructs in Ecosystem Diagnosis and Evaluation). These antecedents, defined in Table 11-5, become the focus of intervention. Once the analysis is complete, evidence-based strategies are identified to act on the modifiable conditions and bring about positive changes in lifestyle and the environment (Proceed: Policy, Regulating or Resourcing, and Organizing for Educational and Environmental Development and Evaluation).

The following section illustrates the steps of the precede–proceed analytic process described earlier. The example identifies the predisposing, enabling, and reinforcing factors that affect physical activity in school-aged children and youth. For a more in-depth understanding of the process, please review the text by Green and Kreuter (1999).

Quality of life issues

People in your community tell you they value good health and fitness. Parents want their children to play with friends, take part in sports, and grow up strong and happy. They feel that if children are involved in local activities as they grow up, they will be less likely to get involved in vandalism and petty crimes. Physical activity is seen as being essential to learning and health, and there is an expectation that healthy students will become fit and healthy adults.

Recent social planning documents from your community show that although the size of the child population has been stable for several years, there continues to be a need for services for children. Social trends, such as the rising numbers of single parent families resulting from an increase in divorce rates and the breakup of partnerships, low minimum wages, an increasing number of working poor with children, and the lack of stability in the labor market, all contribute to increases in the number of children in need of services.

Health issues

There is compelling evidence that physical activity is an important determinant of the health and quality of life of children and that the effects extend into adulthood. Two guidelines on recommended levels of activity for children are provided in Table 11-6.

Obesity is a growing problem among young children, and population health approaches are required to increase activity levels in school-aged children to control weight, reduce blood pressure, raise levels of high-density lipoprotein (HDL) ("good") cholesterol, and reduce the risk of diabetes and some kinds of cancer. Physically active children and adults show improved psychological well-being, including gaining more self-confidence and higher self-esteem (American Heart Association, 2003). Because the majority of children

TABLE 11-6	*Physical Activity Guidelines*	
	CANADA'S PHYSICAL ACTIVITY GUIDE FOR HEALTHY ACTIVE LIVING (HEALTH CANADA, 2002)	**PHYSICAL ACTIVITY GUIDELINES (AMERICAN HEART ASSOCIATION, 2003)**
Age of child	6–9	5 and older
Types of activities recommended	90 minutes of physical activity daily—increase activity each month until the child has reached the target. Promote activities to build endurance, flexibility, and strength.	At least 30 minutes of enjoyable, moderate-intensity activities every day. Children should also perform at least 30 minutes of vigorous physical activities at least 3–4 days each week to achieve and maintain a good level of cardiorespiratory (heart and lung) fitness.
Contextual factors	Activity can take place at school, at play, inside or outside the home, and on the way to school and might involve family and friends. Physical activity should be fun.	If your child or children do not have a full 30-minute activity break each day, try to provide at least two 15-minute periods or three 10-minute periods in which they can engage in vigorous activities appropriate to their age, gender, and stage of physical and emotional development.

and youth can be reached at school and spend a lot of their day at school, the school provides a channel for reaching children and youth.

Lifestyle and environmental factors and their antecedents

A national survey examined the physical activity of Canadian children and youth aged 5 to 19 years from their parents' perspective (Canadian Fitness and Lifestyle Research Institute [CFLRI], 2002). The report described children's physical activity patterns, preferences for physical activities, the physical activity opportunities available to them through daycare programs and the school system (including physical education and other opportunities), the kind of activities children do after school, the use and availability of facilities in the local community for children's physical activity, safety concerns, and the influence of income-related factors on their participation in physical activity. An important study finding was that the levels of physical activity in schools varied considerably by region and by age of the child.

National data from the United States confirm that physical activity declines dramatically over the course of adolescence, and girls are significantly less likely than boys to participate regularly in vigorous physical activity (U.S. Department of Health and Human Services, 2002). Comparative data are not available for Canada, but the CFLRI (2002) study found that more than one third of young people in grades 9 through 12 do not regularly engage in vigorous physical activity. Furthermore, 43% of students in grades 9 through 12 watch television more than two hours per day.

One factor that makes it difficult to interpret the available research is that physical activity is defined in different ways by different studies. Having a standard accepted definition would aid interpretation. In the CFLRI (2002) study, the term *active enough* is defined as the equivalent of an energy expenditure of at least 8 kilocalories per kilogram of body weight per day (KKD). Based on this definition, a half-hour of martial arts plus walking for a total of at least one hour throughout the day would be sufficient activity for a child.

Clearly, the CFLRI (2002) study provided detailed information on a health issue that is important to the community and to health providers—physical activity in schoolchildren. In addition to generating information that can be used to design change, the data yield a baseline measure, which can serve as a benchmark for measuring change once interventions are implemented to increase the level of activity in schoolchildren.

Predisposing, reinforcing, and enabling factors

Systematic reviews identify several factors that determine lifestyle choices and environmental support for physical activity in young people. These factors suggest points of intervention that might be considered when lifelong physical activity is being promoted:

Predisposing factors:
- Enjoying different forms of physical activity and developing the skills to participate
- Understanding the relationship between physical activity and health
- Valuing physical activity

Reinforcing factors:
- Parental support for participation in physical activity

- Parental role models and involvement of parents and guardians in physical activity instruction and programs for young people
- Promotion of lifelong physical activity by health providers

Enabling factors:
- Policies that promote enjoyable, lifelong physical activity
- Physical and social environments that encourage and enable physical activity
- Physical education curricula and instruction in schools
- Health education curricula and instruction in schools
- Extracurricular physical activity programs that meet the needs and interests of students
- Personnel training
- Health services for children and adolescents
- Developmentally appropriate community sports and recreation programs that are attractive to young people
- Regular evaluation of physical activity instruction, programs, and facilities (CDC, 1997)

The preceding information is summarized in Figure 11-2, based on Green and Kreuter's (1999) Precede–Proceed model.

Developing and carrying out a plan of action is a complex undertaking that benefits from broad involvement. Although communities and public health may appear to focus on different issues or look at issues from different angles, they have many common concerns. The community understands health from lived experience and brings a vision of a community as a place to live well and raise families. Public and community health workers understand the science of causal mechanisms, modifiable risk and protective factors, and the theoretical and research evidence for potential interventions. They know about health promotion. The two perspectives do not need to be at odds with each other. McKnight (1997) suggested that professionals can best contribute to community capacity building by respecting the wisdom of the community and working in partnership rather than trying to exert control, by providing access to information and resources, and by using professional skills to strengthen the power of community associations (McKnight, 1997). At the same time, community health workers should feel justly confident of their role in bringing professional knowledge and skills to the table, but they must listen to communities and, most important, act on the information that they hear instead of disregarding it (Kreuter, Lezin, Kreuter, & Green, 1998).

DISCUSSION QUESTIONS

1. How might parents engaged in shift work be helped to participate in child activities at home and school?
2. Parents are constantly telling you they want their children to be able to take advantage of the summer weather to play outdoors. You read the following statements in the newspaper.

A dermatologist says: "Everyone is responsible for their own health, and one of our key mandates is to encourage people to adopt a healthy lifestyle by wearing adequate

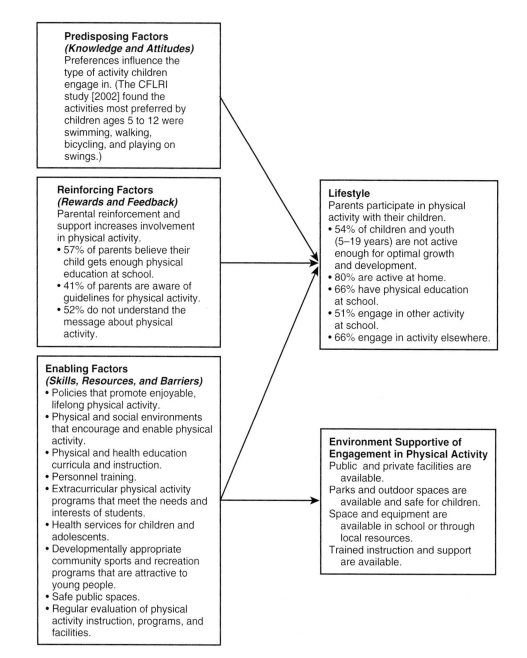

FIGURE 11-2. Example of predisposing, reinforcing, and enabling factors that precede lifestyle choices and environmental support for physical activity programs for children and youth.

sunscreen, protective clothing, or finding a shady spot that safeguards them from the sun while allowing them to enjoy the outdoors."

How could you build these ideas into an action plan to increase physical activity in school children?

Evaluating the formation of coalitions

One of the main reasons given to support coalitions is that they bring together the diverse resources required to change the health of populations. Yet, after reviewing the literature, Kreuter and Lezin (1998) concluded that few coalitions can claim to have done this successfully. They identify three reasons: 1) most coalitions find the task is just too difficult and complex; 2) achieving health status change through collaborative efforts is an unrealistic outcome, no matter how well the coalition performs; and 3) even if a change in health status was achieved it would be difficult to detect and attribute to the efforts of a particular coalition because of the technical difficulties posed by evaluation. On the other hand, Kreuter and Lezin observed that despite the lack of evidence, other perceived benefits, such as community capacity building, may be sufficient incentive for the funding to continue.

Given the difficulty in proving that coalitions have an impact on health, it becomes even more important to demonstrate that a coalition operates effectively and thereby contributes to community capacity. Francisco, Paine, and Fawcett (1993) set out a framework for evaluating the work of coalitions at all stages of their development from formation through collaborative assessment, planning, and implementation. They reasoned that a coalition must successfully complete the early stages of development before it can hope to effect more remote changes in health status. The framework identifies indicators that can be used to monitor the formation of coalitions, described earlier in this chapter. Many evaluation tools are now available to monitor coalitions and other collaborative efforts (Brown, 1997; Goodman, Wandersman, Chinman, Imm, & Morrissey, 1996; KU Work Group, 2003b; National Association of County and City Health Officials, 2000).

Some examples of evaluation questions that might be asked in relation to the developmental tasks of a coalition, discussed earlier, and the type of data required to answer the questions are provided in Box 11-2. The questions address how the coalition is structured; its policies and procedures for recruiting, retaining, and socializing members; and its achievements. (For a more comprehensive checklist, see Brown, 1997.)

PHYSICAL ACTIVITY IN SCHOOL-AGED CHILDREN AND YOUTH SCENARIO (continued)

Over the last month, Mary has completed the literature review and has collaborated with the national sports and recreation association survey team to develop the presentation on physical activity in school-aged children and youth. Thanks to the foresight of the health department, who contributed additional funds to

BOX 11-2	**Selected questions for evaluating coalitions**

The questions below may be asked about the developmental tasks of a coalition. The information needed to answer the questions appears below too.

Does the Coalition Have Appropriate Membership and Committed Members?

■ Document the number and type of coalition members.
■ List members by the community sectors they represent; determine whether the key sectors are represented.
■ Ascertain what percentage of committee members attend meetings regularly; that is, are present for at least 50% of committee meetings.

Does the Coalition Have Adequate Resources? Is There Evidence That the Community Is Willing to Invest in the Partnership?

■ Document the resources obtained through the partnership.
■ Money or in kind donations (e.g., space, computers) are equally significant.
■ Determine the number and type of trained volunteers who have been recruited, trained, and are donating time to assist with implementation of the coalition plan.

Are Members Satisfied with the Coalition?

■ Is meeting time used effectively? (Appendix A provides an example of a questionnaire that can be used to evaluate the effectiveness of coalition meetings.)
■ Do you feel that, on the whole, members have an equal voice within the coalition? Please explain.
■ How satisfied are you with the way decisions are made in the coalition? How is leadership exercised? Does one person, or a small group, make decisions for the coalition? (Usually, Sometimes, Rarely)

Does the Coalition Conform to the Standards of Good Partnership?

■ Ask coalition members for their perceptions of whether there is shared commitment of resources, shared decision making, efficient use of time, and a high level of productivity.
■ Do all coalition members make an equal contribution to the partnership?
■ Are the program and policy initiatives undertaken cooperatively?
■ Has the coalition produced valued outcomes?
■ Do the benefits of the partnership outweigh the costs?

Is There Tangible Evidence of Coalition Planning?

■ Terms of reference developed
■ Mission and goals identified
■ Plan of action drawn up
■ Logic model developed
■ Subcommittees formed
■ Funding proposal developed

the survey team to increase the size of the sample in the region, they are able to draw on local data. The four months have flown by, but Mary now feels confident in her understanding of the issues related to the promotion of physical activity in children and youth and has increased her understanding of coalition building. She can see the pieces starting to come together. The school-aged physical activity team members have been named—she knows two of them quite well—and the team will start planning soon. Also, there will be opportunity to participate in research because a professor doing research in exercise physiology has requested a joint appointment with the health department and plans to develop a research agenda for physical activity in school-aged children. The best news is that Jean will be the team leader. Mary has enjoyed working with her over the past months and looks forward to continuing the relationship. Jean is equally happy with the arrangement and has already started to think about how they can improve the process of building a coalition.

When Jean asks her to put together a package of information for discussion at the first team meeting, Mary knows exactly what she will include. She suggests to Jean that they use the meeting effectiveness questionnaire to evaluate their process (Application 11-1). "Yes," agreed Jean. "Let's set the standard and encourage open communication."

Summary

Coalitions are an important mechanism for creating the conditions for health in a community. However, they require a lot of effort to set up and maintain. Given the reservations expressed by Kreuter and Lezin (1998), it is important to choose the issues carefully with the full cooperation of the community, to agree to specific and attainable goals, and to design multilevel interventions based on evidence. Without a strong conviction that the issue is of importance to the community and health providers and that the potential results are worthwhile, it will be hard to justify the effort. A coalition must complete key developmental tasks to be effective. Monitoring and evaluating the coalition will help to ensure success.

PRACTICE AND APPLICATION

1. Your health center is the lead agency of a coalition with new funding to prevent alcohol, tobacco, and other drug abuse in urban youth. List four or five points that you would address when seeking to engage the following community groups in the coalition:
   a) A sports club run by the community police
   b) The local business group, which includes restaurant and bar owners
   Role play the interview with a partner.

2. Identify two community groups attended mainly by women—one health related, one not health related. Obtain a copy of their terms of reference or attend a meeting. Identify how you might engage this organization in a community coalition on women's health.

3. Attend a community coalition meeting. Evaluate the effectiveness of the meeting using the tools described in this chapter.

REFERENCES

American Heart Association. (2003). *Exercise (physical activity) and children.* Retrieved May 19, 2003, from http://www.americanheart.org/presenter.jhtml?identifier=4596.

Bracht, N., Kingsbury, L., & Rissel, C. (1999). A five-stage community organization model for health promotion: Empowerment and partnership strategies. In N. Bracht (Ed.), *Health promotion at the community level: New advances.* (2nd. ed., pp. 83–104). Thousand Oaks, CA: Sage.

Brown, C. R. (1997). Appendix 3: Coalition checklist. In M. Minkler (Ed.), *Community organizing and community building for health.* (pp. 359–365). New Brunswick, NJ: Rutgers University Press.

Butterfoss, F. D., Goodman, R. M., & Wandersman, A. (1993). Community coalitions for prevention and health promotion. *Health Education Research, 8*(3), 315–330.

Canadian Fitness and Lifestyle Research Institute (CFLRI). (2002). *Results of the 2001 physical activity monitor.* Retrieved May 19, 2003, from http://www.cflri.ca/cflri/pa/surveys/2001survey/2001survey.html#kids.

Centers for Disease Control and Prevention (CDC). (1997). Guidelines for school and community programs to promote lifelong physical activity among young people. *Morbidity and Mortality Weekly Report (MMWR), 46*(No. RR-6), 1–36.

Centers for Disease Control and Prevention (CDC). (1998). *Principles of community engagement. Part 1—Community engagement: Definitions and organizing concepts from the literature.* Retrieved May 11, 2003, from http://www.cdc.gov/phppo/pce/part1.htm.

Chambers, L. W., Underwood, J., Halbert, T., Woodward, C. A., Heale, J., & Isaacs, S. (1994). 1992 Ontario survey of public health nurses: Perceptions of roles and activities. *Canadian Journal of Public Health, 85*(3), 175–179.

Cottrell, L. S. (1976). The competent community. In B. H. Kaplan, R. N. Wilson, & A. H. Leighton (Eds.), *Further explorations in social psychiatry* (pp. 195–209). New York: Basic Books.

Edwards, N., Murphy, M., Moyer, A., & Wright, A. (1995). *Building and sustaining collective health action: A framework for community health practitioners* (No. DP95-1). Ottawa, ON: Community Health Research Unit.

Francisco, V. T., Paine, A. L., & Fawcett, S. B. (1993). A methodology for monitoring and evaluating community health coalitions. *Health Education Research, 8*(3), 403–416.

Goodman, R. M., Wandersman, A., Chinman, M., Imm, P., & Morrissey, E. (1996). An ecological assessment of community-based interventions for prevention and health promotion: Approaches to measuring community coalitions. *American Journal of Community Psychology, 24*(1), 33–61.

Green, L. W., & Kreuter, M. W. (1999). *Health promotion planning: An educational and ecological approach* (3rd ed.). Mountain View, CA: Mayfield.

Green, L. W., & Kreuter, M. W. (2004). *The Precede-Proceed Model of health program planning & evaluation.* Retrieved June 9, 2004 from http://www.lgreen.net/precede.htm.

Green, L. W., Richard, L., & Potvin, L. (1996). Ecological foundations of health promotion. *American Journal of Health Promotion, 10*(4), 270–281.

Hawe, P. (1994). Capturing the meaning of "community" in community intervention evaluation. *Health Promotion International, 9*(3), 199–210.

Hawe, P., Noort, M., King, L., & Jordens, C. (1997). Multiplying health gains: The critical role of capacity-building within health promotion programs. *Health Policy, 39*, 29–42.

Health Canada. (2002). *Canada's physical activity guide for children.* Ottawa, ON: Minister of Public Works and Government Services Canada.

Kaye, G. (1997). Appendix 6: The six "R's" of participation. In M. Minkler (Ed.), *Community organizing and community building for health* (pp. 372–373). New Brunswick, NJ: Rutgers University Press.

Kreuter, M., & Lezin, N. (1998). *Are consortia/collaboratives effective in changing health status and health systems? A critical review of the literature.* Atlanta, GA: Health 2000 Inc.

Kreuter, M. W., Lezin, N. A., Kreuter, M. W., & Green, L. W. (1998). *Community health promotion ideas that work: A field-book for practitioners.* Sudbury, MA: Jones and Bartlett.

KU Work Group on Health Promotion and Community Development. (2003a). *Organizational structure: An overview* (Community Tool Box: Part 1, Chapter 9, Section 1). Retrieved June 10, 2004 from http://ctb.ku.edu/tools/en/sub_section_main_1092.htm.

KU Work Group on Health Promotion and Community Development. (2003b). *Coalition building I: Starting a coalition.* (Community Tool Box: Part B, Chapter 5, Section 5). Retrieved May 17, 2003, from http://ctb.ukans.edu/tools/en/sub_section_main_1057.htm.

Labonte, R., & Robertson, A. (1996). Delivering the goods, showing our stuff: The case for a constructivist paradigm for health promotion research and practice. *Health Education Quarterly, 23*(4), 431–447.

McKnight, J. L. (1987). Regenerating community. *Social Policy, Winter*, 54–58.

McKnight, J. L. (1997). Two tools for well-being: Health systems and communities. In M. Minkler (Ed.), *Community organizing and community building for health* (pp. 20–29). New Brunswick, NJ: Rutgers University Press.

McLeroy, K. R., Kegler, M., Steckler, A., Burdine, J. M., & Wisotzky, M. (1994). Community coalitions for health promotion: Summary and further reflections. *Health Education Research, 9*(1), 1–11.

Minkler, M. (1990). Improving health through community organization. In K. Glanz, F. M. Lewis, & B. K. Rimer (Eds.), *Health behavior and health education: Theory, research and practice*. San Francisco: Jossey-Bass.

Minkler, M. (1997). *Community organizing and community building for health*. New Brunswick, NJ: Rutgers University Press.

Mittelmark, M. B. (1996). *Centrally initiated health promotion: Getting on the agenda of a community and transforming a project to local ownership*. Retrieved June 17, 2004, from http://elecpress.monash.edu.au/IJHP/1996/6.

Moyer, A., Coristine, M., MacLean, L., & Meyer, M. (1999). A model for building collective capacity in community-based programs: The elderly in need project. *Public Health Nursing, 16*(3), 205–214.

National Association of County and Health Officials. (2000). *Organize for success and partnership development*. Retrieved June 10, 2003, from http://mapp.naccho.org/ofsapd/index.asp.

Nyswander, D. (1956). Education for health: Some principles and their applications. *Health Education Monographs, 14*, 65–70.

Ostrom, C. W., Lerner, R. M., & Freel, M. A. (1995). Building the capacity of youth and families through university-community collaborations: The development-in-context evaluation (DICE) model. *Journal of Adolescent Research, 10*(4), 427–448.

Parker, E., Margolis, L. H., Eng, E., & Henríquez-Roldán, C. (2003). Assessing the capacity of health departments to engage in community-based participatory public health. *American Journal of Public Health, 93*(3), 472–476.

Plough, A., & Olafson, F. (1994). Implementing the Boston healthy start initiative: A case study of community empowerment and public health. *Health Education Quarterly, 21*(2), 221–234.

Robertson, A., & Minkler, M. (1994). New health promotion movement: A critical examination. *Health Education Quarterly, 21*(3), 295–312.

Schoenfeld, B. M., & MacDonald, M. B. (2002). Saskatchewan public health nursing survey: Perceptions of roles and activities. *Canadian Journal of Public Health, 93*(6), 452–456.

Stokols, D. (1996). Translating social ecological theory into guidelines for community health promotion. *American Journal of Health Promotion, 10*(4), 282–298.

Thompson, B., & Kinne, S. (1999). Social change theory: Application to community health. In N. Bracht (Ed.), *Health promotion at the community level: New advances* (2nd ed., pp. 29–46). Thousand Oaks, CA: Sage.

U.S. Department of Health and Human Services. (June 20, 2002). *Physical activity fundamental to preventing disease*. Retrieved May 20, 2003, from http://aspe.hhs.gov/health/reports/physicalactivity/.

Wandersman, A., Valois, R., Ochs, L., de la Cruz, D. S., Adkins, E., & Goodman, R. M. (1996). Toward a social ecology of community coalitions. *American Journal of Health Promotion, 10*(4), 299–307.

WEB SITE RESOURCES

Many of the Web sites provided in Chapter 10 also apply to this chapter.

Keyword search: For specific coalitions precede the word "coalition" with issues or populations such as "tobacco," "poverty," "multicultural," or "youth" and you will find numerous examples of coalitions.

EVALUATION OF COALITION MEETING

Date: _____

Please circle the number that best represents your view regarding the process and content of the coalition meeting.

PROCESS	DISAGREE				AGREE
1. The objectives of the meeting were clear to me.	1	2	3	4	5
2. The atmosphere created by the chairperson was conducive to exploring ideas and sharing experiences.	1	2	3	4	5
3. I was provided with opportunity to share my views and participate fully during the meeting.	1	2	3	4	5
4. The number of participants was conducive to exploring and sharing ideas.	1	2	3	4	5
5. The length of time allotted for discussion was appropriate.	1	2	3	4	5
6. The decisions were made by the group as a whole, not just by a few people.	1	2	3	4	5
7. I was able to participate in decision making.	1	2	3	4	5
8. Group members worked well with each other and were not antagonistic.	1	2	3	4	5
9. The group made good use of its time and accomplished its objectives.	1	2	3	4	5
10. The meeting was well organized and ran smoothly.	1	2	3	4	5
11. Was there conflict present at this meeting?	No_____		Yes_____ (please describe)		

PROCESS	DISAGREE	AGREE
12. If there was conflict present, was it resolved?	No_____	Yes_____
13. If the conflict was not resolved, please check why:		

_____ Conflict avoided, not discussed.

_____ Members argued with one another.

_____ Other (specify)_____

CONTENT	1	2	3	4	5
14. The discussion centered on issues that were relevant to the purpose of the meeting.					
15. The discussion centered on issues that were relevant to the coalition.					
16. The discussion centered on issues that were related to health and healthcare.					
17. The ideas were specific and relevant to the purpose of the coalition.					
18. The ideas were specific and relevant to my area of knowledge and skill.					

What could have been done to make the meeting more effective?
_____

Please add any additional comments about the meeting you would like to make:

_____
_____
_____
_____

Thank you for participating and completing this evaluation.

12

Population Health and Policy Change: Managing Multiple Projects

ALWYN MOYER

FOUR BREASTFEEDING PROJECTS

Lillian is sending an email with the draft breastfeeding policies to the Health Department Policy and Procedures Committee when Janet pops her head around the door. Both are public health nurses in the Health Department: Lillian works in the Healthy Children's Team and Janet is with the Workplace Health program. That program links with large and small businesses in the region to foster healthy workplaces and promote the health and well-being of employees. Janet is seeking advice.

The Workplace Health program is meeting with two large employers in the area—an Information Technology (IT) firm and the new airport authority—to discuss ways of increasing support for women in the workplace. Both firms are concerned about absenteeism and retention of employees. The IT firm has always seen itself as a leader in promoting employee health and is a member of the Healthy Heart coalition. More than half of its employees are women with the majority in the child-bearing and child-rearing years. The IT firm laid off staff last year because of a downturn in the economy but is optimistic for the future and sees early signs of recovery. If this continues, the firm will begin rehiring in the coming months. The airport has just completed an expansion and is hiring new staff. In addition to improving conditions for employees, it wants to improve services for travelers with small children.

Both firms employ occupational health nurses, recreation staff, and counselors. Under discussion is the possibility of providing emergency daycare, with a room for breastfeeding. Janet brought with her an article describing such a program offered by a large bank and asks Lillian if she knows anything about it, or if she has other ideas. As an aside, Janet explains she is supervising two community health nursing students for the next 12 weeks and sees this as an opportunity for a student project.

Lillian is excited at the thought of increasing support for breastfeeding in the community. She is a member of the coalition that is seeking baby-friendly status for the city. This is associated with a World Health Organization (WHO) initiative to create support for mothers and children. Support for breastfeeding is an important element of the initiative.

Janet's idea also fits well with the Healthy Children program goals—to increase to 50% the percentage of infants breastfed up to six months by the year 2010. The Health Department, Healthy Children's team, has a mandate to advocate for and assist in developing policies to support breastfeeding in the workplace, restaurants, shopping malls, and other public places. The team also works with health professionals to enhance their knowledge and skills related to breastfeeding.

After Janet leaves, Lillian thinks to herself, "This is an opportunity that can't be missed, but my plate is full already. When I joined the program as a public health nurse last year after graduation, I was spending nearly two days with the well baby clinics. Now that we have a new community nurse, maybe I can taper off. This would give me the time I need for my breastfeeding projects. I will miss the mothers and babies, but I would like to learn more about policy change. Thank goodness I have Jake as my supervisor. He has a lot of experience with policy development related to tobacco and alcohol use and has many contacts in the business community. When I talk to him on Friday about my workplan for the next six months, I will propose that I drop the well baby clinics for the next three months and take on this new project. I really want to increase my skills in policy development now that I see what is possible. Maybe I can negotiate some time with him. I will prepare another draft of my workplan (Table 12-1) to see if this new project will fit."

OBJECTIVES **After reading this chapter and answering the questions throughout the chapter, you should be able to**

1. Discuss policy as a health promotion strategy in community health nursing practice.
2. Identify the nursing role in creating healthy public policy.
3. Discuss the policy change process.
4. Describe how the community health nursing process is used to assess readiness for change.
5. Conduct a force field analysis and document the results.
6. Identify ways to increase community involvement in policy initiatives.
7. Coordinate work in more than one interdisciplinary team.

KEYWORDS **force field analysis ▪ health policy ▪ healthy public policy ▪ policy**

Nurses and policy

Policy is a course or principle of action. It is exemplified in the formal and informal rules and understandings that are adopted on a collective basis to guide individual and collective behavior (Schmid, Pratt, & Howze, 1995). All of these various rules and guidelines can have a profound influence on daily life; however, this chapter is concerned mainly with formal, written policies, communicated in position papers, standards, guidelines, and policy statements, which have an impact on health.

National, provincial, and local (regional) policies provide a framework for community health practice. In common with other health providers, community health nurses must understand the legislation, regulations, and policies that govern their professional practice and client relationships. They also need to be familiar with the health policies that guide the selection and delivery of community health programs and services (Ontario Public Health Association [OPHA], 1996).

Advocates for change

Of equal, or perhaps more significance, community health nurses have a social and professional mandate to speak out for health in its broadest sense. Not only are they well placed to observe the impact of policy decisions on health, community health nurses have opportunities to raise policy issues in many different arenas through their work with diverse client groups, disciplines, community organizations and businesses. Community nurses' long history of concern with issues of equity and access (Canadian Nurses Association, 2000; Kang 1995) shows they take this responsibility seriously. As policy change becomes an increasingly important part of community health practice (Chambers

TABLE 12-1	*Lillian's Draft Workplan*

CHILDREN'S HEALTH
Lillian Smith   Draft WORKPLAN 2005–6
Revision date: 21 July 2005

ACTIVITIES	TIMELINES (RESPONSIBILITY)	RESULTS AND COMMENTS
1. Revision of departmental breastfeeding policy guidelines in line with Baby-Friendly Initiative (BFI)		
a. Revise policies.	Aug. 20, 2005 (work group)	Work group met three times and completed the revisions.
b. Submit revised policy to Policies and Procedures Committee for approval.	Sept. 23 (LS)	Revised policy submitted
c. Develop training resources.	Dec. 16 (work group)	
d. Provide training session for all staff.	Jan.–Feb. 2006 (work group)	
2. Baby Friendly Coalition project for baby-friendly status for city	September 2005, ongoing	—Attend monthly meetings. —Coalition formed. —Consultant hired to conduct an environmental scan to determine where each member organization is at with regard to meeting BFI requirements.
a. Assist consultant with environmental scan of department.	Oct. 30 (LS)	
b. Chair coalition work group and prepare presentation on model breastfeeding policies.	Nov. 21 (LS, work group)	
3. Preparation of Health Committee proposal seeking funds to maintain breastfeeding support in Leeland, a rural community with limited resources	Oct. 23, 2005	
a. Prepare first draft of report and provide input to final draft	Sept. 12 (LS) Oct. 23 (Jake, LS)	First draft prepared.
4. Workplace Health (WH) Proposal for breastfeeding resources in two workplaces		
a. Assist WH team to prepare breastfeeding component of the proposal, including breastfeeding policies.	December 2005	
b. Collaborate with WH to recruit businesses to the BFI coalition.	March 2006	

et al., 1994; Schoenfeld & MacDonald, 2002), community health nurses will need to continue to hone their skills in this area.

Nursing process in policy change

The community health nursing process can be used to assess need and plan for policy change, as was discussed in Chapter 6. Usually, nurses will undertake this work as part of a multidisciplinary team or coalition that brings together community members and different sectors of the community. The collaborative assessment process is appropriate for policy projects, and Table 11-1 from Chapter 11 can be modified slightly to fit the timescale and stage of policy development. Some examples of how community health nurses become involved in policy change are shown in Table 12-2.

Policy as a health promotion strategy

Policy is one of several approaches used to promote environments in which the "healthy choices are the easy choices" (Milio, 1989). Related interventions include education and awareness and environmental support. Traditional education and awareness activities are rooted in the belief that failure to make healthy choices results from lack of information (Wallack, 1998). Education, tailored to particular target groups, is designed to fill the knowledge gap and lead to health seeking behavior. Prenatal classes are examples of education activities with the aim of preparing families for healthy pregnancy, childbirth, and parenting. Similarly, social marketing aims to decrease the information gap by changing attitudes and social norms. Social marketing campaigns try to increase public awareness of health risks and build support for policy change strategies (Public Health Nursing Section, 2001). As the name suggests, environmental support entails providing resources that will enable healthy behavior. For example, public parks with climbing frames, trails, bicycle paths, and outdoor skating rinks enable year-round, physical activity for all age groups (Stokols, 1996).

As illustrated in the policy formation model (OPHA, 1996), policy, education and awareness, and environmental support are linked and are nonhierarchical strategies (Figure 12-1). In any given situation, one may be more appropriate than another. The choice of one, or any combination of the three, should be based on which is most likely to meet the health goals.

How policies affect health

Significant health gains were made in the last century in developed countries through the introduction of legislation to provide food subsidies, safe drinking water, and better sanitation (McKeown, 1979). These policy measures, enacted through programs and services and legislative, regulatory, or organizational mechanisms, were a key factor in reducing the occurrence of infectious diseases and improving community health (Schmid et al., 1995). Attention is now turning to policy as a means of influencing healthy personal lifestyle choices—for example, related to tobacco and seat belt use—that are implicated in

| TABLE 12-2 | The Community Health Nursing Role in Policy Change | |

COMMUNITY HEALTH ISSUE	NURSING ACTION
Women living in a seniors' apartment building take part in an exercise group held in a common room where other residents smoke. One member leads the group, with support from the community health nurse and the city recreation department. The women complain that the benefits of exercise are outweighed by their exposure to second-hand smoke. The room is exempt from city smoking by-laws, and the group wants this changed.	The nurse offers to provide information on the health impact of second-hand smoke.
Several recent incidents of threats and physical assault have left nurses providing care in the home feeling vulnerable. Often little information about new clients is available.	The nurses feel their agency could do more to protect them and ask for a review of organizational policies related to home visiting safety.
Women attending prenatal classes receive tokens for milk but cannot afford to buy winter clothing or equipment such as baby strollers.	The multidisciplinary team organizes a clothing exchange, and the manager develops a partnership with a citywide coalition on poverty that is advocating for increased maternal health benefits.
A community group running a drop-in center for young men living and working downtown, offers bar workers a Smart Serve training program in support of municipal alcohol policies. The training course provides information and techniques on how to prevent alcohol-related incidents but lacks information on what to do when incidents occur.	Public health nurses indirectly support the alcohol policy by working with the community group to help them develop training on how to intervene when alcohol-related incidents do occur.
Following up on a missed appointment for TB monitoring, the PHN finds the family huddled in coats and blankets trying to keep warm. It is –20° C (–5° F) outside. In contravention of the law, the landlord turns down the heat in the apartment during the day.	The nurse advises the family on housing policies and helps the parents file a report with housing authorities.
Community health nurses collaborated with the local school board to provide resources and workshops on increasing classroom physical activity. Their efforts are appreciated, but they realize that not all students will benefit because physical activity is not emphasized in the school curriculum.	The nurses develop a resolution directing their nursing association to lobby the government to introduce system-wide regulations on regular physical activity in schools.

the development of chronic disease and occurrence of accidents and injuries (Brownson, Newschaffer, & Ali-Abarghoui, 1997; Minkler, 1999; Schmid et al., 1995; Stokols, 1996).

This shift in thinking is based on a growing recognition that personal life choices are strongly influenced by the socioeconomic environment. Reviewing the evidence, Minkler (1999) showed that individual behavior change strategies work well under some circumstances, but their impact is limited when there is no policy reinforcement. Others support Minkler's argument for a balanced approach of individual and environmental interventions that complement and reinforce each other (Brownson et al., 1997; Flynn, 2000).

Policies support community health by changing the range of choices people can make (OPHA, 1996). They do this in different ways. Some policies reduce exposure to health

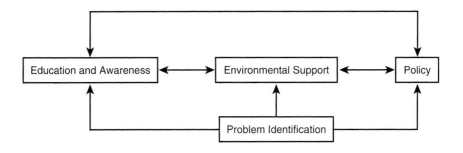

FIGURE 12-1. Policy formation model (OPHA, 1996). Adapted with permission from Ontario Public Health Association. (1996). Making a difference in your community: A guide for policy change (2nd Ed., p.10). Toronto: Ontario Public Health Association.

hazards by severely restricting opportunities to engage in unhealthy behavior, such as tobacco use or by requiring people to follow proven, safe practices, such as using seat belts. With these so-called passive strategies, individuals do not have to take the initiative. The monitoring and enforcement of such legislation is an important issue, which must be addressed.

Policies also play a part in creating environments that support certain behaviors and discourage others, as with by-laws that specify the use of green space in housing developments or restrict smoking in public places to reduce exposure to secondhand tobacco smoke.

On a broader scale, policies can increase control over the resources for health by guaranteeing minimum wages, welfare support, and entitlement to essential health care (The Health Communication Unit [THCU], 2000).

Healthy public policy refers to the broader role of policy in promoting health, in contrast to **health policy**, which has as its goal an efficient and effective healthcare system (or, as some would say, illness care system). Healthy public policy advocates that all government sectors—labor and business, justice, transportation, agriculture, and education—should formulate policy with a view to its potential health impact. Flynn (2000) identifies three types of healthy public policy categorized by which determinants are addressed. The first category addresses the traditional health concerns of health promotion, disease prevention, and the provision of health services; the second category is concerned with social, educational and cultural policy; and the third category is concerned with the broader economic and environmental policies, including industrial development, transportation, and housing, that determine health. Governments and organizations can initiate these policies. Government legislation and regulatory practices have a wider reach than organizational policies, which only apply within the organization. See Table 12-3 for examples of healthy public policy for each category as applied to governments and organizations.

An advantage of healthy public policy over some other strategies is that policies are likely to have a broader reach than individual behavior change strategies, and, unlike community capacity building, can be directed to specific and tangible ends. Furthermore, policy is likely to have a long-lasting effect on the community, mainly because, once implemented, it is difficult to change, in contrast to community programs and services, which can be withdrawn. On the other hand, the evidence to support policy intervention is often lacking. Even in well-researched policy areas such as youth smoking, there has been limited

TABLE 12-3	*Categories of Healthy Public Policy and Examples*	
CATEGORY OF HEALTHY PUBLIC POLICY	**POLICY FOCUS**	
	LEGISLATIVE/REGULATORY	**ORGANIZATIONAL**
Health services	Promotion of safe food handling practices in restaurant and public gatherings	Workplace health and safety policies
Social, educational, and cultural policies	Liquor License Act	Workplace or school policy on use of alcohol on the premises
Economic and environmental policies	Maternity leave to provide women with time to develop a relationship with their infants	Policies governing extended leave allowances without penalty

evaluation of the effectiveness of policy in changing behavior (Multicultural Advocates for Social Change on Tobacco, 2004), and there are few well-controlled studies designed to assess the effects of interventions on health inequalities (Macintyre, Chalmers, Horton, & Smith, 2001). Also, there is some apprehension within the health promotion field that policy interventions, such as the promotion of self-care, are viewed by government as a means of conserving health dollars through the withdrawal of costly individual services (Minkler, 1999).

On a cautionary note, Labonte (1997) points out that it is difficult for communities to introduce meaningful policy change because most economic and social policy is national and transnational in nature. This is an advantage when one is addressing the broad determinants of health—trying to make an impact on issues such as poverty at the level of community can be overwhelming. However, it leaves communities vulnerable to shifts in national priorities and cuts in health care spending, unable to protect community programs or secure funding for local policy initiatives.

DISCUSSION QUESTIONS

1. From your experience, identify two or three informal organizational policies that potentially have an impact on health.
2. Identify policy changes in your community that might lead to an increase in breastfeeding. Explain how you might support these changes, both as an individual and through your professional organization.
3. Discuss how food-labeling policies promote health.
4. Discuss the following statement: "Once a strategy for health and measurable health goals have been struck, then healthy public policies and the health system become tactics for the achievement of that strategy" (Hancock, 2001; Rachlis, 1989).

FOUR BREASTFEEDING PROJECTS SCENARIO (continued)

Three months later, Lillian's working group is scheduled to report back to the baby-friendly city coalition on breastfeeding policies. The coalition has representatives from all the major hospitals and the various community agencies, public and private, who provide breastfeeding support across the region. A sales representative, employed by a company selling baby formula attends the bimonthly meetings and there has been discussion about involving other businesses and other sectors of the community.

Since the last coalition meeting, the working group gathered breastfeeding policies from all the member agencies and compared them with the WHO's Baby-Friendly Initiative (BFI) standards. This had proven to be a much more onerous task than they anticipated. It had taken several weeks and many phone calls to collect the policies, despite assurances they would be dispatched within one week of the previous meeting. Then summer holidays reduced the time available for meetings, leaving them with only two weeks to complete the analysis. Lillian and her copresenter Mona had worked late for the past two nights to complete the presentation.

BOX 12-1	**Slide 1—ten steps to successful breastfeeding**

Every facility providing maternity services and care for newborn infants should:
1. Have a written breastfeeding policy that is routinely communicated to all health care staff.
2. Train all health care staff in skills necessary to implement this policy.
3. Inform all pregnant women about the benefits and management of breastfeeding.
4. Help mothers initiate breastfeeding within a half-hour of birth.
5. Show mothers how to breastfeed, and how to maintain lactation even if they are separated from their infants.
6. Give newborn infants no food or drink other than breast milk, unless medically indicated.
7. Practice rooming-in—allow mothers and infants to remain together—24 hours a day.
8. Encourage breastfeeding on demand.
9. Give no artificial teats or pacifiers (also called dummies or soothers) to breastfeeding infants.
10. Foster the establishment of breastfeeding support groups and refer mothers to them on discharge from the hospital or clinic

From World Health Organization (1998).

BOX 12-2	**Slide 2—criteria for evaluating breastfeeding policies**

1. There are appropriate policies on all practices concerning breastfeeding agreed between relevant authorities.
2. Those policies are made explicit in a written document.
3. All staff and patients are made aware of the policies.

From World Health Organization (1998).

BOX 12-3   **Slide 3—findings**

1. All agencies have some breastfeeding policies
2. The policies range in length from 2 to 22 pages; some agencies have a global policy, some are organized by themes.
2. No two policies are the same on a particular topic—even within an organization.
3. Close to two thirds of hospitals are able to support rooming-in and all are moving toward that goal.
4. There is significant variation in training plans and resources.
5. Only two organizations have policies that contain a communication strategy.
6. All the organizations have plans to update the policies.

Mona began the presentation with a review of the Ten Steps to Successful Breastfeeding, which are the foundation of the BFI (Box 12-1). Lillian presented the evaluation criteria and the findings (Boxes 12-2 and 12-3).

The chairperson thanked Lillian and her team for their hard work and invited questions. This was the first working group of the baby-friendly coalition to present a report, and members were eager to discuss the findings. Several members thanked the group for their sensitivity in presenting the findings, which showed that there was much work to be done. One health unit nurse agreed there was a need to review policies: "Our agency was restructured last year and we are employing more part time staff—there is never any time to update policies. I am embarrassed to think when we last looked at them. This really gives us an incentive to do it." Another member said: "We know our policies and practices are inconsistent across units and have been meaning to tackle this for some time. Some units are more enthusiastic about the BFI than others and rooming in seems to work more smoothly in those units." Generally, members found the WHO evaluation criteria useful and acknowledged that policies were just the tip of the iceberg. More than one said that they expected to find considerable variation in the way the policies were implemented if they took a closer look. Everyone agreed there was no point in making excuses; it was time to make changes.

As a next step, the working group agreed to identify model policies on breastfeeding, rooming in, staff training for breastfeeding support, and a discharge policy for linking women to breastfeeding support groups.

At the end of the meeting, Lillian recalled the meeting with Jake, during when they had agreed that she assign one-half day each week to this project for the remainder of the year and then review. The time allocation had appeared adequate then, allowing for some juggling of projects to meet deadlines. "Life just gets more complicated," she thought, "I will have to take another look at my commitments."

Guide to policy change

There are several, easy-to-follow, guides to changing health-related policy. Some are written primarily for nurses, and others are directed to a broader audience of healthcare providers and community groups (Ewles & Simnett, 1999; Flynn, 2000; OPHA, 1996; Public Health Nursing Section, 2001). All the guides describe a systematic, problem-solving approach that is similar to the community health nursing process and encompasses the four steps of assessment, planning, implementation, and evaluation. All advocate broad community involvement at all stages of the process and recommend that decision-making should be transparent, involve all the key stakeholders, and draw on evidence-based knowledge. Minor variation occurs in the number of steps, the terms used to describe them, and the level of policy change addressed—local or national—however, the process

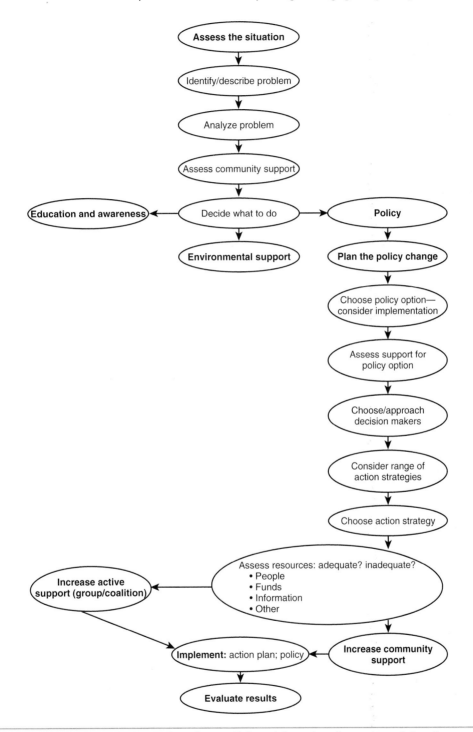

FIGURE 12-2. Process involved in policy change. (Adapted from http://www.thcu.ca/infoandresources/road map.htm and The "Road Map" for Policy change found in Ontario Public Health Association. (1996). *Making a difference in your community: A guide for policy change.* (Second ed. p. 30). Toronto, ON: Ontario Public Health Association.)

described is applicable to policy change at any level. The following discussion uses the OPHA (1996) "road map" for policy change (Fig. 12-2), with some modifications. The reason for choosing this guide is that it addresses policy change at the local level, which is likely to be the major focus for community nurses; it also provides useful tools. Furthermore, the Health Communication Unit (THCU) at the Centre for Health Promotion, University of Toronto (2000, 2004) has developed workshops using this guide. The OPHA road map is organized into four sections. These sections are the following:

- Identify the problem and decide what to do.
- Develop an action plan for a policy change intervention.
- Implement the action plan.
- Evaluate the results.

Identify the problem and decide what to do

The road to policy change starts when an issue or problem, such as those shown earlier in Table 12-2, has been identified. Community nurses can play a key role here. The purpose of this first step is to gain a comprehensive understanding of the issue for the defined population and to determine that policy change is a viable solution to the problem. There are two parts. The first is to conduct a preliminary assessment to document the issue, get a sense of how big it is, and learn who is affected and why. Once it has been determined that this is an issue the community is concerned about, the second part is to perform a detailed analysis of the problem and search for evidence to establish whether policy change offers a feasible solution. Policy change takes considerable time and effort; it should not be undertaken lightly.

Much of the foundation work of documenting community needs and strengths will have been carried out as part of a situational assessment. As discussed in Chapters 3 to 5, this includes setting priorities and developing action statements to guide the choice of interventions for a particular issue. Before deciding on policy change, the following questions need to be answered:

- How likely is it that policy change will solve the problem?
- Is there evidence that policy change has worked before in similar situations?
- Are there other solutions that might be more appropriate?

Look for evidence that has already been compiled in systematic reviews and position papers. "Toward a Healthy Future: Second Report on the Health of Canadians" (FPTACPH, 1999b) provides statistics on a range of health determinants linked to health status and identifies policy options. For example, data show that smoking rates have dropped significantly over the past 20 years, but are dropping more slowly in young women and women and men with low incomes. In part, this is attributed to a period of low cigarette prices, which is thought to encourage smoking. Citing promising evidence that links early onset of smoking to heavier smoking and difficulty quitting, the report recommends as a priority the use of strategies to delay the onset of smoking, particularly in young girls.

There is evidence to support the use of policy to discourage teenage smoking. Primarily this involves policies related to the price of cigarettes. Health Canada estimates that a 10% increase in the price of cigarettes will decrease smoking by 4% among adults and up to 14% among youth (THCU, 2000, Slide 14). This is supported by a recent review of youth smoking prevention and control efforts (Lantz et al., 2000), which provided cautious support for increasing cigarette prices. While many strategies have had mixed results, this is identified as one of several types of strategies that warrant additional attention and evaluation. The other promising strategies included aggressive media campaigns, teen smoking-cessation programs, social environment changes, and community interventions, especially if the strategies are coordinated to take advantage of potential synergies across interventions.

It takes time and effort to sift through the weight of information on health issues and assemble evidence to justify policy initiatives. Familiarity with the literature helps, and this is an area for which health workers can make an important contribution. Before starting out on policy change, it is important to determine that it is a realistic option associated with proven success.

Develop an action plan for a policy change intervention

The purpose of this phase of policy development is to develop a plan that will lead to implementation of the selected policy. Several interlocking pieces have to be eased into place to make this happen. Herein lies the challenge. It is important to remember that policies are an expression of values and beliefs. In addition to being grounded in empirical evidence and research, they should reflect accumulated wisdom and public opinion. Public input has been likened to the second arm of a nutcracker, enabling the community to influence decision makers and take control of the process (Labonte, 1997).

Central to the plan is a policy that is scientifically sound, politically and socially acceptable; it should also be economically feasible and administratively and technologically possible (THCU, 2000). Key planning elements include tailoring the selected policy to the local situation, building a climate of acceptance and support, and crafting the policy statement and a guide to implementation. This phase requires broad input, a range of talents and abilities, and commitment. It is crucial to have adequate resources, people, funds, and information. The many facets of the operation, all proceeding at the same time, are why a group or coalition is best suited to undertake this work.

Assess the local situation

In a democratic society it is very difficult to enforce policies unless communities are ready for them. This fact is clearly illustrated by the statistics on smoking policies. Smoking has been clearly identified as a risk factor for many chronic diseases and as the main cause of premature death in Canada—more than 50% of deaths before age 70 are estimated to result from smoking (FPTACPH, 1999a). Yet there are significant interprovincial differences in the implementation of municipal smoking by-laws, with some provinces being more restrictive than others. In 1995, a mere 3% of the population was covered by smoking by-laws in Newfoundland compared with 81% of Ontarians (FPTACPH, 1999a).

Furthermore, the data show some settings were more likely to be covered by no smoking by-laws than others, with schools being more likely to be covered by smoking restrictions than daycare centers and healthcare institutions. For example, in British Columbia, which had the highest rate of school coverage, there were policies in 65% of schools, 51% of daycare centers, and only 29% of hospitals and other health care institutions. These statistics illustrate the fact that the political will to ban smoking in public places varies across the country and across settings.

Conduct a force field analysis

An important part of laying the groundwork for policy change is to ensure that sufficient support for the policy option to drive the process exists. A **force field analysis,** a process initially developed by psychologist and change theorist Kurt Lewin, can be undertaken to identify driving and restraining forces associated with policy change. To start, identify all key stakeholders, that is, those who will be affected by the problem and by the way it is resolved, both positively and negatively. In determining whether a person or group is likely to support the policy or act against it, ask what they stand to gain or lose if the problem is resolved in a certain way. Unfortunately, this is easier said than done.

Positions on an issue are not always stated explicitly, and it is easy to fall into the trap of thinking that people share identical views just because they agree on one point. Stakeholders may be motivated by different and sometimes conflicting reasons or allegiances, some of which may be concealed. Silence does not necessarily signify consent (Ewles & Simnett, 1999). As with any assessment, it is important to review published material. For example a review of council minutes will tell you how council members vote on smoking-related issues.

The next step is to list the driving forces and restraining forces, describing them as completely as possible and determining how likely they are to influence the process. For example, the tobacco manufacturers have been a powerful lobby against the introduction of smoking by-laws, whereas health promoters have mounted aggressive campaigns to support them. Gathering this information may require a more detailed enquiry. This can take several forms: informal discussions with key informants, focus groups, surveys, or public meetings. As discussed in Chapter 4, all have their advantages and disadvantages in terms of how representative the views are and the time required to gather the information.

By understanding the issue from many different viewpoints—the experts, opinion leaders, and various subpopulations—it is possible to devise strategies to increase the positive forces, decrease the restraining or negative forces, and formulate creative solutions that are acceptable to a wide range of people.

Build support; engage decision makers

Broad public support and the support of key decision-makers are both important. Talking to people (either one-on-one or at public meetings), media interviews, and newspaper articles are all ways to raise awareness about an issue, generate discussion, and create support for policy options. If there is little interest in the topic, it may be necessary to conduct a social marketing campaign to influence public opinion before policy change can be attempted.

Early on, it is necessary to identify the agencies or departments responsible for policy related to your issue, the process for setting policy, and the key decision makers. For example, if the aim is to influence school policy, then you need to know how school policy is formed. Does each school have a policy committee or is there a regional committee? How often does the committee meet? What is the process for placing an item on the agenda? Who chairs the committee and who are the members?

The decision makers, both political and bureaucratic, steer the policy through the political process, so they need to be on your side. It is important to gain their support and work closely with them. There is good reason to think that bureaucratic decision making is influenced by many factors other than systematic, empirical evidence. Macintyre and colleagues (2001) list several factors that might have equal weight:

- Cogent argument
- Scale of likely health benefits
- Likelihood that the policy will bring benefits other than health benefits
- Fit with existing or proposed government policy
- Possibility that the policy might do harm
- Ease and cost of implementation

In addition to these rational arguments, decision makers may be motivated by personal needs, such as gaining public approval and status, values, and a sense of duty (THCU, 2000). Hence the importance of balancing persuasive evidence with community campaigns to sway public opinion and influence key decision makers.

Make contact. Establishing contact is the first step. A range of strategies can be used to do this: letters, telephone calls, or face-to-face meetings are the usual ways to approach elected officials. No one method is necessarily any better than another, and elected representatives often have a preferred approach that works best for them. Networking through professional associations, interest groups, and less formal channels offers another approach to gain access to opinion leaders. For those who wish to pursue this topic further, there are several guides with practical advice on how to make the first contact effectively (e.g., Nagy, 2003, 2004; THCU, 2000). Regardless of the initial approach, the aim is to build relationships and create alliances with decision makers and opinion leaders.

Exercise power. Exercising power, or the ability to influence others, is the second step. Ewles and Simnett (1999) describe four types of power: position power, resource power, expert power, and personal power. Position power is conferred through position in an organization; resource power stems from being able to allocate resources; in senior levels of management, these powers go together. Expert power arises from specialized knowledge or expertise and is a potential source of power for community health nurses. Personal power comes from personal attributes or leadership qualities such as intelligence, initiative, self-confidence, and charisma. Since persuading, negotiating, and making deals are a fundamental part of the process, community health nurses need to understand the different sources of power at their command and develop the appropriate influencing skills.

Plan for adequate time and resources

Achieving the goal of policy change takes time, adequate resources, and endurance. There are many aspects to the work and like any project it will benefit from careful planning and coordination. Effective time management is essential to meet deadlines. Flexibility is also important to take advantage of opportunities and respond quickly when there is a change of plan. Policy change can be a slow process with many roadblocks; once underway, it is important to maintain the momentum and keep the process moving.

DISCUSSION QUESTIONS

1. Accidents and injuries are major contributors to present day mortality and morbidity in youth. Identify key stakeholders in developing policies related to water safety in a seaside community and describe possible driving and restraining forces.

2. Increased rates of smoking among girls and women are described as a national priority and policies related to tobacco prices look promising (FPTACPH, 1999b). Discuss how you might influence the driving and restraining forces for such policies in Aboriginal communities.
3. Legislation on the registration of firearms has had mixed success in Canada and is strongly opposed in the United States. Locate newspaper articles presenting different aspects of the issue and suggest how the approach to policy development might be influenced.

FOUR BREASTFEEDING PROJECTS SCENARIO (continued)

The last hour of the December meeting of the baby-friendly community coalition was devoted to the force field analysis. A consultant, Sylvie, led a brainstorming exercise to identify key stakeholders in the region. Moving round the circle, participants were asked to supply one name and or a title, which was recorded on a flip chart. The facilitator kept the process moving quickly so they had a long list in less than 10 minutes. The stakeholders included: mothers, families with parents in their child-bearing and child-rearing years, health professionals (nurses, lactation consultants, dietitians, physicians, and obstetricians). formula manufacturers and sales representatives, hospital administrators, and hospital and community health boards. Rather than waste meeting time, the consultant planned to send out the list for additional names that came to mind and completion of contact information, where needed.

Sylvie then asked the group to identify the barriers and facilitators for policy change, using the same process. Lillian appreciated the wisdom of employing an external consultant. Sylvie kept the group on track and discouraged discussion and debate, reminding them that this would come later. Once or twice, participants tried to edit the list saying things like: "There's no point in listing the contracts with formula manufacturers because they are set in stone," and "Why write that down; I don't think it is relevant to our community." This was in response to a suggestion from the manager of the airport, who had joined the group on Lillian's invitation. He drew attention to a special supplement on food in The Economist *in 2003 entitled "Spoilt for choice: A survey of food," which addressed the issue of fast food, low activity levels, and obesity dating back to early childhood and identified the perceived health benefits of breastfeeding as a driving force. The group agreed with Sylvie that it was better to get all perspectives down and analyze them later. A preliminary list of the forces appears in Table 12-4.*

All members were assigned the task of reviewing the driving and restraining forces and ranking them in order of importance by an agreed date. This would set the stage for the next meeting when the group would develop a strategy for influencing the forces and develop a plan for drafting a policy and building community support. Echoing Sylvie, the committee chair thanked the group for their efforts and drew the discussion to a close saying, "We are learning just how many angles there are to the issue. It will be a challenge to sort out the different points of view. Thank goodness the WHO has provided clear guidelines and some resources, because they have set high standards."

The next day, Lillian thought about what she had agreed to do before the next meeting. The coalition chair had suggested they should include the results of the survey of breastfeeding policies in an introductory presentation to senior management in the various agencies. The coalition executive felt it was time to confirm they had management support for the BFI across the city. While pleased that her work was valued, Lillian felt a little nervous at the prospect. Luckily, the focus of the next meeting with Jake was how to work with business leaders, using the workplace health project as a launching point.

At Jake's suggestion, Lillian had started to keep a reflective journal on her work in the various teams. Looking at her notes from the last meeting, she realized she had learned a lot from the consultant and was beginning to appreciate the contributions made by other disciplines and was starting to understand their different priorities. This would be the topic for a future meeting.

However, seeing Janet at the coalition meeting with her students had made her realize how far she had come in the last year. The students were compiling an inventory of public places in the city where women could breastfeed, which would provide useful information for the coalition. They were keen to learn more about policy development and had many questions for Lillian about different aspects of policy change. With

| TABLE 12-4 | Forces for Change |

DRIVING FORCES—FACILITATORS	RESTRAINING FORCES—BARRIERS
Most women want to breastfeed	Decreased revenue for hospitals and community boards from contracts with formula manufacturers
Increased demand for baby-friendly settings by women with higher education	Decreased support from formula companies for health provider educational activities and client teaching tools
BFI well documented, successful in many countries, easy to follow instructions, training programs, strong evidence base	Cost of restructuring in-patient settings to accommodate rooming in
Increased media coverage of childhood obesity, reported links to lower rates of breastfeeding	Opposition from staff who resist changes to work assignments
Increased media coverage of nurturing mother	Reduced hospital stay and cuts to community-based programs offering breastfeeding support
Extended maternity benefits enable women to stay at home for one year	Social circumstances that deter breastfeeding, e.g., women, who have to return to work when maternity benefits run out and are more likely to be employed in jobs without facilities to breastfeed
	Opposition from community members who believe that choices around breastfeeding should be left to women

some satisfaction, Lillian realized she was looking forward to the time when she would orient a student group to a policy development project. Closing the journal, Lillian made a mental note to look back at these entries six months from now.

Construct a draft policy

Clear goals and objectives help to focus the policy document. They should state which particular aspect of the problem is to be addressed and the expected health outcomes. For example, the policy could start with the following statement: "This policy aims to reduce smoking among young girls by increasing the price of cigarettes." Specific, measurable objectives further define the content of the policy.

A policy is likely to go through several iterations before it is approved. The draft policy serves a number of purposes:

- It gets ideas down on paper for discussion and debate.
- It forms a succinct statement of intent to inform others and negotiate support.
- The draft reduces later effort because it is easier to modify something that is already written than to construct a policy from scratch.

The approach to developing a policy is no different from that for designing any intervention. There should be evidence to show that the policy, when implemented, will bring about the desired changes. (You may find it helpful to refer to Chapters 5 and 6.) In many cases this evidence will be lacking for several reasons:

- Sensitive measures to evaluate the impact of policy change on key target groups may not be readily available (Davidoff, 2004).
- Decision makers have failed to evaluate the impact of health policy (Macintyre, 2003).
- A policy change to affect the determinants of health may take years to achieve its goals (Leon, Walt, & Gilson, 2001).

Assembling the strongest evidence possible and a plausible argument for why one option is preferred over another offers a way forward.

Formal policy and its parts

Formal policy has several parts: the rationale or preamble, which explains why the policy is needed; definitions; the components, which explain how the policy is implemented; the communication strategy; and the plan for enforcement and monitoring (THCU, 2000). A sample municipal alcohol policy is provided in Application 12-1.

Rationale

This is a succinct statement explaining the reason for the policy and what it is trying to achieve. Sometimes the reasons are contained in statements beginning with "Whereas. . . ."

Definitions

A definition of key terms using clear language helps to prevent ambiguity. For example, the following definition makes it clear that merely holding a lit cigarette qualifies as smoking: "*Smoking* includes carrying a lighted cigar, cigarette, pipe or any other lighted smoking instrument and *smoke* has a corresponding meaning." Often, it is necessary to define the setting where a specific policy is in force. For example, in the smoking policy below, "Enclosed Public Place" requires definition.

Components of the policy

The components of the policy explain where, when, and how the policy will be implemented. For example, a smoking policy gives the following directions:

- No person shall smoke in any enclosed public place within the city whether or not a No Smoking sign is posted.
- Every proprietor of an Enclosed Public Place shall post signs at every entrance to the Enclosed Public Place in accordance with Section 4.1 of this by-law.

The municipal alcohol policy example of Application 12-1 is more complex and requires careful reading because it has many components.

Communication strategy

The purpose of the communication strategy is to explain how the policy will be made known to those who are likely to be affected by it. An important consideration is that everyone touched by the policy understands what it is about, knows when it will come into effect, and can determine how it will affect daily life. It also flags where advance preparation, such as training, may be necessary. The sample "Municipal Alcohol Policy"

(Application 12-1) contains training implications. The policy dictates that bartenders (alcohol servers) must undergo special training in order to meet their new responsibilities. When planning the implementation, sufficient time should be allowed to spread the key messages. This allows the necessary supports to be put in place so that the implementation will run smoothly.

Another aim of the communication strategy is to prepare the public and create acceptance of the policy before it is introduced so the majority will comply. Policy that is likely to affect many people, for instance, car seat belt legislation, is often introduced through a media campaign, with television and radio advertisements, talk show discussion, and Web sites. Public officials and managers will probably be responsible for policy implementation, including the preparatory work, but these aspects need to be considered at the planning stage. Community health nurses have a role to play in creating awareness of policy change, for example, by advising clients, participating in talk shows, and writing letters to the editor in support of the policy.

Plan for enforcement and monitoring

This section of the policy states how the policy will be enforced and lays out the consequences of failure to comply. The penalties need to be sufficient to act as a deterrent but may start with a warning and escalate for repeated offenses. The Municipal Alcohol Policy (Application 12-1) provides an example. The advantages of compliance can be used as an incentive. For example, by promoting moderate alcohol use and protecting patrons from intoxication, alcohol servers may avoid brawls and liability in case of accidents.

As with evaluation, the plan for monitoring should be in place before the policy goes into effect. Monitoring helps to identify situations for which the policy is unclear or difficult to apply. It can also provide information on whether the policy is being applied as intended and consistently. Such feedback can be used to improve implementation and thereby help to attain the long-term goals. Keep in mind that no policy will be completely flawless, especially when it is being implemented for the first time.

Implement the action plan

Community health nurses may or may not have a direct role to play in the implementation of policy, depending on where the responsibility for implementation lies and the nature of the policy. They may, however, play a valuable role in providing education to support policy change. Some examples of how nurses might do this: offer smoking cessation programs; provide telephone advice and resources to help smokers quit; organize support for car seat installation at well baby clinics; and provide training on breastfeeding support. Another possible area of involvement is informal monitoring in places where nurses practice. For instance, in the case of smoking, this could be in community settings such as schools and day care facilities, where nurses practice.

Evaluate the results

As discussed earlier, evaluation is a step in policy work that is often neglected. The question of ultimate importance is "Did the policy achieve the desired impact on health?" This is a difficult question to answer for many reasons: baseline data before policy change may be unavailable or nonexistent; it is difficult to distinguish the impact of policy change from that of the many other factors influencing health behavior, and there is often a time lag between innovation and change in health status.

As a result, evaluation often looks for clues that policy change is moving in the right direction: Was the policy implemented as planned? How well is it accepted? Are there measurable effects on attitudes, if not behavior? Are there beneficial effects that were not anticipated?

It is also useful to reflect on the process of policy development: Did it go as planned? What tips can be shared with others starting on a similar journey? What lessons have been learned about the issue or about the policy change process? This learning can guide future policy initiatives or be applied in other situations. The Policy Evaluation Checklist in Application 12-2 can be used to evaluate the policy change process (THCU, 2000).

Summary

Healthy public policy is an important strategy for influencing the health of populations. Community health nurses can make a contribution to policy change in many ways by collaborating with community members to identify issues that lend themselves to a policy solution; providing evidence that policy change is effective, joining the policy development team, and monitoring the impact of policy change.

PRACTICE AND APPLICATION

1. Select a health issue for policy intervention; identify the goals of the intervention, and put together a plan to determine the feasibility of the intervention.

2. Assess the support in your community for a municipal alcohol policy (Application 12-1).

3. Compare and contrast organizational policies pertaining to employee safety from two types of community agency from which clients receive visits in the home. Develop a model policy for a new clinic in a neighborhood with high crime rates.

REFERENCES

Brownson, R.C., Newschaffer, C.J., & Ali-Abarghoui, F. (1997). Policy research for disease prevention: Challenges and practical recommendations. *American Journal of Public Health, 87*(5), 735–739.

Canadian Nurses Association. (2000). Nursing is a political act—The bigger picture. *Nursing Now: Issues and Trends in Canadian Nursing*(8), 1–4.

Chambers, L.W., Underwood, J., Halbert, T., Woodward, C.A., Heale, J., & Isaacs, S. (1994). 1992 Ontario survey of public health nurses: Perceptions of roles and activities. *Canadian Journal of Public Health, 85*(3), 175–179.

Davidoff, A. (2004). Identifying children with special health care needs in the National Health Interview Survey: A new resource for policy analysis. *Health Services Research, 39*(1), 53–71.

Ewles, L., & Simnett, I. (1999). *Promoting health: A practical guide* (4th ed.). Edinburgh: Baillière Tindall.

Federal Provincial and Territorial Advisory Committee on Population Health [FPTACPH]. (1999a). *Statistical report on the health of Canadians, 1999. Prepared for the meeting of Ministers of Health, Charlottetown, P.E.I. September 16–17, 1999.* Ottawa, ON: Ministry of Supply and Services.

Federal Provincial and Territorial Advisory Committee on Population Health [FPTACPH]. (1999b). *Toward a healthy future: Second report on the health of Canadians. Prepared for the meeting of Ministers of Health, Charlottetown, P.E.I., September 16–17, 1999.* Ottawa, ON: Ministry of Supply and Services.

Flynn, B.C. (2000). Health policy for healthy cities and communities. In E.T. Anderson & J. McFarlane (Eds.), *Community as partner: Theory and practice in nursing* (3rd ed., pp. 137–149). Philadelphia: Lippincott.

Hancock, T. (2001). People, partnerships and human progress: Building community capital. *Health Promotion International, 16*(3), 275–280.

Kang, R. (1995). Building community capacity for health promotion: A challenge for public health nurses. *Public Health Nursing, 12*(5), 312–318.

Labonte, R. (1997). Community, community development and the forming of authentic partnerships: Some critical reflections. In M. Minkler (Ed.), *Community organizing and community building for health* (pp. 88–102). New Brunswick, NJ: Rutgers University Press.

Lantz, P.M., Jacobson, P.D., Warner, K.E., Wasserman, J., Pollack, H.A., Berson, J., et al. (2000). Investing in youth tobacco control: A review of smoking prevention and control strategies. *Tobacco Control, 9,* 47–63.

Leon, D.A., Walt, G., & Gilson, L. (2001). International perspectives on health inequalities and policy. *British Medical Journal, 322*(591–594).

Macintyre, S. (2003). Evidence based policy making. *British Medical Journal, 326,* 5–6.

Macintyre, S., Chalmers, I., Horton, R., & Smith, R. (2001). Using evidence to inform health policy: Case study. *British Medical Journal, 322,* 222–225.

McKeown, T. (1979). *The role of medicine: Dream, mirage, or nemesis.* Princeton, NJ: Princeton University Press.

Milio, N. (1989). Making healthy public policy; developing the science by learning the art: An ecological framework for policy studies. In B. Badura & I. Kickbusch (Eds.), *Health promotion research: Towards a new social epidemiology* (pp. 7–27). Copenhagen, Denmark: World Health Organization Regional Office for Europe.

Minkler, M. (1999). Personal responsibility for health? A review of the arguments and the evidence at century's end. *Health Education Quarterly, 26*(1), 121–140.

Multicultural Advocates for Social Change on Tobacco [Mascot]. (2004). *Smoking prevention and control strategies for youth.* Retrieved January 15, 2004, from http://www.mascotcoalition.org/education/youth_smoking.html.

Nagy, J. (2004). *Changing policies to increase funding for community health and development initiatives.* Retrieved February 4, 2004, from http://ctb.ukans.edu/tools/en/sub_section_main_1280.htm.

Nagy, J. *Writing letters to elected officials.* Retrieved February 4, 2004, from http://ctb.ukans.edu/tools/en/sub_section_main_1238.htm.

Ontario Public Health Association. (1996). *Making a difference in your community: A guide for policy change.* (2nd ed.). Toronto, ON: Author.

Public Health Nursing Section. (2001). *Public health interventions: Applications for public health nursing practice.* St. Paul, Minnesota: Minnesota Department of Health.

Rachlis, M. (1989, May 17–19). *Health and health care for Ontario in the 1990's: Will the crisis of the 1980's spell danger or opportunity?* Paper presented at the Healthy populace/Health policy: Medicare toward the year 2000, Kingston, ON.

Schmid, T.L., Pratt, M., & Howze, E. (1995). Policy as intervention: Environmental and policy approaches to the prevention of cardiovascular disease. *American Journal of Public Health, 85*(9), 1207–1211.

Schoenfeld, B.M., & MacDonald, M.B. (2002). Saskatchewan public health nursing survey: Perceptions of roles and activities. *Canadian Journal of Public Health, 93*(6), 452–456.

Spoilt for choice: A survey of food. (2003). *The Economist,* 1–16.

Stokols, D. (1996). Translating social ecological theory into guidelines for community health promotion. *American Journal of Health Promotion, 10*(4), 282–298.

The Health Communication Unit (THCU) at the Centre for Health Promotion University of Toronto. (2000, June 13 2002). *Policy Powerpoint Slideshow.* Retrieved November 15, 2003, from http://www.thcu.ca/infoandresources/policy_resources.htm#tp.

The Health Communication Unit (THCU) at the Centre for Health Promotion University of Toronto. (2004, March 31, 2004). *Developing health promotion policies.* Retrieved May 24, 2004, from http://www.thcu.ca/infoandresources/policy_resources.htm#tp

Wallack, L. (1998). Media advocacy: A strategy for empowering people and communities. In M. Minkler (Ed.), *Community organizing and community building for health* (pp. 339–352). New Brunswick, NJ: Rutgers University Press.

World Health Organization. (1998). *Evidence for the ten steps to successful breastfeeding.* Retrieved January 22, 2004, from http://www.who.int/child-adolescent-health/publications/NUTRITION/WHO_CHD_98.9.htm

---

APPLICATION 12-1

EXAMPLE OF A MUNICIPAL ALCOHOL POLICY

Municipal alcohol policy

Rationale (Why the policy is needed)

It is the intention of the Municipality of Summerland to provide for the **safe and responsible use of alcohol** in municipally owned properties, to **minimize the legal responsibility** for users as well as the Municipality's broad legal liability, and to **foster awareness of the responsibilities** of the Special Occasion Permits to the Users so that they in turn may encourage the responsible consumption of alcohol.

Components (Explains how the policy is implemented)

- **A special permit is required** for special occasion events where alcohol will be sold.
- **Events can be held only in designated locations**. Responsibility for the event is assigned to a designated person or "event User." The Liquor License Act of Ontario clearly states that the event User has a **"duty of control,"** that is, to protect participants from foreseeable harm to themselves and others. The Act also states that the server of alcohol is responsible for intoxicated individuals until they regain sobriety, not only until they arrive home safely. Be aware that you and your group can be held liable for injuries and damages arising from failure to adhere to the Liquor Licence Act of Ontario. Infractions to the Act include the following:
  —Serving someone to intoxication
  —Serving someone who is already intoxicated
  —Serving minors
  —Failing to prevent impaired individuals from driving
- **The User must provide proof of insurance** (at least 1 million dollars) for alcohol-related events (e.g., Carnival, rock concert, or any event with attendance over 500 people) and indemnify the municipality.

- **Minors are prohibited from attending unless accompanied by a responsible adult**; it is forbidden to serve alcohol to minors who do attend.
- **The User must follow sensible alcohol marketing practices** (no oversized drinks, double shots of spirits, drinking contests, volume discounts, or unlimited free alcohol, which encourage increased immoderate consumption).
- **An appropriate number of properly educated servers should be present.**
  —Bar, floor, and door supervisors, 19 years of age or older; numbers based on estimated attendance on permit
  —Certified by a recognized alcohol server training course such as Smart Serve (a four-hour training course that provides the event workers with information and techniques on how to prevent alcohol-related problems from occurring and how to intervene when they do occur.) Monthly training sessions are held at City Hall [*contact person named*]. A Smart Serve Resource Bank has been created for persons wishing to hire the services of certified Smart Serve event workers. A list is available at the Parks and Recreation Department.

If Users fail to adhere to the policy guidelines and controls, the following enforcement procedures will be taken:

- **First infraction:** The User will be sent a Registered letter outlining the consequences of further infractions.
- **Second infraction:** The User will be sent a Registered letter stating that he or she will lose all scheduled privileges for a three (3)-month period including all monies related to the rental and are suspended from all functions at any municipal property for the same period of time.
- **Third infraction:** The User will be sent a Registered letter stating that he or she will lose all rental privileges for one (1) year and are suspended from all functions at any municipal property for the same length of time. Before the end of the suspension period, the User must meet personally with a municipal representative to discuss how he or she will ensure that all rules will be followed in the future so that similar incidents do not occur.

The municipality will report any infraction of this policy to legal authorities, including the Liquor License Board, whenever it believes such action is required.

Policy monitoring and revision

Municipal staff will monitor the events where alcohol is served in municipal facilities.

Minor variations to the policy can be approved, on an event-by-event basis, by the Commissioner having jurisdiction over the facility/location, for events requiring exception to the policy.

The Municipal Alcohol Policy will be reviewed annually and updated to reflect any subsequent legislative changes.

Guidelines and controls

The User must acknowledge intent to observe and comply with the controls of the policy, specified below, by initialing the facility permit or rental agreement.

Obtain and display the necessary permit; provide evidence that event workers are properly trained, and purchase liability insurance.

Be present at the event, support staff, refrain from using alcohol, and be in charge of decision-making.

Employ appropriate numbers of trained staff, advise them of their legal responsibilities, ensure that they are present at all times and that they refrain from using alcohol and ensure adequate security staff.

Observe that alcohol is sold under safe conditions and consumed on premises.

Restrict sale of alcohol to reasonable amounts—four tickets at a time; sell none to underage youth, check identification (unmask if participating in masquerade events).

Provide nonalcoholic drinks and low-alcohol beverages at lower cost than alcohol.

Serve sufficient, appropriate food; avoid salty snacks.

Take steps to discourage excessive drinking; for example, if tickets are used, allow them to be cashed at any time; do not flag closing time to avoid stocking up; stop on time; and clear up and remove liquor from premises swiftly.

Provide a safe physical setting, monitor exits, and ensure there are safe transportation options; take immediate action to prevent the outbreak of disturbances.

APPLICATION 12-2

POLICY EVALUATION CHECKLIST

1. Have you identified and analyzed the issues your policy needs to address?
2. Do you have sufficient information about these issues to support and justify the implementation of your policy?
3. Are your policy goals reasonable and your policy objectives measurable?
4. Do you have the required support and approval of key decision makers? If not, how will this be obtained?
5. Have you selected your policy components and prepared a written policy that describes these components and a strategy for implementation?
6. Do you have an accurate estimate of the resources (time, money, person power, and expertise) needed to implement and monitor your policy?
7. Is the timeline for implementation realistic?
8. Does your policy specify who is responsible for doing what?
9. Have you identified the barriers to implementation you are likely to encounter?
10. Do you have a plan for dealing with these barriers?
11. Have you shared your draft policy with other key stakeholders who will be responsible for implementation?
12. Is this the appropriate time to start implementing your policy?

Adapted with permission from The Health Communication Unit (THCU) at the Centre for Health Promotion, University of Toronto. (2002) *LH Policy Slides* (Slides 104–106).

Community Health Programs and Evaluation

ALWYN MOYER

INFECTIOUS DISEASE CONTROL: INFLUENZA PREVENTION FOR OLDER ADULTS

A poster catches Mai's eye as she enters the Public Health Department building. The message says "Get your flu shot now." Mai exchanges a guilty look with her classmate Fadma. On the way to this first meeting with the project team, they chatted about the scramble they had to complete their immunizations and present proof of up-to-date immunization status before the start of their clinical course.

Cora, the program manager, welcomes them to the team meeting and makes introductions. Millie, a public health nurse and the team leader, asks, "Why did you choose to join the communicable disease team?" Laughing, she adds, "Most students think that communicable disease is boring." Fadma explains that for the past two summers she had volunteered at a community health center, which is well attended by women from the Somali community. She was surprised that many of the women expressed fears and misunderstanding about immunization. For example, one day she heard women working at the food bank discussing the idea that it was better for children to catch measles so that they would develop a stronger natural immunity; another day one woman left the women's clinic saying angrily that she did not need tuberculosis (TB) testing because she came from a region where there was no TB and her family had always been healthy. These situations made Fadma realize that she needed to better understand issues related to immunization and communicable disease control.

Mai explains that she wants to learn about the planning and organization of mass immunization campaigns. She is also attracted by the opportunity to learn more about program evaluation, which she understands will be a major focus of her assignment.

At the meeting Mai learns that planning for the influenza, or flu, program usually starts in June so that the annual campaign is ready to launch at the end of September. "Just in time for the flu season" says Millie. Cora provides a package of material on the influenza program, including a program logic model, and suggests that everyone read this to become familiar with the program. Moving to the student project, she explains that the health unit promotes a community-wide influenza campaign each year and ensures that residents who need it have access to government funded vaccine. Several other agencies are involved, including community health centers, resource centers, home health provider groups, and a number of ethnic groups. Millie reviews the organization of the campaign to bring Mai and Fadma up to date.

Last year, the community health centers were dissatisfied with the participation in the immunization program compared with that in the previous year. Although the number of clinics had increased, not as many older adults had been reached as expected. Particularly disappointing was the lower than expected turnout at the sessions held in seniors' centers. This year, the team wants to conduct a stronger evaluation of the flu clinics with the help of the students.

347

OBJECTIVES   **After reading this chapter and answering the questions throughout the chapter, you should be able to**

1. Describe how the community health nursing process is adapted for an evaluation project.
2. Create a program logic model to describe a community program.
3. Discuss how the program logic model is used to guide program evaluation.
4. Identify ways to increase community involvement in program evaluation.
5. Develop an observation checklist.
6. Document and communicate observations.

KEYWORDS   **cold chain** ▪ **community health program** ▪ **program logic model** ▪ **directly observed therapy (DOT)** ▪ **program evaluation** ▪

Evaluation in ongoing programs

A project that deals only with evaluation may make you feel that you can skip all the previous steps of the community health nursing process. That is not the case. Your team will still progress through the steps to ensure that the evaluation is appropriate to the situation. Some adaptations of the substeps are necessary to accommodate program evaluation. Table 13-1 shows the adaptations.

Community health programs

In previous chapters we discussed how small groups can effectively undertake a community health project by systematically applying the community health nursing process. These projects provide an opportunity for students and new practitioners to apply the principles of primary health care, perfect problem-solving skills, and hone communication techniques while addressing a community health issue of significance. It is important to view the projects in perspective: each project is conducted over a relatively short time in the life of a community and is embedded in a complex web of community health programs and services. You need to understand and appreciate how your project fits with and contributes to existing community health programs.

A **community health program** is commonly defined as a series of activities, supported by a group of resources, intended to achieve specific outcomes among particular groups (Porteous, Sheldrick, & Stewart, 1997). This definition translates into the questions that provide a framework for understanding the dimensions of a specific program:

- What is the goal of the program?
- Which population group is specified by the program?
- What resources (e.g., people or money) are required to deliver the program?
- What activities are carried out to achieve the program goal?

Programs to control infectious diseases are an example. The overarching goal of infectious disease control programs is the reduction or elimination of infectious diseases within the population as a whole. Typically, there is a program providing general guidelines

TABLE 13-1	Adaptation of Collaborative Assessment Process with Groups or Communities for Evaluating Ongoing Program
STEPS OF PROCESS	**ADAPTATION FOR EVALUATION OF A COMMUNITY PROGRAM**
1. Establish relationships within project and community	Review mandate, policy, and procedures of agency and particular program. Identify the program evaluation team.
2. Assess secondary data	Review literature, epidemiology, and socio-demographics related to program. Review program needs assessment. Review program description and program logic model to identify program goals and activities. Review program statistics (if available).
3. Initiate assessment of community	Interview key informants: program providers, partners, and recipients. Determine availability of similar or related programs and services.
4. Conduct specific assessment	Observe program delivery at two or more sites.
5. Determine action statements	Agree on the goals of the evaluation.
6. Plan	Plan the evaluation. Describe the program as it is being delivered. Clarify the purpose of the evaluation and define the questions to be answered. Develop the evaluation plan. Develop evaluation measures or tool.
7. Take action	Conduct pilot of evaluation measures. Carry out the evaluation.
8. Determine results/impact	Similar to communities and groups. Provide report in format that is useful to agency.
9. Evaluate teamwork	Similar to communities and groups.

for the management of reportable and communicable diseases and for the emergency response structures required to manage outbreaks. In addition, there are programs focused on controlling the potential for disease in food and water, together with programs to control specific diseases such as tuberculosis (TB) and certain diseases that can be prevented by vaccination. Other programs define requirements for ensuring that effective infection control techniques are in place in institutions, day care centers, and personal service settings. Usually, public health departments are responsible for the infectious disease control budget, and they employ program staff to perform activities that include surveillance, case-finding, contact tracing, immunization, infection control, and risk assessment. Together, these programs ensure effective control of infectious diseases (Ontario Ministry of Health, 1997).

Even though the infrastructure for infectious disease control has been in place for a long time in developed countries and the programs usually run smoothly, they must constantly adapt to changing conditions. For example, new and improved vaccines entail changes in immunization schedules. Periodically, internationally orchestrated strategies to eliminate common diseases such as polio and measles demand a shift in resources.

Changing patterns of infectious disease outbreaks present an ongoing challenge. In North America, TB is reemerging as a public health problem with the burden of illness being concentrated more and more in the foreign-born population. Two reasons for this are the ineffective identification of persons with active TB at the time of immigration and the poor adherence to medical surveillance (Chang, Wheeler, & Farrell, 2002; Uppaluri et al., 2002). Furthermore, treatment effectiveness has been compromised by the inappropriate use of antitubercular drugs, which produced an increased prevalence of resistant strains of bacteria (Cowie, Field, & Enarson, 2002). In addition, the high levels of poverty and homelessness in some cities are creating vulnerable populations with low levels of protection against infection. The situation is further complicated by outbreaks of new diseases such as severe acute respiratory syndrome (SARS), which can travel around the globe with breathtaking rapidity because of international travel. As a result, the control of infectious disease is under continuous scrutiny and program managers and community boards must routinely evaluate local programs to make sure they are effective and synchronous with national and international standards.

Program logic model

A **program logic model** is a useful tool for understanding how a program is expected to work. Applicable to almost any program, a program logic model provides a visual representation of program activities, in a flow chart or table, and links them to the stated program goals (Wong-Reiger & David, 1995). The main value of the program logic model, as the name implies, is that it illuminates the underlying logic or causal reasoning that connects program activities to the expected results. An example given in Box 13-1 describes an innovative TB prevention program offered in conjunction with English as a second language (ESL) classes to new immigrants (Moyer, Verhovsek, & Wilson, 1997). The program is first described and then is used to illustrate a program logic model.

Example: TB prevention program

 A public health nurse (PHN) attends English as a Second Language (ESL) classes to administer the tuberculin skin test to participating students. After a 48- to 72-hour wait, the nurse returns to assess the results and provide counseling. When the results are positive, the nurse refers the student for treatment at a community health clinic. The PHN traces and screens contacts and provides case management until treatment is completed. The program is offered at a variety of times and places throughout the week in ESL classrooms throughout the region so that it is available to as many students as possible. Sessions are offered in English and French, and, if numbers of students are sufficient, in other languages. The PHN undertakes a range of activities to increase awareness, knowledge, and referrals to the program. Some examples follow:

- Placing advertisements in grocery stores, shopping centers, pharmacies, etc.
- Writing articles for community newspapers
- Sending letters to physicians to let them know about the program

To create support for treatment, the PHN works with teachers of ESL classes, the school board, and immigrant organizations to provide educational materials on TB prevention and control and healthy lifestyles. Additionally the PHN provides information on community resources and devises strategies to help students build an informal support network with other students in the group.

The TB prevention program aims to

- Increase students' knowledge of the risk of TB and the benefits of treatment.
- Increase knowledge of community resources.
- Increase links with other students undergoing treatment.

This program is expected to increase the number of students who present themselves for TB testing and complete the screening process. It should increase the number of persons with active TB who are accurately identified, who initiate and complete treatment, and whose contacts are traced, screened, and, if necessary, treated. Ultimately, the program will decrease the number of persons with active TB and increase those with optimal health.

Elements of the program logic model

The three main elements of the program logic model are: 1) program activities, 2) short-term outcomes, and 3) long-term outcomes. The program activities are expected to bring about the short- and long-term outcomes.

The next section explains the program elements and discusses how they are assembled into a program and depicted in a program logic model. The previously discussed TB prevention program in Box 13-1 is used to illustrate the elements as an example. To make the discussion easier to follow, the elements are addressed in reverse order: long-term outcomes, short-term outcomes, and program activities.

Long-term and short-term outcomes

The outcomes of the program describe what the program is trying to accomplish. They are usually divided into results that can be expected in the long-term, or ultimately, and results that can be expected in the short-term, or more immediately. The long-term outcomes are usually envisioned as changes in health status and the short-term outcomes as the changes in knowledge, skills, attitudes, and intentions that act as stepping stones to the long-term outcomes (see Objectives, Chapter 6). For example, intending to register for a smoking cessation program is a precursor to registering, which is a precursor to learning techniques to help stop, which is a precursor to stopping. When research evidence links the different levels of outcome, there is good reason to believe that a short-term outcome will lead to the long-term outcome, and this assumption is often made (Israel et al., 1995). For example, the links between smoking and lung cancer are well-documented, and so smoking cessation programs are assumed to prevent lung cancer, although it would probably be more accurate to say that they reduce the risk that the disease will develop.

In the TB prevention program described earlier, the identification of persons with active TB represents a short-term or immediate outcome of screening activities. The long-term outcome of reduced incidence of TB depends on many interrelated factors including the prescription of the right medication and completion of a full course of treatment, both of which can be more or less successful. From these examples, it can be seen that long-term and short-term represent points on a continuum rather than a defined period of time.

Program activities

The choice of program activities is based on evidence that the activities will produce the desired outcomes. To continue with the previous example, it is well known that new immigrants encounter many barriers to TB treatment. Some fear that discovery of disease may cause them to be deported, and many lack medical insurance to cover immediate health care costs (Uppaluri et al., 2002). A case management approach using **directly observed therapy (DOT)** has been successful in ensuring that persons with active TB complete the full course of antitubercular drugs required to bring the disease under control. With DOT, health and community workers and trained volunteers observe and record that patients have swallowed the drugs over the duration of the treatment. The treatment course takes six to eight months, and incomplete treatment is associated with the risk of secondary drug resistance (Chaulk, Moore-Rice, Rizzo, & Chaisson, 1995). Because close contacts of a person with active TB are at high risk for developing the disease, tracing and assessing contacts and, if necessary, providing prophylactic treatment will prevent latent TB from progressing to active TB. The two steps together contribute to the ultimate goal of decreased incidence of TB.

The links between the elements are then specified to show which activities will lead to which outcomes. Figure 13-1 shows a diagram of a completed program logic model.

Service delivery outcomes

Program activities may be further defined in the program logic model to provide a measure of service delivery. These service delivery outcomes specify the types and frequency of service to be delivered for each activity (Wong-Reiger & David, 1995). In other words, they prescribe the "dose" to be administered. For example, one of the activities described in the TB program plan was that program staff would submit articles to ethnic community newspapers on the importance of TB testing and control. A service delivery outcome might be to submit a monthly 1000-word article to three local English language newspapers and one foreign language newspaper read by the specific community. Of course, there are many practical considerations to take into account when these targets are set, such as the readership, distribution, and frequency of the newspapers.

The program logic model may be developed as part of program planning, or it can be constructed at a later date on the basis of descriptions by knowledgeable staff of how the program is actually offered. Information provided in program proposals, annual reports, and operating data can be used to complete the picture. If done as a part of program planning, defining the program goals—what the program is intended to achieve, as indicated by the needs assessment—is the starting point followed by determining how best to do it. In reality, this usually involves an iterative approach. It is similar to the process of linking interventions and outcomes discussed in Chapter 6.

Program Activities with Short and Long-term Outcomes

Activities	1. Recruitment	2. Screening and Follow-up	3. Case Management	4. Support
	• Place articles in ethnic newspapers about risk of TB and importance of testing for new immigrants • Distribute leaflets to physicians' offices	• Screen ESL students and contacts of positive cases • Refer ESL students with positive test to physicians for full assessment, diagnosis, and treatment	• Case management using directly observed therapy (DOT) initiated	• Assemble resource materials on TB control and healthy lifestyle for ESL teachers • Work with ESL teachers, school board and immigrant groups to increase opportunities for building social networks (impacts awareness of ESL TB prevention program in recruitment)
	⬇	⬇	⬇	⬇
Short-term Outcomes	• Increased awareness of importance of TB testing in new immigrant groups • Increased awareness of ESL TB prevention program • Increased uptake of TB screening	• Positive cases identified and referred for treatment • Accurate diagnosis established, and appropriate treatment initiated	• Treatment completed • Latent cases do not become active cases	⬅ • Increased links to formal and informal support networks (impacts successful completion of treatment)
	➡ **impacts screening**	➡ **impacts case management**	⬇	⬇
Long-term Outcomes			• Reduced incidence of active tuberculosis in new immigrants	• Increased community support for TB prevention and control

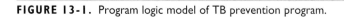

FIGURE 13-1. Program logic model of TB prevention program.

Advantages of a program logic model

Program logic models take time to complete but are worth the effort because of the advantages described below.

- Drawing the model requires that you show the connections between program elements, which helps to clarify the program logic.
- The model identifies duplication of activities or weak links before the program is implemented.
- The model promotes a common understanding among program staff and stakeholders and thereby facilitates involvement.
- Practitioners can see which program activities are crucial for attaining the long-term goals.
- The definition of activities assists the program manager to calculate the resources that will be required at different stages of the program.
- If the logic model is constructed during program planning, evaluation is a focus up front: the program outputs and outcome indicators are explicit from the outset, which makes it easier to set up systems to gather critical operational data.

DISCUSSION QUESTIONS

1. Identify the number and type of resources required to carry out the TB prevention program described in Box 13-1.
2. Identify three short-term outcomes that might be used to evaluate the success of a television commercial to raise parents' awareness about the importance of physical activity for schoolchildren.
3. Public health nurses are training volunteers to answer queries about healthy lifestyles at a Health Fair that is focusing on women who intend to become pregnant in the near future. Give an example of an appropriate service delivery outcome.

INFECTIOUS DISEASE CONTROL: INFLUENZA PREVENTION FOR OLDER ADULTS SCENARIO *(continued)*

Mai and Fadma were dismayed when they saw the pile of the documents they had to review. It was not easy reading—Public Health Program Guidelines, several articles on influenza immunization, a report on best practices, and the previous year's statistics for the region, as well as the program report. "We are never going to get through this in one morning" said Mai. After a few minutes griping, Fadma said, "What we need is a plan. Let's make a list of what we need to know to get started." Quickly, they generated the following questions:

1. *What is the public health mandate regarding influenza immunization?*
2. *How does the influenza program operate?*
3. *When was the last needs assessment carried out?*
4. *What are the key facts on influenza and influenza prevention*
   a. *Who should be immunized—what is the schedule?*
   b. *Are there side effects to the immunization?*
   c. *What proportion of the population is immunized; who does not get immunized but should?*
   d. *Are there other health measures that help to prevent influenza?*
5. *What are the statistics on the number of cases of influenza?*
6. *Where were the outbreaks of influenza last year?*

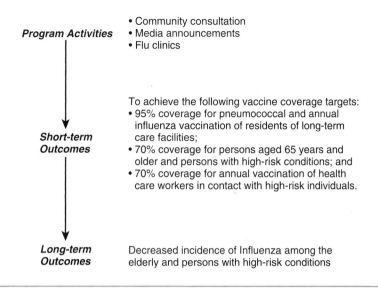

Program Activities
- Community consultation
- Media announcements
- Flu clinics

Short-term Outcomes

To achieve the following vaccine coverage targets:
- 95% coverage for pneumococcal and annual influenza vaccination of residents of long-term care facilities;
- 70% coverage for persons aged 65 years and older and persons with high-risk conditions; and
- 70% coverage for annual vaccination of health care workers in contact with high-risk individuals.

Long-term Outcomes

Decreased incidence of Influenza among the elderly and persons with high-risk conditions

FIGURE 13-2. Draft of influenza program logic model.

Fadma elected to quickly read through the program documents to get a better sense of the influenza program. Mai agreed to find out more about influenza and its prevention. They wrote their key findings on the blackboard as they went along. At the end of two hours they reviewed what Fadma had recorded:

- *The previous year's influenza campaign was directed to three groups: adults 65 years of age and older, adults with chronic disease, and formal and informal caregivers. This is consistent with the regional mandate.*
- *The program maintains effective working relationships with community health centers, the school board, ESL teachers, and family practitioners through an annual community consultation plus individual meetings. This year, representatives from the ethnocultural community resource centers were invited to participate to better meet their needs.*
- *Influenza prevention resource materials were disseminated through the media (television, radio, and newspapers) and agencies, including ethnic group–specific media and agencies.*
- *Educational material was disseminated to family practice/medical centers, e.g., Ministry of Health influenza fact sheets in eight languages were distributed in the community and 1794 prescription note pads with a message about getting flu vaccine were sent out to physician's offices.*

Mai said, "As you can see (Figure 13-2), I've started to put this into a logic model. I have put in arrows to indicate how the program activities lead to the short-term objectives but I am not certain how this actually happens."

Millie explained how the various activities contributed to the outcomes. "The community consultation fulfills several functions. It brings together the key provider groups for an update on this year's campaign. We review changes to the vaccines and the immunization protocol, reinforce the importance of maintaining the "cold chain," and discuss reporting and documentation. This helps to ensure a consistent approach and good records. Also, we have to ensure that everyone in the region has access to the government funded vaccine, so the meeting provides an opportunity to talk about the clinics."

*"What is the **cold chain**?" asked Fadma. Millie explained that it was vitally important to store vaccines at the correct temperature to maintain their potency. The vaccines should not be too hot or too cold (World Health Organization, 2002). In this area, it was the Health Department's responsibility to ensure that proper conditions, i.e., the cold chain, were maintained, wherever vaccines were stored.*

Millie continued, "Most people go to their family doctor or a health clinic for their flu shot, but this year the community health centers (CHCs) are offering clinics in other locations to try to increase the uptake. Last year, we conducted a needs assessment in the Italian and Chinese communities and found that many older adults did not attend the flu clinics because they did not speak English. So this year one CHC will offer clinics at a seniors' residence serving the Italian community where they have interpreters available.

"The fact sheets, newspaper articles, and public announcements promote immunization in two ways. First, we use articles, fact sheets, and local television shows to disseminate factual information on influenza and to explain why it is important to prevent flu in older adults and others whose health is compromised. The general public hears the message, not just the at-risk group, and we know that informal support networks are an important influence on health behavior. Second, throughout the campaign we advertise where and when the clinics are held each week."

The students began to see how the program activities contributed to the short-term outcome of increasing uptake of flu vaccine and agreed to expand the description of program activities in the logic model drawing. They also agreed to identify some service delivery outcomes, such as the number of clinics to be held at each site.

Millie helped the students to interpret the previous year's clinic statistics and showed Mai how to log on to FluWatch—the Health Canada influenza Web site—to compare regional statistics with provincial and national statistics. The incidence had been lower than that during in the previous year across the country. Mai followed the links to the World Health Organization (WHO) FluLine and was excited to find so much information with so little effort. The FluLine tabulated weekly influenza statistics from around the world, identified the causal agents, plotted the outbreaks on a world map, and allowed a comparison of rates between regions and countries and against the rates for previous years.

At the end of their second day in the program, the students agreed that they had completed the first five steps of the community health nursing process and were ready to start thinking about program evaluation for the planning meeting next week. Before the meeting, though, they want to see the flu clinics in action.

Millie says, "You can visit the Sunnyside health clinic any time—I told the nurses to expect you." They decide to visit Sunnyside together and then each will go to another site. Mai will attend the clinic at the seniors' center and Fadma will go to the Italian resource center.

Evaluation of community health programs

Program evaluation is the systematic inquiry to generate information about a program that will be used to guide decision making (Porteous et al., 1997). Evaluation shares some common features with research, such as the careful framing of the questions and the methodical approach to seeking answers. However, rather than seeking to create new knowledge—which is the hallmark of research—program evaluation has a more practical orientation and seeks information to guide program development. It addresses the following questions (Health Canada, 1996):

1. Did we do what we said we would do?
2. What did we learn about what worked and what did not work?
3. What difference did we make?
4. What could we do differently?
5. How do we plan to use evaluation findings for continuous learning?

Program evaluation used to be seen more as a specialist activity carried out by program evaluators and researchers, following strict scientific method. More recent writings caution against trying to impose evaluation strategies and methods suitable for quantitative sciences on community situations (Nutbeam, 1998; Pirie, Stone, Assaf, Flora, & Maschewsky-Schneider, 1994; Rootman, Goodstadt, Potvin, & Springett, 2001).

Natural settings are more complex and difficult to control than laboratories. Many community programs are offered in a range of settings, from health clinics to schools, shopping malls, and homes, where the delivery of health programs is just one of the many activities carried out. Sometimes, several program activities are combined in a way that makes sense for the participants. For example, a resource center might offer a well baby clinic and include a session on parenting (family health program) and offer immunization (infection control program), free milk, and access to a food bank (food security program), all at the same time. This makes it difficult to isolate cause and effect.

Currently, more attention is being paid to the context in which community health programs operate, and evaluation is being approached as a collaborative inquiry, conducted as part of program delivery. The recommended approach is to conduct program evaluations in a way that is true to the principles that govern the way the programs are delivered. This means involving stakeholders, adopting empowering processes, and considering the multiple dimensions and time frame of program activities (Love, 1995). All of which adds to the complexity of program evaluation.

Evaluation serves a different purpose at different stages of program development. In the early stages of program implementation, evaluation is concerned with how the program is being delivered. Later on, the focus of evaluation turns to whether the program is achieving the desired results. These types of evaluation are termed process evaluation and outcome evaluation, respectively.

Process evaluation

Process evaluation provides information on progress toward the achievement of the short- and long-term outcomes and permits midcourse adjustments (Israel et al., 1995). Broadly speaking, it answers the question: Are we doing what we said we were going to do? For example, in the TB prevention program described earlier, suppose after 6 weeks of a 12-week series of ESL classes, the program data show the number of students screened at each site ranges from a low of 4 students at site A to a high of 60 students at site Z. Process evaluation might be used to determine: Why is there such a difference? Is the program being offered the same way at all the ESL sites? What factors explain the difference in attendance?

Process evaluation is particularly important in community programs for which the health outcomes are not likely to be observed for many years. Process evaluation helps to distill learning: What is working and why? Such information can be used to improve the way the program is delivered by identifying which aspects of the program can be improved and which aspects can be continued without change (Pirie et al., 1994).

Outcome evaluation

Outcome evaluation examines what change has been brought about as a result of the program. It answers the question: What difference has the program made? Both the immediate effects, such as changes in knowledge, attitudes, or behavior and the longer-term effects such as changes in health status are of interest. The findings from a process evaluation can contribute to outcome evaluation by helping to interpret why the

TABLE 13-2	Types of Evaluation
TYPE OF EVALUATION/ ALTERNATIVE TERMS	**QUESTIONS**
Process evaluation/Formative evaluation	How is the program delivered by the program team to address issues of continuity, coordination, sequencing (Donabedian, 1987)? What activities were provided, where, under what conditions, by whom, to what audience, and with what level of effort? What are the differences between program sites? Who participated—is the program reaching the specified audience? Who does it fail to reach and why? What is the nature of staff-client interaction? What did participants experience—are they satisfied? Which activities worked and which did not? What are the strengths and weaknesses of the program?
Short-term (immediate) outcome evaluation Short-term impact evaluation/ Summative evaluation	What changes occurred in knowledge, attitudes, beliefs and behavior of participants, programs and policies of organizations and governments as a result of the program?
Long-term (ultimate) outcome evaluation/Long-term impact evaluation/Summative evaluation	What changes occurred in health status, morbidity, and mortality as a result of the program?

outcomes were or were not achieved (Israel et al., 1995) and by providing clues to what might be done differently (Health Canada, 1996).

Adapted from the work of Israel and colleagues (1995, p. 368), Table 13-2 compares the different types of evaluation, identifies alternative terms used to describe them, and provides sample questions pertinent to the type of evaluation.

DISCUSSION QUESTIONS

1. Identify potential short-term and long-term outcomes of the following program activities: promotion of alcohol-free high school graduations; Heart Health grocery tours to promote healthy food choices; distribution to physicians' offices of tear-off message pads with a prescription of daily exercise targets.
2. Discuss how the multiple resource center activities described above (well baby clinic, parenting sessions, immunization, free milk, and access to a food bank) might interact to produce a single outcome such as increased immunization.

Conducting a program evaluation

Program evaluation can be broken down into several steps. These steps, listed below, serve to organize the discussion, but it is worth noting that the first three are not entirely independent and do not proceed in a lock-step fashion. Usually there is movement backward and forward, and the evaluation plan is refined in stages. Once the evaluation questions are agreed upon, the plan begins to take on its final form.

- Assemble the evaluation team and clarify the purpose of the evaluation.
- Prepare the evaluation plan.
- Describe the program.
- Determine the evaluation questions.
- Decide on the methods and tools.
- Conduct the evaluation.
- Document the evaluation in an evaluation report.

Assemble team; clarify purpose

More and more, evaluation is considered to be part of the role description of community health nurses (Chambers et al., 1994; Schoenfeld & MacDonald, 2002) and other community health care providers. A team approach helps to bring together those with an interest in the program and the range of skills required to conduct the evaluation. Depending on the scope and complexity of the evaluation, persons with specialist knowledge such as health planners, epidemiologists, and measurement experts may be included in the evaluation team or used as consultants. As with all teamwork, it is important for team members to agree on their roles and responsibilities at the outset.

Bear in mind that evaluation is rooted in values, and members of the evaluation team may have different priorities for what should be evaluated. For example, health providers may want to show the value of their work and let other health providers know which health promotion strategies work with which communities, managers at different levels in the health system require information to make informed decisions about the use of resources, community leaders look for guidance on policy development, academics are interested in developing the body of knowledge of health promotion theory, funding agencies want to know what has been accomplished with project funds, and community members want to know that community health programs are improving health and offer value for money.

Fundamentally, program evaluation is about making program decisions, so it is helpful to clarify at the outset the general nature of the decisions to be made and when the results are expected. This may seem obvious, but it is easy to assume that everyone has the same agenda when they do not. The initial, broad direction will probably come from the program manager or a program steering group. Knowing whether the main purpose of the evaluation is to improve program delivery, provide evidence of cost effectiveness, or determine whether or not to continue to offer a program provides a context for the inquiry and gives a sense of the intended scope of the evaluation. An explicit agenda, even if it holds the prospect of program closure, can be used to build cooperation. In addition, it is helpful to confirm the level of management support for conducting the evaluation and determine what resources are available. Bear in mind that as planning proceeds, some of the evaluation parameters may change.

Prepare evaluation plan

Once the broad purpose and scope of the evaluation is established and the evaluation team is assembled, the next step is to develop the evaluation plan. The plan provides a blueprint

TABLE 13-3	Evaluation Plan	
TASK	**EVALUATOR(S)**	**WHEN**
Assemble evaluation team, clarify the purpose of the evaluation (including budget).	Evaluation team leader	September 10
Prepare the evaluation plan.	Evaluation team leader with team input	September 10
Describe the program.	Team members	September 16
Determine what questions the evaluation will answer.	Team	September 30
Identify key stakeholders.	Team	September 30
Interview stakeholders.	Team member	October
Define the methods and tools.	Team members	October
Conduct the evaluation.	Team	November
Write the report.	Team members	December 1–14
Present results.	Team members	December 18

for conducting the evaluation. It lays out the main tasks, sets timelines, and allocates resources. Often the plan is developed as a working document, starting with a skeleton outline of the main tasks, which are then elaborated on. A simple format is shown in Table 13-3. As you can see, the process is similar to that provided in the time line and Gantt chart in Chapters 6 and 7. When student projects are integrated into a larger program evaluation, the project team will contribute to the team plan but will also need to maintain a project plan.

Describe the program

A current program description is essential for program evaluation. As discussed earlier, a program logic model may have been developed as part of program planning but programs can drift away from their original form and some elements are planned but never implemented for various reasons. Lack of funds, a change in priorities, and timing conflicts are among the possible explanations. Given the settings in which community programs operate, variations from the plan are not unexpected. Before an evaluation is started, it is important to ensure that the logic model reflects the program being delivered and describes what is really happening rather than what the program should ideally look like. At this point, it helps to have someone who is not intimately involved in the program asking questions and seeking clarification. If necessary, the program logic model can be redrawn until there is consensus that it accurately captures reality.

Determine questions to be answered

After the program logic model is established as the framework for the evaluation, the next step is to determine the specific questions the evaluation will answer about the program activities and/or outcomes. What kinds of information are needed to aid decision making now?

Obtain stakeholder input

There is growing recognition of the importance of involving multiple stakeholders in all phases of program development, including program evaluation (Israel et al., 1995). Stakeholders may be internal or external to your organization. Examples of internal stakeholders are program staff, the program manager, health planners, and senior managers. External stakeholders include steering committees, boards of health, agencies with similar or related programs, program participants, and volunteers.

Many different levels of input are possible. At one end of the spectrum, stakeholders can merely be asked what questions they would like answered. This input can be obtained equally well through key informant interviews, surveys, or possibly a group meeting. At the other end of the spectrum, multiple stakeholders can be directly involved in all phases of the evaluation, including the design, conduct, and writing of the report. The more participatory the approach, the more likely it is that the evaluation will meet the information needs of all stakeholders. The time and resources required, as well as the strengths and weaknesses of the various approaches, need to be considered. (It may be useful to review the section on key informant interviewing in Chapter 4 at this point.) Participatory approaches tend to take a longer time because of the high level of interaction required.

Porteous and colleagues (1997) cautioned that for an evaluation to be useful, it is better to focus on the needs of key users. While acknowledging that program evaluation, especially of mandated programs tends to be dominated by professional interests, evaluators are well advised to remember that program decisions are best made in collaboration with the community (Nutbeam, 1998; Rootman et al., 2001).

Synthesize stakeholder feedback; agree on evaluation questions

As with any data, the input from stakeholders must be collated and summarized for analysis. One way to do this is to use the program logic model as a guide and organize the feedback in relation to the elements of the model, i.e., by specific program activities and short-term and long-term outcomes. Evaluation questions for each element can then be determined.

For example, all of the following concerns expressed about the TB-prevention program discussed earlier relate to program activities and the way the program is being offered across the sites:

1. Program manager, program staff, volunteers, and ESL students say many clinics are being canceled at two sites because the clinic space is needed for other activities.
2. All stakeholders say that the number of students attending the clinic is too many for one nurse. The ESL students say there is not enough time to complete the testing before class or during breaks.

3. Two female students tell the interviewer that in their culture it is not considered appropriate for women to receive health care from men. They say when the clinic is run by a male nurse, women will not attend.

4. Many participants report, "Some clinics are very busy and others are empty."

The final selection of the evaluation questions rests with the evaluation team and may involve some negotiation. Explicit criteria can be used to decide which questions have the highest priority. For example, one approach would be to set priorities based on the relevance of the information to immediate decision-making needs and the importance of the question to more than one stakeholder. Inevitably, other considerations, such as time and resources, will play a part in the final selection. Once the questions have been decided, then they can be reformulated so that answers can be specific and measurable (see SMART objectives in Chapter 6).

Determine methods and tools

Ask yourself what data is required to answer the questions and where the data can be obtained—who has the information. Then determine the most appropriate method for data collection and identify specific instruments. Using the worksheet in Table 13-4 as an example, you can see that the first question to be answered is: Were the scheduled TB screening clinics in ESL classes implemented as planned across the city? The evaluators will consider that this activity has been carried out successfully if 90% of the clinics are held as scheduled. The question will be answered by auditing clinic site records to determine which scheduled clinics were held and which were canceled. The clinic nurse holds the records. The percentage of canceled clinics can then be calculated for each site and the percentages for the sites can be compared.

TABLE 13-4	Worksheet for Success Indicators			
QUESTION	**PLANNED PROJECT ACTIVITY**	**INDICATOR OF SUCCESS**	**EVALUATION TOOL**	**WHO HAS THE INFORMATION**
Were the clinics implemented as planned across the city?	Scheduled clinics held across the city, in ESL classes TB screening	90% of clinics were held as scheduled 75% of students were screened	Audit of clinic records	Program staff
How were barriers to access addressed?	Barriers to clinic access are identified and, where possible removed	List of barriers, compiled, efforts to eliminate described and degree of success identified	Audit of "barriers list" Observation checklist to identify barriers	Program staff Independent observer

DISCUSSION QUESTIONS

1. Why is it important to use the "program as delivered" rather than the "program as planned" as the basis for an evaluation?
2. Identify three strategies to increase the involvement of specified populations in the process evaluation of the program activities listed above.
3. Discuss the advantages and disadvantages of community involvement in program evaluation.

INFECTIOUS DISEASE CONTROL: INFLUENZA PREVENTION FOR OLDER ADULTS SCENARIO (continued)

The students eagerly discuss their experience at the flu clinics. The first clinic, which they attended together, was quiet so they were able to observe several immunizations. They also had time to talk to the clients and ask questions of the clinic nurse. Mai had a similar experience at the seniors' clinic. In contrast, only two older women attended the Italian Resource Center clinic but neither was Italian. The clinic nurse told Fadma this low attendance was the norm.

The students met with Cora, the program manager to discuss their project. She explained that the flu program has stable funding, but it is not sufficient to cover the anticipated increase in the older adult population specified by the program. She expects that the evaluation will help to identify ways in which the program can make the best use of current resources.

An evaluation group, which has already been set up, will meet next week to develop the evaluation plan. Tentatively, Cora determines that the students' role will be to assist Millie in preparing the program logic model for that meeting, conduct the stakeholder interviews, and report back to the evaluation team. Depending on progress, they may have time to conduct a small part of the evaluation—the exact focus will be decided in collaboration with the evaluation team once the evaluation questions are agreed on.

Mai and Fadma identify the main stakeholders for the influenza prevention program. They include the community health centers, ethnic groups, and the three specific groups: older adults, persons with chronic disease, and health providers. Millie points out that all are represented on the steering group. They decided to randomly choose one person from each category of stakeholder. Millie provides the contact information to set up interviews.

The students ask interviewees what questions should be addressed by the evaluation and tabulated the answers (Table 13-5).

When the evaluation team reviewed the input, there was consensus that the priority for the evaluation was to determine whether the flu clinics were being implemented as planned across the sites and whether they were reaching the specified group. Four questions were composed, indicators of success were defined, evaluation tools were identified, and the source of the data was noted (Table 13-6).

The evaluation team decided, in consultation with Mai and Fadma, that the students should complete an observation study of the screening clinics to identify facilitators and barriers. With input from team leader Millie, the students developed a workplan to guide their part of the evaluation. The main items are the following:

1. Adapt the clinic checklist (Application 13-1) for observation of the flu clinics (week 6).
2. Select 25% of clinics (ten) and schedule two observation periods at each, as agreed on with the evaluation team (week 6).
3. Conduct four interviews to establish interobserver agreement; Millie, a program volunteer on the evaluation team, Mai, and Fadma each to do three of the interviews. Discuss areas of disagreement to resolve differences (weeks 6 and 7).
4. Conduct observations (weeks 7 through 9).
5. Summarize observations from all sites on an enlarged observation sheet (weeks 9 and 10).
6. Identify barriers to access and cluster by themes, e.g., transportation and parking, hours of operations, or language of service (week 10).

| TABLE 13-5 | Inventory of Stakeholder Questions |

INTERVIEWEE	QUESTIONS AND OBSERVATIONS
Program manager	"According to program staff, the Monday evening clinics are always quiet. I am wondering if we should eliminate that clinic altogether or increase staff another evening." "I would like to know who is attending the clinics. Are we reaching the right group?"
Program staff	"Clinics at the health center are working well. We are getting a lot of older adults we have never seen before. I wish there was more time to talk. The other day, an older man came in. He was very quiet and had soup stains on his shirt. I intended to talk to him, but the clinic was full and he left before I had a chance." "Clinics at the resource center had to be canceled because of other activities going on." "We need more staff at the evening clinics." "Some of the clinics are combined with a drop-in clinic. Usually this is not a problem, but it is difficult to keep track of people when there are many drop-in patients."
Community partner	"There is limited parking at the seniors' center; we get a lot of complaints about this."
Volunteer	"Some clinics are very quiet—no-one there; others are so busy you feel exhausted when you get home." "The handout does not say anything about side effects. A lot of people ask me if they are likely to get mild flu symptoms with the injection."
Participant	"The clinic is convenient, but several women said they had to wait a long time; the clinic is at 6:30 p.m., when they usually eat an evening meal." "The parking is too far from the center; my mother-in-law uses a walker and it tired her to walk so far."

7. Prepare three overheads (methods, overview of clinic sample, and results) for brief (5 to 10 minute) presentation at evaluation meeting (week 11).
8. Write section of evaluation report, incorporating comments from evaluation team (week 11 and 12).
9. Attend debriefing of evaluation team, program team, and project team (week 12).

Determine tools: Observation for collecting data

Between-site variation in program delivery can have a bearing on overall program success. One way of gathering information about possible site differences is to observe and compare activities across sites. Observational data can be used to complement data gathered using other data collection methods, but it can also provide unique insights. For example, through observation, key differences in the physical and social environment and in the clinical context can be identified. The value of the approach is that it does not disturb the natural order of things; life can go on just as it does every day. As a result, the observer has access to what people say and do, which may be different from what they think they say or do. Also, some activities become so ritualized that people perform them without thinking or questioning the need; these habitual activities may be difficult to recall as significant. Without being obtrusive, the observer can view experiences in context, learn what is typical and what is not, and gain insight into what the experience means to people in the place where it happens (Hammersley & Atkinson, 1995; Patton, 1990).

TABLE 13-6	Worksheet for Success Indicators for Flu Clinic Evaluation			
QUESTION	**PROJECT ACTIVITY**	**INDICATOR OF SUCCESS**	**EVALUATION TOOL**	**WHO HAS THE INFORMATION**
Were activities implemented as planned (how many clinics were held, where)?	Scheduled influenza clinics held across the city, in CHCs, seniors centers and resources centers	90% of clinics were held as scheduled	Audit of Project records	Program staff
What are the barriers and facilitators of accessibility?		Barriers and facilitators are identified	Observation checklist	
Were participants satisfied with the program?		At least 50% of participants are satisfied with the service	Satisfaction questionnaire	Specified group
How many people in the specified group have the clinics reached? How many people outside the specified group were reached?		More than 60% of clinic attendees are in the specified group	Audit of project records	Program staff

Observation and description are the first steps in understanding a phenomenon. Things have to be described before they can be measured. Gathering observational data is integral to nursing practice, and the same skills can be applied in collecting observational data for the purpose of evaluating community programs. The approach to observation can be more or less structured, depending on how much is known about the subject of interest. Less structure is an advantage if little is known. However, it is impossible to observe everything when in a natural setting, so it is helpful to have some organizing framework in mind. Patton (1990) identified some options for organizing observations:

- Chronology: Describe events as they happen in time. For example, describe interactions with staff from the time a person enters a clinic setting to the time he or she leaves.
- Key events: Record critical events (e.g., unusual or unexpected events, or events that exceed or do not meet expectations).
- Setting: Describe the physical and social aspects of the environment.
- People: Describe the people and what they say and do, including their nonverbal behaviors.
- Processes: Make note of the key processes that happen in the setting (e.g., for clients in the clinic setting: registration at the clinic, waiting for appointments, and booking another appointment).
- Issues: Questions arising from reflection on the observations.

Another approach is to start with sensitizing concepts. These are concepts known to be fundamental to the issue of concern. For example, the previous discussion on the TB prevention logic model has identified the crucial role of screening. This sensitizes the observer to looking for factors that support or prevent screening at the sites. The factors can be specified in more detail once their salience is confirmed. This type of flexibility in approach is an advantage to using observation as a data collection technique (Patton, 1990). A more structured approach to observation entails the use of an observation checklist. The checklist helps to keep track of observations and promotes a consistent approach, thus enabling comparison. Items on the checklist can be precoded to indicate what response is expected, for example, a yes or no. This is particularly useful when the key variables are already well known. An advantage of using a checklist is that it helps to minimize the degree of inference required by the observer. A disadvantage is the lack of flexibility. Combining a checklist and unstructured observations can remedy this and allow the observer to add items to the list for systematic observation.

A sample checklist, developed to assess the barriers to clinic access, is shown in Application 13-1. The checklist is structured to enter observations from the perspective of a clinic participant, starting with the approach to the clinic. Attached to the checklist you will find a list of tips to help you obtain reliable information.

Conduct evaluation, analyze data, summarize findings

The process is similar to that described in Chapters 6, 7, and 8. For example, if you are collecting observation data with the observation checklist in Application 13-1, use a blank checklist to summarize observations and make comparisons across the settings. Highlight barriers and facilitators and note their frequency, e.g., all clinics offer free parking; only one clinic offers services in French. Another analytical strategy might be to develop a profile of a barrier-free clinic and compare the profiles of other clinics to this one. Whatever the analytical approach, it is important to remember that each set of data collected—observations, audits, and interviews—must be analyzed and synthesized in the final report.

DISCUSSION QUESTIONS

1. Discuss factors that might interfere with the quality of observational data gathered at a screening clinic.
2. How would you measure the success of activities to build the support networks of students attending ESL classes?
3. How might you explain a program logic model to program volunteers?

Summary

It is difficult to grasp all the ramifications of a community health program. Participating in a program evaluation challenges all those involved with a program to pool their wits and work together to provide the information that is necessary to guide decision making. Program logic models are a useful tool. They help evaluators to comprehend the program activities, explain how they work together, and determine whether or not they are successful in bringing about changes that are likely to have an impact on health. Developing the tools and skills for program evaluation is an important part of community health nursing practice.

PRACTICE AND APPLICATION

1. Read the article on tuberculosis in immigrants in Canada (Cowie et al., 2002). Identify the values underlying the proposed solution for eradicating tuberculosis in Canada.

2. Debate the proposal: The decision to immunize children against measles should be left up to parents.

3. Many agencies offer prenatal programs. Working in groups of three, use the questions at the beginning of the chapter to interview program staff. Use the information to draw a program logic model. Compare similarities and differences between the programs.

4. Develop a work plan to conduct an observation study of the appropriate installation of car seats after a workshop attended by two groups of 30 parents.

REFERENCES

Chambers, L. W., Underwood, J., Halbert, T., Woodward, C. A., Heale, J., & Isaacs, S. (1994). 1992 Ontario survey of public health nurses: Perceptions of roles and activities. *Canadian Journal of Public Health, 85*(3), 175-179.

Chang, S., Wheeler, L. S. M., & Farrell, K. P. (2002). Public health impact of targeted tuberculosis screening in public schools. *American Journal of Public Health, 92*(12), 1942-1945.

Chaulk, C. P., Moore-Rice, K., Rizzo, R., & Chaisson, R. E. (1995). Eleven years of community-based directly observed therapy for tuberculosis. *Journal of the American Medical Association, 274*, 945-951.

Cowie, R. L., Field, S. K., & Enarson, D. A. (2002). Tuberculosis in immigrants to Canada: A global problem which requires a global solution. *Canadian Journal of Public Health, 93*(2), 85-86.

Donabedian, A. (1987). *Some basic issues in evaluating the quality of health care.* New York: National League for Nursing.

Hammersley, M., & Atkinson, P. (1995). *Ethnography: Principles in practice* (2nd ed.). London: Routledge.

Health Canada. (1996, 2002-11-29 (Revised: April 17, 2000)). *Guide to project evaluation: A participatory approach.* Retrieved April 6, 2003, from http://www.hc-sc.gc.ca/hppb/phdd/resources/guide/introduction.htm.

Health Canada. (2004, 2004-06-04). *FluWatch.* Retrieved June 11, 2004 from http://www.hc-sc.gc.ca/pphb-dgspsp/fluwatch/index.html.

Israel, B. A., Cummings, K. M., Dignan, M. B., Heaney, C. A., Perales, D. P., Simons-Morton, B. G., et al. (1995). Evaluation of health education programs: Current assessment and future direction. *Health Education Quarterly, 22*, 364.

Love, A. J. (1995). *Evaluation Methods Sourcebook II.* Ottawa, Ontario: Canadian Evaluation Society.

Moyer, A., Verhovsek, H., & Wilson, V. (1997). Facilitating the shift to population-based public health programs: Innovation through the use of framework and logic models. *Canadian Journal of Public Health, 88*(95), 98.

Nutbeam, D. (1998). Evaluating health promotion-progress, problems and solutions. *Health Promotion International, 13*(1), 27.

Ontario Ministry of Health, P. H. B. (1997). *Mandatory health programs and services guidelines* Retrieved April 4, 2004 from www.health.gov.on.ca.

Patton, M. Q. (1990). *Qualitative evaluation and research methods* (2nd ed.). Newbury Park, CA: Sage.

Pirie, P. L., Stone, E. J., Assaf, A. R., Flora, J. A., & Maschewsky-Schneider, U. (1994). Program evaluation strategies for community-based health promotion programs: Perspectives from the cardiovascular disease community research and demonstration studies. *Health Education Research, 9*(1), 23.

Porteous, N. L., Sheldrick, B. J., & Stewart, P. (1997). *Program evaluation toolkit: A blueprint for public health management.* Ottawa, Ontario: Ottawa-Carleton Health Department, Public Health Research, Education and Development Program.

Rootman, I., Goodstadt, M., Potvin, L., & Springett, J. (2001). A framework for health promotion evaluation. In I. Rootman, M. Goodstadt, B. Hyndman, D. V. McQueen, L. Potvin, J. Springett & E. Ziglio (Eds.), *Evaluation in health promotion: Principles and perspectives.* Geneva, Switzerland: World Health Organization.

Schoenfeld, B., M., & MacDonald, M. B. (2002). Saskatchewan public health nursing survey: Perceptions of roles and activities. *Canadian Journal of Public Health, 93*(6), 452-456.

Uppaluri, A., Naus, M., Heywood, N., Brunton, J., Kerbel, D., & Wobeser, W. (2002). Effectiveness of the immigration medical surveillance program for tuberculosis in Ontario. *Canadian Journal of Public Health, 93*(2), 88-91.

Wong-Reiger, D., & David, L. (1995). Using program logic models to plan and evaluate education and prevention programs. In A. J. Love (Ed.), *Evaluation methods sourcebook II* (pp. 120-135). Ottawa, Ontario: Canadian Evaluation Society.

World Health Organization. (2002, 26-Nov-2002). *The cold chain.* Retrieved June 8, 2004, from http://www.who.int/vaccines-access/vacman/coldchain/the_cold_chain.htm.

WEB SITE RESOURCES

The Health Communication Unit at the Center for Health Promotion, University of Toronto: *Evaluating health promotion programs.* Available at http://www.thcu.ca/infoandresources/evaluation.htm.

World Health Organization FluNet: http://rhone.b3e.jussieu.fr/flunet/www.

World Health Organization Fact Sheet on Influenza: http://www.who.int/mediacentre/factsheets/2003/fs211/en/

APPLICATION 13-1

CLINIC—OBSERVATIONAL ASSESSMENT

Observation Date/Time (ddmmyy/start and stop time):_____ Observer

Clinic Name	Sunnyside CHC Clinic #1	Sunnyside CHC Golden Age Club Clinic #2	William Street Community Center	Family Medicine Center
Location	212 42nd Street East	Corner of 5th Avenue & Market Street	9 William Street	Corner Main & 2nd Avenue
Accessibility				
Parking available —Yes/no —Cost/hour				

(continued)

Transport nearby —Bus stop —Subway stop				
Building signs —Yes/no				
Wheelchair access —Yes/no				
Waiting Area				
—Seating available				
—Average waiting time				
—Educational matter on display related to clinic focus, e.g., flu posters and pamphlets				
Language spoken —English —French —Other				
Staffing Numbers —Nurses —Volunteers				
Observations				
Clinic Operations				
—Days/hours of week				
Appointment system —Yes/no				
Attendance Record (previous month)				
—Average per clinic —Largest attendance —Smallest attendance —Total clients				
Number of clinics cancelled per month				

Tips for making reliable observations

1. Try to minimize your impact on the setting. Let people get used to your presence before the observation starts. Remember, the presence of an observer may have an impact on behavior. Think about the impact of a police car parked on the side of the road—people slow down and do things "by the book" to show themselves in the best light.
2. Spend enough time in the setting to differentiate the typical from the atypical.
3. Vary observations with regard to people, place, and time; try to capture the full range of possibilities, e.g., do not always observe the same person at the same time each day.
4. Weigh the advantages and disadvantages of staying in one location or moving around. With the former, you can blend into the background; with the latter you can choose to focus on particular events.
5. Schedule observations for manageable periods of time to avoid fatigue, e.g., 10 minutes on and 10 minutes off. What we see, what we attend to, is influenced by our expectations, by our emotions, and by our physical state.
6. Collaborate with another observer to avoid selectivity and bias; check that your observations are in agreement.
7. Clarify the need for ethical clearance. Generally speaking, conducting observations at clinical sites does not present ethical issues any different from those that might arise in the course of clinical practice. However, health provider–client interactions are considered confidential, and observations for the purpose of evaluation may require informed consent.
8. Think about how you will respond if you are asked to help out at the clinic when it gets busy during your observation period.

14

Using the Community Health Nursing Process in Practice

ELIZABETH DIEM

TWO YEARS AFTER THE FINAL PRESENTATION (continued from Chapter 1)

Two years ago, Ellen and Fatima were baccalaureate nursing students, Khiem had completed his degree the previous year after working for several years in the emergency department of a hospital, and Maria had just graduated from another nursing program. They had come together originally to gain experience in community health nursing by working on a project at a community health center (see Chapter 1). Now they were together again as participants in a study on community health nursing education. (Note: During the project, all four closely followed the community health nursing process described in this text.)

The purpose of the present study is to determine what influence their participation in the community health nursing project had on their beginning practice in the community. In preparation for their focus group with the researcher, they were asked to review the description of their project (Chapter 1), their project report, and the questions that would be used in the focus group. The focus group questions were the following:

1. Give an overview of your present practice including the organization for which you work, population served, teamwork, and satisfaction.
2. Describe a situation that you found challenging in your practice and explain what influence, if any, the project had on your approach to the situation in terms of a) assessment, b) planning, c) taking action, and d) evaluation.
3. What are your future plans?

The researcher, Dana, explained that the subparts of question 2 could be divided up among the team members. After giving them this direction, Dana left the meeting room to allow the team time to discuss among themselves what they would like to do.

Khiem jumped right in by saying, "I like the idea of dividing it. Otherwise we could go on forever. What do the rest of you think?"

"Yes, I agree," stated Ellen. "I know that I have lots to say about each of them. It doesn't matter to me which one I address."

"Well, I didn't think that I would have anything to say because I haven't been working in community health nursing," declared Fatima, "but I have been making waves! I would like to talk about taking action."

Maria said that she wanted to talk about planning, and Khiem preferred assessment.

Ellen summarized by stating, "Well, we haven't changed. We can still work things out together. I'll take evaluation. I'm looking forward to hearing what everyone has been doing for the last two years. Imagine, Fatima making waves!"

OBJECTIVES   **After reading this chapter and answering the questions throughout the chapter, you should be able to**

1. Reflect on practice to identify the steps in the community health nursing process.
2. Compare the skills, knowledge, and abilities learned during the community health nursing process with projects needed in practice.
3. Identify the skills, knowledge, and abilities learned during work on projects that can be transferred to other areas of nursing.
4. Determine the influence of teamwork, collaboration, Primary Health Care, determinants of health, and working at multiple levels on community health nursing practice.

KEYWORDS   **community health representatives (CHRs)** ■ **emergency measures organization** ■ **transferable skills** ■ **triage**

Using the community health nursing process in practice

The emphasis of this text has been on using the community health nursing process to work as a team and collaboratively with community members to complete a project that is relevant to them. A project is defined as a time-limited, team task to accomplish a specified goal and objectives. The main purpose of the text is to encourage the development of the skills, knowledge, and abilities needed in community health nursing practice by working on a project. In this chapter, situations from practice are analyzed to identify the principles of Primary Health Care and how the skills, knowledge, and abilities learned during the project are transferred to practice.

In practice, projects may not be clearly defined from the beginning or people may not be designated as team members. One community health nurse may identify an issue and start working on it; a manager may ask for preliminary work on an issue; or a policy, services, or funding may be changed and require a team of people to take action. Professional nursing organizations can also decide to take action on an issue.

Although the situations or issues may differ in practice, the community health nursing process provides a framework and direction to take action to make a difference in the health of people in the community. The use of the community health nursing process provides both process measures, such as the number of activities completed or people seen, and outcome measures, such as the reduction of illness and disability, and increases in health and well-being to keep practice in line with the health needs of community groups.

Because this chapter is focusing on practice, a scenario from practice will precede the discussion of the transferable skills, knowledge, and ability during the four generic stages of the community health nursing process: assess, plan, take action, and evaluate.

TWO YEARS AFTER THE FINAL PRESENTATION ASSESSMENT SCENARIO

Dana, the researcher, asked Khiem to give an overview and describe a challenging situation in his present practice. Khiem began, "Soon after we finished our project, I applied and was accepted for a position in a nursing station serving a First Nation community in the north. As you know, I had been working in the hospital emergency department for several years and managed to get my degree part time. I am good at my job. I didn't want to lose that, but could see that what I was doing was 'downstream,' rescuing people when they were ill rather that working with them to stay healthy. I wanted a nursing position where I could make use of my degree, use my skills in emergency nursing, and work with community members. Outpost nursing would give me that opportunity. I chose the north because I enjoy the wilderness: the quiet, the lakes, rivers, and endless bush. I also have to admit that I love fishing.

"In the nursing station, which is funded by the federal government, I worked with two female nurses to provide treatment in medical clinics, and health promotion and disease prevention in the school. For the first six months that I was there, I was scrambling to get used to making decisions largely on my own without the backup of a medical team.

"The clinic was available for emergencies '24/7,' and we all had to share in being on call. I found most of my time being taken up with treatment. It was difficult finding time for health promotion, let alone community capacity building. Also, I realize now that I was experiencing culture shock both in dealing with the First Nations people and living in an isolated community.

"It took me a while to identify the differences in culture and understand how culture affects the health of the community. The challenging experience that I had involves smoking. I noticed what seemed like a high number of children with asthma and respiratory infections. I did a quick chart review for all patients seen in two different weeks in January and February, and my suspicions were confirmed. Because one of the factors contributing to these conditions is second-hand smoke, I asked the parents if they smoked, but they were not willing to talk about it. My nursing colleagues were aware of a high number of smoking-related diseases, but felt that trying to take action on smoking would turn people away.

"I started talking to an older fellow who was one of the **community health representatives (CHRs)** working at the nursing station. A CHR is usually a band member who has received some government sponsored training in the medical and social aspects of health. He told me that tobacco was an important part of traditional ceremonies and, therefore, had a strong cultural significance. I also struck up a friendship with some young men and went fishing with them. Literally everyone smoked but me. They took smoking for granted. Throughout the community, I realized that there were no restrictions on smoking except in the nursing station, school, and church. At the band council meetings, dances, and gatherings everyone smokes.

"Knowing the dangers of smoking, I felt that I should say something, but did not know what. I realized that possibly because I was male, was Vietnamese, and went fishing with them, the men were more willing to explain things to me. However, they were very angry at 'white men' for things that had been imposed on them in the past, such as sending their parents to residential schools. They felt that they had a right to smoke, especially because it was part of their heritage.

"I wasn't prepared to give up on trying to reduce tobacco use, but I knew that I had to find a process that would work. I had access to the Internet and found a study on the health status of Aboriginal, First Nations, and Inuit people (Health Canada, 1999) that confirmed everything I was noticing in my practice. For example, the study reported a smoking rate of 62%, which is more than twice the national average for the same time period. The study found that children started smoking as early as age 6, and pregnant First Nations women, in at least one province, had a higher rate of smoking than pregnant women elsewhere. Children had twice the rate of bronchitis and a slightly higher rate of asthma than other Canadian children.

"The First Nations and Inuit people study (Health Canada, 1999) was organized according to the determinants of health and indicated how much the determinants, especially the poor socioeconomic environment, affected the subjects' health. Although I wasn't able to directly address unemployment, low education, or poverty, I could work with the people in my community to let them know how environmental tobacco smoke affected the health of their children. Although all cultures care for their children, I noticed that the community, even young men, showed great care and concern for children. I also learned that I had to work with the people on their time schedule.

"I started with one family who was very concerned about their 4-year-old daughter who had asthma. The girl was constantly being brought into the nursing station in respiratory distress. So far, the nurses had not given the girl's mother any suggestions on how to improve the situation. Apparently that is not unusual. In my review, I came across two studies that described the encounters of First Nations women with mainstream healthcare professionals as racist, discriminatory, and inadequate (Browne & Fiske, 2001; Sokoloski, 1995). I do not like to be critical of my colleagues, but I found that many concentrated on tasks rather than trying to understand situations.

"When I asked the First Nations woman about smoking in her family, she stated that practically everyone in the family smoked, even the older children. After I explained to her that reducing smoke in the house would probably reduce the occurrence of asthma attacks, she was ready to start working on getting her family to smoke outside.

"We decided to use a calendar to show the number of times the girl had been to the nursing station over the previous year. The woman told the family that she wanted everyone to smoke outside. Thank goodness it was summer! She kept marking the calendar with the girl's emergency visits to the nursing station and could show her family how the number of visits was decreasing since they were smoking outside. This woman has become my ally: She has organized a women's group and helped with a presentation to the band council. That presentation didn't go too well. They listened to us politely and said that they wanted a copy of the national study, but that was it for them. I suppose I shouldn't have been surprised. Often in the north, communities on and off reserves are male-dominated and have other concerns than meeting the needs of women and children (Leipert, 1999). On the other hand, the families with children are starting to listen to us."

Dana then asked Khiem, "What specific aspects of your previous project have influenced your present practice, particularly related to assessment?" Khiem responded, "In reflecting about my experience, I realize that I followed all the steps of the assessment process and the principles of Primary Health Care. I must have learned it well or it is a logical process. I reviewed the demographic and epidemiologic data and made sure that I was informed about the effects of smoking. At the same time, I learned about the community by observing and asking questions about their lives and concerns. I realized that changing smoking behavior would be a real challenge in a community in which the majority of members smoke.

"When we worked on the original project, we really learned about the importance of collaboration with the women in the community. I found that learning to collaborate is a transferable skill, because I have been able to apply that skill in my present practice. I looked at the issue from the perspective of the community members and worked with them rather than trying to impose a solution. I talked with the mother of the girl with asthma to find out how I could support her in getting her family to smoke outside. She suggested using the calendar. I also realized from the project that community action can start with one person or a few people and will build up to groups and the community if they believe that the action will benefit them or their families. I found during the previous project that some people, particularly managers, like to have numbers or figures related to health status; others just want to see the benefit to their family. On the reserve, the band council wanted the figures about the smoking rates from the national study, and the women wanted to hear how the 4-year-old girl did not need to go to the nursing station as much now that the family wasn't smoking inside. I have enjoyed observing how the thinking is changing in the community.

"The importance of culture was really reinforced. In our project two years ago we worked with women from many different cultures who spoke different languages. At first I didn't think that culture was a big issue in the native community because most people, except the elders, spoke English. It was only when I met such resistance when talking about smoking and learned about the resentment against 'the white man,' especially those from the south, that I realized that I needed to take the culture into account if I wanted to have any influence."

Assessment in practice

In this practice situation, Khiem took an issue that he identified from his practice in the nursing station and started to work on it. He definitely wanted to move more into illness prevention and health promotion and away from a focus on the treatment of disease.

His knowledge and skill were displayed in knowing and using the steps in collaborative assessment in the community health nursing process. He had the ability to form a relationship with people in the community so he could learn what was important to them and they would work with him. From his analysis of the secondary assessment data from the individual and community levels, he decided that the best approach was to start small with an issue that was important to the community—children's health—rather than with the issue of smoking.

The choice of an issue is also affected by gender. Often in small northern and resource-based communities, men control the decisions (Leipert, 1999) such as smoking by-laws. In most cultures, issues related to health and children are usually in the women's domain. Recognizing this situation, he framed the issue in terms of a smoke-free home for an asthmatic child. In that way Khiem was able to support the mother's and family's concern for the child and work with them to start changing ideas about smoking within the broader community.

Although Khiem mentioned the band council, he did not mention other organizations or professionals in the community. For example, a highly respected teacher, priest, or minister could work with the women's group. That intersectoral collaboration could help to increase awareness in the community.

Although nursing services were available "24/7," the community did not have access to health practitioners familiar with their culture. By working with the community on reducing children's exposure to smoke, Khiem was also demonstrating how to work within cultural beliefs (Houston, 2002) and hopefully increasing the desire of his colleagues to do the same (Campinha-Bacote, 2003). This aspect of accessibility is particularly important in promoting the health of groups with a culture different from that of the healthcare practitioners.

Khiem demonstrated through his description and reflection how he was able to use his experience with the project and incorporate most of the principles of Primary Health Care in his practice.

DISCUSSION QUESTIONS

1. What other practice situations can you think of in which the ability of practitioners to work on health promotion or illness prevention can be greatly hampered by a lack of cultural competence?
2. Are you aware of practice situations for which poor outcomes were the result of a superficial or narrow assessment?
3. What practice situations would warrant the quick formation of teams to conduct an extensive assessment?
4. Which principles of Primary Health Care are particularly useful in providing direction for a thorough assessment?

TWO YEARS AFTER THE FINAL PRESENTATION PLANNING SCENARIO

Dana, the researcher, asked Maria to explain her practice and why planning was important to her. Maria provided the following account: "If you remember, I had just graduated when I joined the rest of you on the project two years ago. I decided to volunteer for the project at that time because I wanted to get more experience in community development. In my nursing program, we had a short community health clinical experience doing home visits with middle-class mothers of new babies. That really did not give me a sense of how the healthcare system worked or didn't work for people who were vulnerable. Soon after the project, I started working as a home care nurse.

"Most of the people on my caseload are elderly women. I am constantly amazed at how they overcome their limitations. A large part of what I do is to help the women plan and carry out necessary changes to their routines so they can remain in their own homes. Often I help them to connect to resources in the community. This experience has really reinforced the importance of planning. Anyway, on to talking about my situation.

"I was working that evening in August 2003 when the blackout occurred. The office was just swamped with calls. I had my usual clients to see, but I was asked to look in on others in the area. Many were really anxious and didn't have any way of finding out what was happening or how to get help. Some were immobilized on the top floors of apartment buildings. They couldn't get down the stairs. They didn't have any water either.

"I started thinking that everyone should have an emergency kit that included a light and battery or hand-powered radio. The light couldn't be from candles because of the fear of fires and couldn't be too heavy. I also wondered if there was a system for checking on people in emergencies. That was the time when we were also hearing about the thousands of elderly dying of heat stroke in France. That experience made me realize that while I helped my clients plan changes to their lives, I had not given any thought to planning for emergencies.

"A few of us started talking about what should be included in the emergency kit and how a system for identifying vulnerable people could be organized. We did some planning around both ideas, and management heard about it. They had been contacted by the emergency measures association and were asked to identify a representative to work on a team with Public Health to update a system of identifying vulnerable people in the community. Each municipality usually has an **emergency measures organization** to prepare the community to deal with various potential disasters. Well, I became the 'rep.' They liked my idea about the emergency kit and formed a small technical committee to work on identifying safe, lightweight items. They planned to promote the kits as the perfect Christmas gift for grandma or grandpa.

"I spent considerable time planning with the Public Health nurses. In the old disaster plan, the home visiting nurses were expected to report to the hospitals because of their medical and surgical skills. The public health nurses were to triage people in their homes to determine whether they needed to be moved to a shelter. **Triage** is a procedure that sorts people experiencing difficulties into categories according to how quickly they need care. This sounded all right in theory, but although the Public Health nurses were good at organizing, many of them had very little experience doing home visits with the elderly. At the same time, the elderly were reluctant to open a door to someone they didn't know. We are working on a plan that combines Public Health and home visiting nurses into teams to cover geographical areas. It's a lot of work, but it makes the best use of both sets of expertise."

Dana asked Maria, "What specifically have you learned during the project that was useful in your practice?" Maria responded, "Well, it's obvious, isn't it? I don't think I would have thought about the bigger picture if I hadn't done the project. I would just have been killing myself trying to go and look after everyone. In the project, I learned that planning took considerable time and effort but eventually paid off. Back then it took a while to write our goal and objectives so the manager understood them. The same thing happened in the disaster planning. When others questioned us on early drafts of our plan, we were annoyed at first. Then we started joking about how the number of revisions was sharpening our thinking and collaboration. We had decided quite early in the process that the plan had to be based on the KISS principle, 'Keep It Simple, Stupid.' If people didn't understand it or if it was complicated, the disaster plan would be a disaster itself.

"Another thing that has just occurred to me is that I learned about working on a team. There were four of us on the original project, and six of us are working on the disaster plan. In both situations we have come together from different backgrounds and experiences. Because I didn't have previous links with people, I found it fairly easy to speak up immediately when I was not happy. For example, although I didn't know people that well, I challenged the idea in the disaster team that we would take a vote to make decisions. I said that we should discuss things until we had a consensus. I felt that if we couldn't reach a creative solution to differences, what we produced might not be relevant to nurses working in different areas. The rest of the team were quite surprised at my comment, but eventually agreed with me. Both teams that I have worked with have taken time to listen to everyone and made decisions only after everyone had their say. That sometimes has meant extra meetings, but all of us are proud of what was produced."

Planning in practice

When Maria was working with the women before the major blackout, she was working at the individual level and was using a narrow scope on the zoom lens. After the blackout and deaths from heat stroke in Europe, her scope expanded to consider vulnerable people in the community. The broader scope also meant that other decision makers such as Public Health and the emergency measures organizations needed to be included in the disaster planning.

Planning at the community level started with an assessment of the previous plan and the strengths and weaknesses of various options. The plan included a goal and objectives and definitely was a collaborative effort. The only part that was not mentioned was evaluation.

Teamwork was particularly important in both the original project and this scenario. As well as getting their work done, both teams adopted a principle to keep them on track. In the first project the team adopted the guiding principle that they would "work in collaboration with the community women." In the disaster planning project, Maria's team concentrated on keeping the plan simple and straightforward. Other indications of good teamwork in both situations are the use of humor, pride in their work, and recognition of each other's contributions.

A contribution to the success of both teams could be the size and diversity of members. Teams of four to seven are the most likely to provide a positive experience for members (Feichter & Davis, 1984–85) and have a diversity of opinions (if heterogeneous) to produce creative results (Brower, 1996; Watson, Jonahson, & Zgourides, 2002). The results from a team with a diversity of views and experience is also going to be more readily accepted by others.

This scenario is a good example of intersectoral collaboration because emergency measures organizations usually include representatives from ambulance services, hospitals, police, and fire fighters. Presumably the draft plan was reviewed by people in these various sectors to ensure that it was feasible. Important decision makers that are not mentioned are the elderly community members.

The scenario also demonstrates the appropriate use of resources by organizing a team of people with technical expertise to determine the components of the emergency kit. In addition, people with expertise in social marketing would probably prepare material to market the kits.

In practice, planning will not always involve the formal preparation of goals, objectives, and evaluation measures for changes within a brief timeframe or involving few people. However, for most initiatives, the use of all aspects of planning will ensure that community health nurses will produce the desired results.

DISCUSSION QUESTIONS

1. What situations are you aware of for which the appropriate decision makers were not doing the planning?
2. What principle of Primary Health Care is not being applied when the appropriate decision makers are not involved in the planning?
3. Why is it important to develop evaluation measures during planning?

4. What size or composition of teams could compromise the ability of the team to work well together?

TWO YEARS AFTER THE FINAL PRESENTATION TAKING ACTION SCENARIO

Dana, the researcher, asked Fatima what challenges she faced in her practice. Fatima gave the following account:

"Ellen and I graduated six months after we finished the project. I was thrilled to get a job on a maternity floor right after graduation. I have always wanted to work with mothers and infants.

"At work I heard about and joined a regional association of perinatal nurses. I liked the group because it brought together nurses working in Public Health, home health, maternity, and labor and delivery. There also were midwives and lactation consultants. The discussions at meetings kept me informed about what was happening to mothers and infants in the community and in the hospital.

"About a year ago, the word was out that the government was planning to replace home visits to teen mothers with well baby clinics. We were all really angry. The government had cut back the length of time women stayed in the hospital after birth, and now they were taking away individual support for single mothers. I saw these teen mothers in the hospital every day, and they could barely cope with their infants there. Six of us who worked in different areas were asked to draft a resolution that could be used by our professional nursing association to lobby the government against the change. I explained to the group the process we had used in our project, and they decided to follow it. We decided that if we were going to march for women's health, we wanted to have our facts and figures ready!

"Others looked at government policies or talked to nursing leaders in the area. My job was to do a literature search. There was plenty to find. Large-scale, randomized, controlled studies with pregnant women and mothers (Kitzman et al., 1997, 2000; Olds et al., 1997, 1998) consistently found benefits for mothers and their children receiving home visits. The women in the studies had two or more sociodemographic risk factors of being unmarried, unemployed, or having less than 12 years of education. The benefits included a reduction in the number of pregnancies, less use of welfare, less child abuse and neglect, and less criminal behavior (Kitzman et al., 1997, 2000; Olds et al., 1997) and extended to reduced adolescent criminal behavior after 15 years (Olds et al., 1998). These benefits were mainly apparent when the visits were conducted by a nurse rather than a lay home visitor (Olds et al., 2002). A summary of the literature to determine evidence to reduce abuse and neglect of children stated that the strongest evidence was for an intensive program of home visits by nurses that begins prenatally and extends to the second year to first-time mothers with one or more of the following characteristics: age younger than 19, single parent status, and low socioeconomic status (MacMillan & Canadian Task Force on Preventive Health, 2000). A systematic review also found that professional home visits increased exclusive breast feeding by mothers and reduced the incidence of diarrhea (Sikorski, Renfrew, Pindoria, & Wade., 2003). Another review found some evidence that professional or social support was effective in postpartum depression (Ray & Hodnett, 2003).

"The team was really excited by what I found, and I thought that I would be finished. They wouldn't let me! I had to prepare the material to present to the large group and then to our professional association. By this time, the nursing association was forming a nursing task force to advise them during their negotiations with other professional associations, such as Public Health and the medical association and women's groups. They wanted to place concerted pressure on the government.

"Well, I got appointed to that group and worked with nurses from all parts of the province! I really got to build on my presentation skills and learned that I had to speak up to advocate for nursing home visits rather than lay home visiting. I found the courage to speak from knowing that what I found in the literature was reflected in my practice on the maternity floor and in the practice of my colleagues in the community. The task force has prepared a preliminary report and is continuing to collaborate on the full report. So far, the government has not reduced the home visits. We don't know if they will increase the number of nurses doing the home visits.

"It has been an amazing time for me. Two years ago I would not have imagined that I would be working on healthy public policy and speaking up for nursing and low-income women and their children!"

Dana asked Fatima what specifically she had learned during the project that was useful in her practice. Fatima responded, "Well, I already explained that I used my skills in doing a literature search and presentations. More that that, though—which surprised me when I reflected on what has happened—I learned that nursing can only do so much by itself. Each of us can strive to do the best we can with the clients we work with, but so much of the health of people depends on other factors, such as how much money they make or what services are provided by the government. I learned from our project two years ago that the best way to help people was for us to help them help themselves. I saw how their strength and confidence grew as more people were involved. I also learned about the importance of teamwork and working toward a common goal. Those **transferable skills** carried over into collaborating on a regional team.

"As an additional point, I asked the chairperson of our perinatal nursing group recently why I was chosen as one of the representatives. I didn't have the experience of most of the others and didn't have a lot of confidence about speaking in public. She told me that the group was impressed with how clearly I explained and followed through with using the community health nursing process and presented the literature review. Apparently I conveyed a sense of purpose and quiet confidence that encouraged people to listen to me. That could only have come from my experience of working on the project.

"For my future, I feel that I will soon apply to Public Health. I just do not get enough time in the hospital to develop a relationship with the mothers or to look at the system overall."

Taking action in practice

Fatima's work on the perinatal task force was definitely at the system level using healthy public policy. Healthy public policy activities work on changing rules, guidelines, operating procedures, laws, by-laws, and legislation that have an impact on health (The Health Communication Unit, 2002). Once the potential issue of the loss or reduction of home visits to teen moms was determined, the regional team turned it into a policy issue by asking what could or should be done (Public Health Nursing Section, 2001) and then turned to research, experts, and their own experience to find the answers. All nurses, not just those working in the community, have a responsibility to work on policy issues that affect the health of the population. Often nurses have considerable credibility with the public and need to lend their voice to issues that affect the health of the population.

Fatima's previous experience in teamwork gave her courage to state her views and realize that negotiation was possible. Although previously she had been fairly quiet, she had learned from her experience and was able to now speak with confidence, even in front of an audience.

Fatima gained credibility from her peers because she knew where to look for evidence in the literature and was able to relate the evidence to her own practice and to the practice of her colleagues in the community. This demonstrates action based on research evidence and the Primary Health Care principle of appropriate technology. The professional nursing association was working intersectorally to bring pressure on the government.

Community health nurses have a repertoire of health promotion strategies to take action at all levels. They will be the most effective when they collaborate with others to use research evidence and theory and work at multiple levels.

DISCUSSION QUESTIONS

1. What is a possible example of healthy public policy in home care?
2. In what other scenarios in this book has action been based on research evidence?

3. What other forms of evidence for action are useful in place of or in combination with research evidence?

4. What theories are relevant for community-level strategies?

TWO YEARS AFTER THE FINAL PRESENTATION EVALUATION SCENARIO

Dana, the researcher, asked Ellen how she found evaluation to be a challenge in her present practice. Ellen gave the following account:

"I never changed my mind about wanting to work in Public Health and luckily got a position in the school health program right after graduation. I quickly found out that the services of the program were basically delivered in two ways: directly through classroom presentations or by provision of resource material to the teacher on request. When I started, I worked with a team doing classroom presentations on various topics. The presentation was all prepared; I just had to go out and give it. I did talk to the teacher to arrange the date and time but really had little time to do either an assessment or an evaluation. After a few months I was switched to responding to and preparing kits for teachers on various topics. I had great conversations with the teachers to determine what they wanted, but rarely got to hear how it worked out. I was feeling cut off from the action and didn't know if anything I was doing was making a difference.

"About a year ago, I met a very experienced Public Health nurse in the school-aged health program. She had worked in a variety of places, including underdeveloped countries in Africa and had learned about the child-to-child approach (Child-to-Child Trust, 2003). She was using the approach with one school and felt that it was much more effective than anything else she had used, although she was spending more time with the kids and teachers. She wanted to write a proposal to get funding to expand to more schools, but didn't know where to start. I told her what we did to evaluate our project two years ago. It wasn't anything complicated, but we had an idea what was working and what wasn't.

"Well, to make a long story short, we both talked to our managers about evaluating what she was doing so we could write a proposal. Both managers felt that there was a need to evaluate all the delivery methods. I became part of a working group to develop and pilot test evaluation measures for what we were doing. Being in that working group was and is quite an experience. You wouldn't believe how threatened people feel about evaluation! It took me a while to understand why they got so upset. I realized that when we did our project, we had evaluation built right into it. Of course, we did it ourselves. We would not have been happy if other people started checking into what we were doing.

"The work group eventually agreed on one topic, bicycle helmets, and to evaluate three delivery methods for the topic. We had presentations, teacher resource kits, and the child-to-child approach. We picked helmets because that was the topic they dealt with in the spring. We didn't have any extra money, so we decided to incorporate measures into what we were doing. Normally we did far more presentations than gave out resource kits, and the child-to-child approach was only being used in one school. We tried to increase the number of resource kits and the use of the child-to-child approach by offering alternatives to teachers when they called to book a presentation. Most wanted to stick to the presentation, but a few were willing to try something new.

"For the outcome measure, we asked the children two baseline questions about their previous and planned use of a bicycle helmet through a show of hands. We did this even if we were simply delivering a resource kit. If we did the presentation or introduced the child-to-child approach, we also asked if they planned to use a helmet after the presentation. If the teacher was using the resource kit on bicycle helmet safety, we asked the teacher to do a count. In June, we tried to get back to every class to ask the students if they were presently using a helmet or planning to use one.

"For the process evaluation, we developed a simple check-off form for ourselves and the teachers. We also documented the amount of time we spent in each type of activity. We are still analyzing the results, and everyone is involved in doing it. The evaluation exercise really opened up people's eyes to different ways of doing things. The presentations are no longer the most favored method. The nurses could see that the presentations weren't having much of an impact on the students, even if they made the program look good

because of the number of students that could be reached. An evaluation component is now being included in everything we do. The teachers have also become partners as we figure out together the best way to engage students in health topics. I feel much more excited about what I am doing. I have been using the child-to-child approach and really enjoy working closely with the kids and teachers."

Dana asked Ellen, "What specifically have you learned during the project that was useful in your practice?" Ellen responded with, "Collaboration. Partnerships. Developing relationships. Focusing on process rather than content. Trying to make a difference. And, yes, how to incorporate evaluation into practice. It is hard to separate them all out. When I started in Public Health doing presentations and then resource kits, I wasn't happy. When I got involved with the work group and was using the child-to-child approach, I felt that what I was doing was useful. That's what drew me to choose Public Health at the end of our project two years ago."

Evaluation in practice

Ellen found that many people, including nurses, are threatened by evaluation. Although professionals probably feel that they are doing meaningful work, the criteria they use to determine the value of the work may not lead to benefits to the population. Evaluation that occurs after a program has been in place for a while or that is imposed by an external authority is more threatening than evaluation that is determined by team members as a part of practice. Evaluation, together with research, theory, and experience, provides a basis for nurses to make a difference in the health of populations. Evaluation is included in the Primary Health Care principle of appropriate use of resources.

One reason that evaluation may not be a part of practice is that many nurses working in public and community health realize that they do not have the skills to conduct an evaluation (Allengrante, Moon, & Gebbie, 2001; Chambers et al., 1994; Schoenfeld & MacDonald, 2002). Evaluation may also be neglected because there is controversy about how and when an evaluation should be conducted or what type of evaluation should be used. Because evaluation in health promotion involves a range of activities and multiple levels of operation, each type of activity requires a different form of evaluation. Evaluation, including process and outcome evaluation and qualitative and quantitative measures, is a challenge to most professionals (Coombes & Thorogood, 2000). However, evaluation that is part of practice and programming does not have the same rigorous requirements of research. Evaluation in practice uses measures that are feasible and timely and will provide some indication of process and impact.

Often one form of process evaluation that counts the number of people who attended a presentation is the only evaluation completed. Although that information is important, other forms of process evaluation, such as how much the participants enjoyed the encounter or their suggestions on how to improve a health promotion product and affect evaluation are necessary to ensure movement toward improving the health of the population.

This scenario also identified the importance of collaboration in teamwork for organizational change. If representatives of the nurses providing the various aspects of the school-aged program had not been included in the evaluation team, the incorporation of evaluation in practice and the change to more interactive methods would be considerably delayed. A high level of participation is important for organizational as well as community change.

Ellen was able to contribute to incorporating evaluation in practice in the school-aged health program because she had previously used evaluation and found it beneficial. She also seemed to understand why more experienced nurses would feel threatened by evaluation. She obviously was committed to improving the health of school-aged children and wanted to be able to determine whether what she was doing was making a difference.

In the scenario, the incorporation of evaluation allowed the nurses to change their practice based on the evidence they collected. They soon saw that the more interactive methods were more effective, whether the interaction was with the students or the teachers. Evaluation provided them the data they needed to make their decisions and a reason to form partnerships with teachers.

DISCUSSION QUESTIONS

1. What skills, knowledge, and abilities used in assessment are transferable to evaluation?
2. What are some reasons that programs may not be evaluated?
3. What are the benefits of including the beneficiaries of programs in the evaluation?
4. How can evaluation affect each of the principles of Primary Health Care?

Using the community health nursing process to make a difference

In this text and chapter, various examples are given on how nurses working both inside and outside of community health nursing can make a difference in their practice. The community health nursing process fully incorporates Primary Health care. This is apparent by encouragement for nurses to look at the broader issues that surround or underlie specific problems faced by community groups; assess for accessibility; plan collaboratively with the community and other health professionals and organizations; take action after choosing an appropriate strategy based on evidence, theory, and previous experience; and incorporate evaluation into individual practice and at the activity and program level.

Although the community health nursing process is designed for use by community nurses, it incorporates transferable skills, which can be used in other situations in which nurses want to make changes. These could include reducing the use of disposable equipment in a hospital or lobbying politicians or remembering that "When every nurse thinks like a community health nurse, we will really make a difference." Collaboration for health is what will make a difference in the health of populations.

PRACTICE AND APPLICATION

1. Identify how the principles of Primary Health Care have been used throughout this chapter.

2. Identify which determinants of health were involved in each of the scenarios in this chapter.

3. In the scenarios in this chapter, describe the situations in which the speaker used or would have used reflection to change what he or she was doing.

4. Compare how nurses working at the direct practice level can assist nurses working at the policy level and vice versa.

5. What skills, knowledge, and ability gained from working on a project with a team are transferable to other areas of nursing practice?

6. How important is it to you and your teammates that what you are doing will make a difference?

REFERENCES

Allengrante, J., Moon, R., & Gebbie, K. (2001). Continuing-education needs of the currently employed public health education workforce. *American Journal of Public Health, 91*(8), 1230–1234.

Brower, A. (1996). Group development as constructed social reality revisited—The constructivism of small groups. *Families in Society, 77*, 336–344.

Browne, A., & Fiske, J. (2001). First Nations women's encounters with mainstream health care services. *Western Journal of Nursing Research, 23*(2), 126–147.

Campinha-Bacote, J. (2003). Cultural desire: The key to unlocking cultural competence. *Journal of Nursing Education, 42*(6), 239.

Chambers, L. W., Underwood, J., Halbert, T., Woodward, C. A., Heale, J., & Isaacs, S. (1994). 1992 Ontario survey of public health nurses: Perceptions of roles and activities. *Canadian Journal of Public Health, 85*(3), 175–179.

Child-to-Child Trust. (2003). *The child-to-child approach.* Retrieved July 21, 2003, from http://www.child-to-child.org.

Coombes, Y., & Thorogood, M. (2000). Introduction. In M. Thorogood & Y. Coombes (Eds.), *Evaluating health promotion: Practice and methods* (pp. 3–10). Oxford, UK: Oxford University Press.

Feichter, S., & Davis, E. (1984–85). Why some groups fail: A survey of students' experiences with learning groups. *Organizational Behavior Teaching Review, 9*, 58–71.

Health Canada. (1999). *A second diagnostic on the health of the First Nations and Inuit people in Canada.* Retrieved Aug. 20, 2003, from http://www.hc-sc.gc.ca/fnihb/cp/publications/second_diagnostic_fni.htm.

The Health Communication Unit (THCU). (2002). *Introduction to health promotion planning.* Retrieved May 29, 2002, from http://www.thcu.ca/infoandresources.htm.

Houston, S. (2002). Aboriginal health: Cultural security as an ethical issue. In Public Health Association of Australia (Ed.), *Ethical debates in Public Health series one* (pp. 2–15). Melbourne, AU: Public Health Association of Australia.

Kitzman, H., Olds, D. L., Henderson, C. R., Jr., Hanks, C., Cole, R., Tatelbaum, R., et al. (1997). Effect of prenatal and infancy home visitation by nurses on pregnancy outcomes, childhood injuries, and repeated childbearing. A randomized controlled trial [Comment]. *Journal of the American Medical Association, 278*(8), 644–652.

Kitzman, H., Olds, D. L., Sidora, K., Henderson, C. R., Jr., Hanks, C., Cole, R., et al. (2000). Enduring effects of nurse home visitation on maternal life course: A 3-year follow-up of a randomized trial. *Journal of the American Medical Association, 283*(15), 1983–1989.

Leipert, B. (1999). Women's health and the practice of public health nurses in northern British Columbia. *Public Health Nursing, 16*(4), 280–289.

MacMillan, H., & Canadian Task Force on Preventive Health. (2000). Preventive health care, 2000 update: Prevention of child maltreatment. *Canadian Medical Association Journal, 163*(11), 1451–1458.

Olds, D. L., Eckenrode, J., Henderson, C. R., Jr., Kitzman, H., Powers, J., Cole, R., et al. (1997). Long-term effects of home visitation on maternal life course and child abuse and neglect. Fifteen-year follow-up of a randomized trial [Comment]. *Journal of the American Medical Association, 278*(8), 637–643.

Olds, D., Henderson, C. R., Jr., Cole, R., Eckenrode, J., Kitzman, H., Luckey, D., et al. (1998). Long-term effects of nurse home visitation on children's criminal and antisocial behavior: 15-year follow-up of a randomized controlled trial [Comment]. *Journal of the American Medical Association, 280*(14), 1238–1244.

Olds, D. L., Robinson, J., O'Brien, R., Luckey, D. W., Pettitt, L. M., Henderson, C. R., Jr., et al. (2002). Home visiting by paraprofessionals and by nurses: A randomized, controlled trial [Comment]. *Pediatrics, 110*(3), 486–496.

Public Health Nursing Section. (2001). *Public health nursing interventions: Applications for public health nursing practice.* Minneapolis, MN: Minnesota Department of Health.

Ray, K., & Hodnett, E. (2003). Caregiver support for post partum depression. *Cochrane Database of Systematic Reviews, 1.* Available from www.cochrane.org.

Schoenfeld, B. M., & MacDonald, M. B. (2002). Saskatchewan public health nursing survey: Perceptions of roles and activities. *Canadian Journal of Public Health, 93*(6), 452–456.

Sikorski, J., Renfrew, M. J., Pindoria, S., & Wade, A. (2003). Support for breastfeeding mothers. *Cochrane Database of Systematic Reviews, 1.* Available from www.cochrane.org.

Sokoloski, E. H. (1995). Canadian First Nations women's beliefs about pregnancy and prenatal care. *Canadian Journal of Nursing Research, 27*(1), 89–100.

Watson, W., Jonahson, L., & Zgourides, G. (2002). The influence of ethnic diversity on leadership, group process, and performance: An examination of learning teams. *International Journal of Intercultural Relations, 26,* 1–16.

WEB SITE RESOURCES

Aboriginal and first nations health

Aboriginal Nurses Association of Canada: http://www.anac.on.ca/. Site provides links to other services and organizations for First Nations People.

First Nations and Inuit Health Branch, Health Canada: http://www.hc-sc.gc.ca/fnihb-dgspni/fnihb/index.htm. Site provides links to related international, provincial, and association sites.

U.S. Department of Health and Human Service, Indian Health Services: http://www.ihs.gov/. Site provides information and links to extensive programs and organizations.

Disaster planning

Centre for Emergency Preparedness, Health Canada: http://www.hc-sc.gc.ca/pphb-dgspsp/cepr-cmiu/. Extensive information and links on disaster planning at a national level.

Columbia University School of Nursing, Local Public Health Competencies for Emergency Response: http://cumc.columbia.edu/dept/nursing/institute-centers/chphsr/cdcppt/index.htm.

U.S. Department of Homeland Security: http://www.dhs.gov/dhspublic/index.jsp. This department is concerned with overall security of the United States. One of its sub–Web sites and associated organizations is ready.gov (www.ready.gov/). This site contains a wide variety of information related to disaster preparedness.

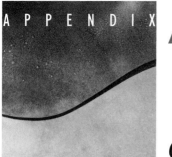

Consultative Presentations

Presentation skills are an important component of community health nursing practice. While using the community health nursing process in your project, your team will regularly need to present ideas in order to obtain feedback and encourage community involvement in the project. At times your presentation will be informal and only involve your organizing teammates; at other times, you may be presenting to very large groups. In all cases, you need to prepare to ensure that your ideas are clearly conveyed.

Before planning a presentation, you need to consider why and when you would give one. In the University of Kansas' Community Tool Box, the following reasons are given for presentations (KU Work Group, 2000):

- To increase community awareness, understanding of you, your group, and your issues
- To garner support for you and your group
- To encourage involvement and action regarding your cause

The KU Work Group also suggests that the best time for a presentation is when community awareness or knowledge about the issue is low, you have new information, the community is interested in the information, and action is needed. The three key elements to a successful community presentation are the right background, the right preparation, and the right delivery (KU Work Group, 2000).

The right background

Before planning your presentation, you need to analyze and determine how to include your potential audience and analyze the setting and equipment.

Analyze the audience

Include your potential audience by analyzing them and ensuring that the people you want are at the meeting. You analyze your potential audience so you can center on their needs rather than on your own (THCU, 2000). This means knowing the audience age range, education level, language ability, values, cultural and ethnic background, and their depth of knowledge about you and the issue (KU Work Group, 2000). Consider the issue from the audience's point of view and provide information that is relevant to them. One formula is to hit them in the heart (with something appealing), hit them in the gut (with a strong message), and hit them in the pocketbook (with something that provides a direct benefit to them) (THCU, 2000).

The gathering of information on your potential audience will differ according to the number of people expected. The Health Communication Unit (2000) at the University of Toronto suggests that, for a small group, you get information on the views of all the people expected and, for a large group, talk to someone who has experience with the group and with group members themselves. The Health Communication Unit also suggests that you imagine what a typical day of an audience member would be like and cautions you not to be misled by those in authority who may have a biased view.

Often the information that you need for a meaningful presentation will come from the key informants and community members who have become involved in the project. They will be part of the planning and possibly part of the presentation. Certainly, you need to ensure that they will be available on the day of the presentation.

Analyze meeting place and equipment

Another aspect of background conditions involves inspecting the room, location, and equipment (KU Work Group, 2000). Visit the room to consider possible seating arrangements and the availability and functioning of equipment, including lighting. Request the type of equipment that is required for the size of the audience and that you will be comfortable using. Also inquire about the availability of technical support should problems occur during the presentation. Be certain that a person is available to open the room at the time of the presentation.

The right preparation

In your preparation, you need to clarify your objectives, develop the speech, select the materials and delivery method, and practice (KU Work Group, 2000).

Clarify objectives

When you clarify your objectives, ask yourself what you want the presentation to achieve. Consider again why and when this was a good time to do a presentation and what message you want to leave with the participants. Because the purpose of the project is to work with people to achieve community benefits, each presentation will have a motivational aspect to encourage participants to join or support the work of the project. Be certain that you are clear on what you want to happen by the end of the presentation. To be the most effective, the presentation needs to do the following (Bender, 2000):

- Inform
- Entertain
- Touch the emotions
- Promote action

Develop the speech

To begin your speech, first prepare an outline. The following gives you the usual components (THCU, 2000; KU Work Group, 2000):

- An introduction (start with an attention-getting device, such as a picture or a story) to inform the audience about what you are going to tell them
- Follow with a transition line to relate the opening to the audience and to explain why you are speaking (THCU, 2000)
- A background to the issue or situation
- A description of the present situation
- Proposed options—include your requests for action
- A summary to reinforce what you have told the audience
- A final point that you want to leave with the audience

The opening of the presentation must grab audience attention in the first few seconds. This can be done in various ways, for example, by 1) creating a strong mental image, such as ships sinking from an overload of people dying from smoking, 2) providing a bottom line message "what's in it for me" from the audience's point of view (e.g., "Why would you want to take part in this? Well, I'll tell you. If you join us you'll have fun and you'll learn job skills such as. . ."), or 3) by citing something that you observed or heard about the audience or their community (THCU, 2000).

In the body of the presentation, follow through what you promised in the opening. Because you are striving for the active involvement, provide the audience with viable options and some pros and cons of each. Encourage members of the audience to offer more.

The ending of the presentation should be stronger than the opening (THCU, 2000). If you had a strong opening theme or quote that worked, repeat it. Summarize your message. To leave the audience with an emotional message, tell them a story that is relevant (e.g., a child died in a house fire from playing with matches) and a call to action.

Be very conscious of the language that you use in the speech and visual aids, such as overhead displays. Presenters stress that fewer, simpler words in the vocabulary used by audience members have the greatest impact (Bender, 2000). Think of the key points that you want to convey and use short sentences to do it. Words with fewer than three syllables are easier to say and are more understandable, especially for audiences whose understanding of English may be limited. One way to ensure that your language is appropriate is to make a list of all the words over three syllables down one side of the page and across from them provide a simpler word or phrase. For example, "collaborate" becomes "working with." Use the time that you spend with community members to identify the vocabulary that they use to express their ideas.

Select materials and delivery method

Definitely use visual devices in your presentation. The combination of telling and showing increases retention after three days by 55% over telling only (Bender, 2000). Examples of visual devices include role playing, printed and illustrated handouts, posters, flip chart displays, overhead projector shows, and a projector or computer-generated slides. The

TABLE A-1	**Visual Aids for Presentations**

TYPE OF VISUAL AID	SIZE OF GROUP	DISADVANTAGES	CONSIDERATIONS
Role play	All	Role play participants need to feel comfortable in front of the group and speak loudly	Especially effective when real situations are portrayed Encourage members of community to enact situations that they face
Handouts	All	Takes time to prepare and proofread	Hand out at beginning or end of presentation Reinforces message
Posters	All	Need to be viewed before or after presentation	Provide a low-tech way to provide information and pictures that can be left in location to reinforce message
Flip chart displays	Up to 40	Needs to be prewritten or requires person with neat handwriting to collect ideas	5 × 5 rule: 5 lines with 5 words each Upper two-thirds of sheet
Overhead transparencies	5 or more	Needs to have backup light for projector	6 × 6 rule: 6 lines with 6 words each Use bullets with key phrases Use large (16+) bold serif-type font
Computer-generated slide presentation	All	System may crash (need to have low-tech backup) Takes time to prepare but then is easy to modify Limit slick "show biz" effects that may distract from the message or overwhelm an audience	Same as overheads Provides opportunity to easily use color, pictures, and graphics

characteristics and effective use of the most available types of visual aids are provided in Table A-1.

After considering the size of the audience and the aids that are available, choose the aid that you are comfortable using, especially for your first presentation. If you have never prepared or delivered a computer-generated slide show, your nervousness about the equipment could greatly distract from the presentation message. Later on in the project you may want to develop your skills in this area. If so, schedule your debut as a computer presenter during a rehearsal with your teammates and have a more experienced person available during your actual presentation.

Another consideration is the use of audiovisual technology such as videos or interactive programs. These add to the complexity of the presentation and could also detract from the message. If you have experience using the technology, certainly consider it, especially with younger audiences who are familiar with multimedia effects.

Practice

Practice is essential for a good delivery. Choose some of the following points to help you practice effectively: rehearse in front of a mirror, in front of your teammates, with a video camera or tape recorder, by reading aloud, by breathing and relaxing, with a clock, while maintaining eye contact, while paying attention to how your words are delivered, or by visualizing yourself doing the presentation (KU Work Group, 2002). Ask a community member to listen to you and identify any ideas or words that were unclear, not understandable, or confusing.

Prepare the presentation material in sufficient time to have a rehearsal in the room and make adjustments before the actual presentation. For example, check that any visual displays or text can be seen easily from the back of the room.

The right delivery

The right delivery involves using notes, convincing your audience, inviting interaction, and following up (KU Work Group, 2000). Experienced presenters advise that you spend 80% of your preparation time on delivery and 20% on content (Bender, 2000). This 80/20 rule is understandable if you consider that you really do know "what" you want to tell the audience; the tricky part is "how" to tell it so that they will understand your message and want to become involved.

Notes

Prepare notes on cue cards with a main point on each card. Use large print and different colors to accentuate points. The cards will give you confidence that you will know what to say from one minute to the next.

Convince the audience

The main purpose of your presentation is to convince your audience to listen to the points you are making. Your credibility begins with first impressions—of your clothing, statements, and manner. Clothing that is informal, neat, and attractive but not distracting adds to a favorable first impression. As discussed earlier, your opening remarks need to grab attention and create the important first impression that you have something significant to say and are concerned about the audience (KU Work Group, 2000). You need to tell them what to expect and then provide your facts and ideas.

By making eye contact with members of the audience, you convey that you are interested in their reaction to your presentation. You will know from their responses if they are following you or if you need to make adjustments. If your audience is not comfortable with eye contact, focus on an inanimate object or the people who are more comfortable.

You also need to speak with personal conviction. Your emotions can show but keep them under control. Repeat and highlight your main ideas. When you want action, show that what you propose is important and possible (KU Work Group, 2000). End on a positive high note.

Interaction

Because the purpose of the presentation is to encourage people to become involved in your project, you need to consider how you can involve them throughout the presentation. To be involved, they must understand you, so provide pauses and provide time to think if you want answers to a question. If you say, "Are there any questions?" you may get no response. You can be more specific by asking what a particular point you have made means to the people in the audience. For example, you could say "I would like to know what you feel about XXX. Take a minute to think about it, maybe write down your ideas. Then I will ask you again."

Another way to obtain responses is to have the audience members first discuss the question with the person beside them. That gives everyone time to think and gain more confidence in voicing their ideas. Also arrange small group sessions, especially when you want the people to consider different options. Distribute team members and key informants from the community among the groups to explain the options in more detail. At the end of the session, each small group would then report their recommendations to the full audience.

Consider the following tips when responding to questions from the audience:

- Listen carefully.
- Repeat the question using the main ideas to ensure that you have heard clearly and so everyone knows what was asked.
- Show respect for the questioner.
- Encourage others to offer a viewpoint.
- Keep your answers short (KU Work Group, 2000).
- When dealing with difficult questions or situations, remain calm, admit when you do not know something and arrange to get back to the person. Identify common areas and the reason for your position if there are differences, and gently steer discussion back to main issues if an irrelevant issue is raised (KU Work Group, 2000).

Encouraging interaction with multicultural audiences can be particularly challenging. The challenge can arise from language difficulties and a culture that does not permit questioning authority (which includes someone who is presenting). Before your presentation, review the information in Appendix B on clear communication. Include all the points about communication with people who have limited knowledge of English, such as speaking slowly, using simple words, and using a lot of pictures. Do not use examples that include activities which audience members may not understand (such as baseball). Instead, use examples from what you have seen or been told about in the community. Because some people understand written language better than verbal language, distribute handouts at the beginning of the presentation.

Having the audience working in small groups during a presentation can be particularly useful for multicultural groups. You can ask them to discuss specific points or list the points you have made in order of importance (THCU, 2000). Although you need to make a special effort to ensure understanding and to obtain feedback from multicultural groups, the effort is also worthwhile for all community audiences. Most community audiences will probably include people with a great range of knowledge and understanding on the issue.

Follow-up

Immediately after the presentation, be certain to capitalize on the enthusiasm that has been generated. Have sign-up sheets that you can circulate or leave at the back of the room. Provide more handouts and information for the next meeting. All team members should circulate among the audience and encourage them personally to sign up for the action you are planning or to come to the next event. You can also leave posters and sign-up sheets in the reception areas of the agencies that are involved with the project. After a successful presentation, the people who were in the audience will be telling others who might want to join. Tell the audience where you will leave the information for others who could not be present.

REFERENCES

Bender, P. (2000). *Secrets of power presentations.* Toronto, ON: The Achievement Group.

The Health Communication Unit, University of Toronto (THCU). (2000). *Strengthening presentation skills.* Toronto, ON: Author.

KU Work Group on Health Promotion and Community Development. (2000). *Making community presentations* (Community Tool Box: Part B, Chapter 4, Section 5). Lawrence, KS: University of Kansas. Retrieved July 15, 2000, from http://ctb.lsi.ukans.edu/tools/en/sub_section_main_1029.htm.

WEB SITE RESOURCES

Presentations

Tutorials and examples of presentations are available online from presentation software manufacturers such as Microsoft, creators of PowerPoint®, and from providers (retailers) of PowerPoint®.

A number of tutorials can be obtained from education sites by typing the following, in parentheses, into a Google search engine window: "PowerPoint tutorial" site:.edu. For example, the University of Kansas provides useful guidelines on what a presentation is, plus why, when, and how you make a presentation. The Web site URL is http://ctb.lsi.ukans.edu/tools/en/sub_section_main_1029.htm.

Plain Language

Canadian Public Association provides The Directory of Plain Language Health Information for North America at http://www.pls.cpha.ca/english/directry.htm. Tips are included in the appendices.

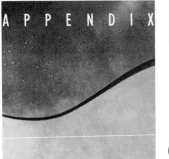

APPENDIX B

Clear Communication

Clear communication is particularly important when one interacts with people who have a limited knowledge of English or the language used in community health meetings with professionals. The most appropriate approach is to use plain language that has no jargon, long words, or complicated concepts. For example, terms such as "collaborate" or "build capacity" can make new members feel like they are hearing another language. Care must be take to use plain language verbally and in documents.

When communicating with community group members who have a limited understanding of English, a most useful approach is to find key informants who understand English to work with you to explain your views to other community members. You would especially want these bilingual key informants to prepare questions with you to ensure that the words, pictures, or symbols can be understood by community members. The key informers can also help you find the approach that works the best with the community.

To simplify the words that you use, make a list of all the words that you would expect to use in a conversation. Identify those with more than three syllables and change them to words with fewer syllables. After you go through this exercise a few times, you will find that you automatically chose simpler words.

When you deal directly with people who speak little English, the following guidelines will assist you in communicating more effectively (Ewles & Simnett, 1999; The Health Communication Unit, 2000):

1. Use simplified language. Speak slowly and clearly without raising your voice or talking down to the audience.
2. Pause while speaking.
3. When not understood, repeat the sentence using the same words.
4. Use simple, short sentences with the active form of the verb. Example: Use "We will start the meeting soon," rather than "The meeting will be started by us soon."
5. State events in the order in which they will occur. Example: "We will eat and then go outside," rather than "We will go outside after we eat." Listeners who miss the word "after" will think that going outside happens first.
6. Do not use slang or sayings such as "bone tired," "fed up," or "raining cats and dogs" or idiomatic verbs such as "Will you go ahead with this project?" or "I will go over it once more."

7. Use pictures, demonstration, and simple written instructions. A checkmark or an "X" on written material may be misunderstood.

8. Humor may not be understood, especially humor derived from the double meaning of some words.

9. When checking to ensure that you are understood, watch for body language and avoid questions with "yes" or "no" answers. People uncomfortable speaking in a new language will say "yes" to "Do you understand?" just to end the conversation.

10. Avoid eye contact if the person seems uncomfortable with it.

REFERENCES

Ewles, L., & Simnett, I. (1999). *Promoting health: A practical guide* (4th ed.). London: Bailliere Tindall.

The Health Communication Unit, University of Toronto. (2000). *Strengthening presentation skills.* Toronto, ON: Author.

WEB SITE RESOURCES

Plain language

Canadian Public Association provides The Directory of Plain Language Health Information for North America at http://www.pls.cpha.ca/english/directry.htm.

Harvard School of Public Health, Health Literacy Studies: www.hsph.harvard.edu/healthliteracy. This site is designed for professionals in health and in education. It provides access to many useful materials including a presentation overview of health literacy, a video entitled In Plain Language and a literature review and annotated bibliography.

National Institute for Cancer Research. (2003). *Clear & simple: Developing effective print materials for low-literate readers.* Includes detailed instructions for calculating a SMOG score. Retrieved June 14, 2004, from http://www.cancer.gov/cancerinformation/clearandsimple.

National Library of Medicine health literacy bibliography site: www.nlm.nih.gov/pubs/cbm/hliteracy.html.

National Institute for Literacy LINCS: www.nifl.gov/lincs. Gateway to the world of adult education and literacy resources on the Internet. Search using "plain language."

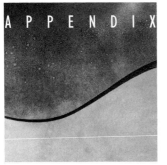

C

Forms for Community and Teamwork

Meeting agenda (for five or more people; simplify if fewer than five)

Date:_____ **Time** (start–finish):_____

Purpose of meeting (relate to workplan):

Meeting objectives:

Agenda (determine time required for each agenda activity and keep to schedule):

1. **Roundtable check- in:**
2. **Key points to discuss:**
3. **Decisions (to be) made:**
4. **Task allocation:**
   - Responsibility for action on decision:
5. **Date and agenda for next meeting** (key issues):
   - Expected reports
   - Expected decisions, activities, strategies. . .
   - Next steps in activities
6. **Premeeting preparation necessary** (if applicable):
7. **Preparation and distribution of meeting summary** (recorder responsible):
      To team members:
      To others:
8. **Reflection on group roles and process:**

Sources: Adapted from KU Work Group on Health Promotion and Community Development. (2001). *Conducting effective meetings* (Community Tool Box, Part E, Chapter 16, Section 1). Lawrence, KS: University of Kansas. Retrieved July 20, 2003, from http://ctb.lsi.ukans.edu/tools/en/ sub_section_tools_1153.htm; and Woods, D. (1994). *Problem-based learning: How to gain the most from PBL.* Waterdown, ON: Author.

Weekly summary

Potential instructions:

1. No more than one page for teams of two or one and one-half pages for larger teams unless an extraordinary event occurred.
2. The weekly summary is to be completed at the end of the clinical day by the full team in 15 to 30 minutes.
3. If some items for activities are consistently the same, such as all the team members and the location, that can be stated at the beginning and not repeated.
4. Most activities will fall into *one of four types:* 1) teamwork, 2) meetings with agency advisor and/or clinical instructor, 3) activities (describe) with community members, or 4) individual work.
5. The weekly summary is to be submitted by _____ (date and time).

Date:_____

Distribution list:_____

A. PURPOSE for week's activities (relate to steps, substeps and activities in timeline and workplan):
B. ACTIVITIES FOR THE WEEK:
    For *each type* of activity provide:
    1. Description of activity
    2. Time involved in activity
    3. Location
    4. Team member(s) and others involved and what they provided
    5. What was accomplished by team
C. PLAN FOR NEXT WEEK:
    For *each type* of planned activity provide:
    1. Description of proposed activity
    2. Expected time required
    3. Location
    4. Team member(s) and others to be involved and what tasks are expected from each
D. Comments or questions on activities or future ideas and plans:
E. Evaluate teamwork according to designated aspects and frequency in team agreement

Individual assessment

Name:_____ Date:_____

Base your responses on your most recent work in a group. If you have been working on a community health nursing team in recent months, base your responses on that experience.

1. What type of groups have you been involved with in the past? (e.g., course work group, community group, work group, or professional group)?
2. Overall, how *positive* would you describe your experience in this recent group?

___ Mostly positive   ___ Half & half   ___ Less than half positive   ___ Not positive

3. What experience have you had in the group that was particularly rewarding to you?
4. What do you feel contributed to your rewarding experience(s)?
5. Using your experience from working in the group, check the characteristics in the following table that apply to you.

TABLE C-1	Individual Assessment			
NO.	**PERSONAL CHARACTERISTIC**	**MOSTLY**	**SOME**	**RARELY**
1	I arrive on time and am prepared to focus on the team task.			
2	I take a turn in roles such as facilitator, recorder, or reporter.			
3	I do a fair share of teamwork.			
4	I admit uncertainty and ask questions to clarify a situation.			
5	I use personal examples to help teammates understand the situation.			
6	I readily use resources such as the preceptor, instructor, and course material to help clarify a situation.			
7	I can be counted on to disclose feelings, opinions, and experiences.			
8	I show respect for others by limiting length of comments, listening to others, and considering their viewpoints.			
9	I encourage teammates by recognizing their contributions and building on their ideas.			
10	I explore different viewpoints and approaches that may not be appreciated at first.			
11	I use logic to challenge the thinking and work methods of the team.			
12	I practice reflective thinking and avoid drawing hasty conclusions.			
13	I listen carefully and respond thoughtfully whenever others disagree or express criticism.			
14	I keep trying even when the task becomes demanding.			
15	I express optimism about the team being able to achieve success.			

Sources: Adapted from Strom, P. Strom, R. & Moore, E. (1999). Peer and self-evaluation of teamwork skills. Journal of Adolescence, 22, 539–553; and Woods, D. (1994). Problem-based learning: How to gain the most from PBL. Waterdown, ON: Author. Woods, 1994.

6. What do you feel are the contributions that you can/do bring to the group? (For example, Do you have previous team or leadership experience, computer skills, presentation skills, ability in a language other than English, cultural perspective, or network contacts?)
7. What has been the most troubling experience that you had with the group?
8. How could you and the team avoid this type of troubling group experience in the future?
9. What do you tend to do when you are faced with differences in a group?
10. What messages have you gotten about the population group that you are working with on this project?
11. What knowledge and skills related to the culture group would be beneficial to you?
12. What rules or guidelines do you like to have about group work? (For example, What are your timelines? How do you like to work?)
13. What personal goals would you like to accomplish by the end of the project? (Indicate at least two; e.g., plan and work to a schedule or express my views when they are different than what is being said.)
14. What would you like the group to accomplish by the end of the project? (Indicate at least one for the group; e.g., we learn to rely on one another and the project, i.e., the people feel that what is produced is worthwhile.)

TABLE C-2	*Ways of Dealing with Conflict*		
REACTION TO CONFLICT	**MOST OF THE TIME**	**HALF AND HALF**	**A FEW TIMES OR NEVER**
Accommodate (do what the other person wants, give in)			
Withdraw (refuse to participate anymore)			
Compromise (find a middle ground that at least satisfies most)			
Collaborate (work together to find something that all believe is important)			
Force (take over decision making and action, leaving little for others but to follow)			
Other_____			

Source: Adapted from Woods, D. (1994). Problem-based learning: How to gain the most from PBL (Box 5-2, pp. 5–7). Waterdown, ON: Author.

Format and questions to develop a student team/partnership agreement

Names:_____

Project Title:_____

Each member of the team/partnership agrees to:

1. *Time:* What amount of time is each person expected to spend on the project each week?
2. *Attendance:* What is expected about attendance at meetings or activities? What is the expected procedure in case of illness or extraordinary occurrence? What will we do if someone is not present?
3. *Work routine for team:* What work routine for the clinical day can we establish to keep us on track? How would an initial meeting to determine an agenda or "to do list" for the day be useful? How can we make sure that we prepare the weekly summary together at the end of the day?
4. *Responsibilities:* What is the expectation about being on time for meetings and completing tasks on time? How are problems dealt with, e.g., a computer problem or information or a person unavailable? What will we do if someone is not fulfilling responsibilities?
5. *Communication:* What type, what is included, who receives it, deadline for distribution, and procedures to follow if unable to meet deadline?
6. *Attitude/behavior:* How will we encourage and monitor a professional attitude and behavior by team members?
7. *Appearance:* How will the team ensure that each member is dressed appropriately for the clinical area? Who can we ask about what to wear on regular and special occasions? What is always inappropriate? What procedure will we use if someone is dressed inappropriately?
8. *Change:* What is the procedure if a change needs to be made in a planned activity? (For example, Who must be contacted and who informs others?)
9. *Feelings:* What is expected about sharing feelings and reflections about the team/partnership with those in the team/partnership and others outside the team/partnership?
10. *Feedback:* What is the expectation about providing constructive feedback to individuals and the team?
11. *Evaluation:* How will we ensure that we are collaborating with the agency contact, instructor, and community in each step of the process? How will we check that we are dealing with the individual needs of members? How will we keep track of our progress and successes? How will we identify and deal with challenges. How frequently (other than the required midterm and final evaluation) will we evaluate these different aspects of teamwork and document results on the workplan?

12. *Other considerations:* What other items will encourage good team work and avoid previous problems?

Signatures:_____ Date:_____

REVISIONS:

Signatures:_____ Date:_____

Format for personal reflection on an event or experience

Name:_____ Date:_____

1. **Describe the event or experience.**
   a. What happened, including when, where, how, and who was involved?
2. **Identify feelings and thoughts.**
   a. What emotion was I feeling as the event happened?
   b. What was I trying to achieve?
   c. Why was this event important to me?
   d. Why did I act the way I did?
   e. What happened to others as a result of my action?
   f. What emotions did the others show?
   g. How did I know that they had those emotions?
3. **Evaluate the situation.**
   a. What was good about the experience?
   b. What was bad about the experience?
4. **Identify main features.**
   a. What features identify my thoughts and emotions before, during, and after the experience?
   b. Did my feelings or beliefs affect what happened before, during, and after the experience?
   c. In what types of situations have I previously responded in the same way?
5. **Consider alternative strategies for the situation.**
   a. What two other approaches could I have taken in this situation?
   b. What are the positive and negative aspects of each alternate approach?
6. **Create an action plan.**
   a. What approach will I use in this type of situation in the future?
   b. How will I prepare for this situation in the future?
   c. Do I feel more confident in supporting myself and others in this situation? If not, what else can I do?

Sources: Brokenshire, A. (1998). Towards reflective practice: Learning from experience. *Registered Nurse, 10,* 7–8; Gibbs, G. (1999). The reflective cycle. In Royal College of Nurses (Ed.), *Realising clinical effectiveness and clinical governance through clinical supervision (Practitioner Book 1).* Oxford, UK: Radcliffe Medical Press; and Johns, C. (1993). Professional supervision. *Journal of Nursing Management, 1,* 9–18.

Key informant contact sheet

I.D.#:_____ Contact date:_____ Written by:_____

Name/position:_____

Address:_____

Phone/fax:_____

Email:_____

Availability:_____

Source of referral:_____

Present and past involvement with issue and community:_____

Interest in project:_____

Suggestions and contact information for additional key informants:_____

Suggestions for timing, location, and assessment methods:_____

Possible involvement in project:_____

Willing to be called again? _____Yes _____No

TO BE COMPLETED AFTER THE INTERVIEW

Impressions of key informant: Describe the quality of the interaction with the key informant including the overall tone of the meeting, the level of interest of the person, and how you would feel about working with this person on the project.
Themes or issues?
How would you approach your next contact with this key informant?
Other information:

Assessment timeline

Revision date:_____

Title of project:_____

STEPS AND SUBSTEPS IN PROCESS	WEEK OF ASSESSMENT											
	1	2	3	4	5	6	7	8	9	10	11	12
1. Establish relationships within project and community												
a. Establish relationship and responsibilities with project organizers												
b. Meet community contact(s)												
c. Define project, population, issue												
2. Assess secondary data												
a. Review national and local policy documents												
b. Review sociodemographic data												
c. Review epidemiological data												
d. Review previous community surveys and program statistics												
e. Review literature and best practice guidelines												
f. Summarize secondary data												
3. Initiate assessment of community												
a. Plan, observe, and map setting, or resources												
b. Plan and interview key informants												
4. Conduct specific assessment												
a. Determine specific methods*												
b. Plan and use _____ (1st method)*												
c. Plan and use _____ (2nd method)*												
d. (as needed)*												
5. Determine action statements												
a. Analyze data and prepare presentation on findings, issues, and possible action statements												
b. Validate findings and devise three action statements with community members and stakeholders												
c. Prepare assessment report												
6. Evaluate teamwork (frequency per team agreement)												

*Choose from progressive inquiry, community meetings, focused discussions, or questionnaires.

Assessment workplan

Revision date:_____

Title of project:_____

STEPS, SUBSTEPS, AND ACTIVITIES (list activities under substeps, number and date activities across columns)	SUMMARY OF RESULTS WITH DATES
1. Establish relationships within project and community	
a. Establish relationship and responsibilities with project organizers	
b. Meet community contact(s)	
c. Define project, population, purpose	
2. Assess secondary data	
3. Initiate assessment of community	
a. Plan, observe and map setting, or resources	
b. Plan and interview key informants	
4. Conduct specific assessment	
a. Determine specific methods*	
b. Plan and use _____ (1st method)*	
c. Plan and use _____ (2nd method)*	
d. (as needed)*	
5. Determine action statements	
a. Analyze data and prepare presentation on findings, issues, and possible action statements	
b. Validate findings and devise three action statements with community members and stakeholders	
c. Prepare assessment report	
6. Evaluate teamwork	

_____

Choose from progressive inquiry, community meetings, focused discussions, or questionnaires.

Collaborative assessment report

[Name of educational institution]
Community health nursing project in collaboration with_____
Date:_____

[Title of collaborative assessment]
Students: **Advisor/project leader:**
Clinical instructor: **Manager:**

Importance of issue/problem (summarize national, provincial, local statistics and literature review; give references and attach reference list)
Agency mandate priority or issue:
Community of interest:
Collaborative assessment purpose:
Assessment methods, timelines (summarize from workplan):
Validated key results/findings with supporting evidence: (Evidence: Do not provide specific details for numbers less than five. Do not include potentially incriminating statements such as the number who smoked or did not exercise. Rather, indicate the number interested in smoking cessation or exercise programs.)
    Issues (barriers to health and preferred health):
    Strengths (assets, previous initiatives, amount of interest, resources, etc.):
    Issue for action:
Limitations:
Possible action statements to address issue for action (three):
Future action proposed:
Attachments (workplan, questionnaires, focused discussion questions, tables of data, excerpts of comments, reference list, etc.):

Action timeline

Revision date: _____

Title of project: _____

STEPS AND SUBSTEPS IN PROCESS	WEEK OF ACTION											
	1	2	3	4	5	6	7	8	9	10	11	12
1. Plan												
a. Assess/reassess												
b. Set priority												
c. Identify goal												
d. Identify strategies, theories, and research												
e. Identify products and activities with timelines in step 2												
f. Identify administrative objectives for pilot test and final products with associated evaluation measures												
g. Identify project objectives and associated evaluation measures												
2. Take action												
a. Prepare for action												
b. Conduct pilot test												
c. Complete action												
3. Determine results/impact												
a. Collect and analyze data for project objectives												
b. Present findings to community												
c. Show appreciation to collaborators												
d. Complete project report												
4. Evaluate teamwork (according to frequency in team agreement)												

Action workplan

Revision date: _____

Title of project: _____

STEPS, SUBSTEPS, AND ACTIVITIES (list activities under substeps, number and date activities across columns)	SUMMARY OF RESULTS WITH DATES
1. Plan	
a. Assess/reassess	
b. Set priority with community and stakeholders	
c. Identify goal	
d. Identify strategies,* theories, and research	
e. Identify products and activities with timelines in step 2	
f. Identify administrative objectives for pilot test and final products with associated evaluation measures	
g. Identify project objectives and associated evaluation measures	
2. Take action	
a. Prepare for action	
b. Conduct pilot test	
c. Complete action	
3. Determine results/impact	
a. Collect and analyze data for project objectives	
b. Present findings to community	
c. Show appreciation to collaborators	
d. Complete project report	
4. Evaluate teamwork	

*List of strategies

1. Mass communication activities
2. Educational activities
3. Counseling/tutoring and skill development
4. Connecting people for support (support groups, buddy system, social networks)
5. Environmental and organizational change activities
6. Community development or capacity building activities
7. Healthy public policy activities

Collaborative project report

[Name of educational institution]
Community health nursing project in collaboration with _____

[Title of project]
[Date]
Students: **Advisor/project leader:**
Clinical instructor: **Manager:**

Importance of issue/problem:
Agency mandate:
Agency priority or issue:
Community of interest:
Collaborative assessment goal:
Assessment methods, timelines:
Validated key results/findings with supporting evidence:
    Issues:
    Strengths:
    Issue for action:
Priority action statement:
Project goal:
Products:
Strategy, theory, evidence base:
Ability objective*:
Accomplishment objective*:
Environmental objective:
Collaborative action:
    Administrative activities and participants (summarize): **Key findings:**
    Process:
    Impact:
Limitations:
Sustainability:
Recommendations:
Attachments:

*Or the two highest objectives achieved.

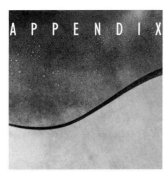

APPENDIX D

Canadian Community Health Nursing Standards of Practice

COMMUNITY HEALTH NURSES ASSOCIATION OF CANADA

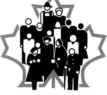

Community Health Nurses Association of Canada

The Community Health Nurses Association of Canada (CHNAC) is a voluntary national association of community health nurses structured as a federation of those provincial /territorial community health nursing interest groups who participate in CHNAC. CHNAC is a recognised Associate Member of the Canadian Nurses Association participating in all the rights and obligations that this recognition allows.

Mission statement

The Community Health Nurses Association of Canada, as a federation of provincial/ territorial community health nurses interest groups, provides a unified voice to represent and promote community health nursing and the health of communities.

The Community Health Nurses Association of Canada gratefully acknowledges the following standards development project funders:

The Alberta Community Health Nurses Association
The Canadian Nurses Association
The Community Health Nurses Initiatives Group of the RNAO
ParaMed Health Care Services
Public Health Department of Health & Wellness, Fredericton, NB
Saint Elizabeth Health Care
The University of Victoria School of Nursing
The Victorian Order of Nurses (Canada)

The Canadian Community Health Nursing Standards of Practice 2003 are reproduced with the permission of the Community Health Nurses Association of Canada (CHNAC). CHNAC is an associate member of the Canadian Nurses Association.

Community Health Nursing Standards Committee

Maureen Best, RN, BN, MEd
Director, Community Health Services
Calgary Health Region, Calgary, Alberta

Claire Betker, RN, MN
Director, Public Health
Winnipeg Regional Health Authority, Manitoba

Shelley Corvino, BScN, IBCLC
Public Health Nursing Orientation Coordinator
Winnipeg Regional Health Authority, Winnipeg, Manitoba

Elizabeth (Liz) Diem, RN, PhD*
School of Nursing
University of Ottawa, Ottawa, Ontario

Rosemarie Goodyear, BN, MSA
Assistant Executive Director, Child, Youth & Family Programs
Health and Community Services Central, Gander, Newfoundland

Rosemary Graham, RN, BScN, MN
Nurse Practitioner-In Charge, Dawson Community Health Center
Dept of Health & Social Services, Yukon Territorial Government, Dawson City, Yukon Territories

Barbara Harvey
Department of Health & Social Services
Government of Nunavut, Kugluktuk, Nunavut

Judith Lapierre, RN, PhD
Université du Québec à Hull, Gatineau, Québec

Jo-Ann MacDonald, BScN, MN
Assistant Professor, School of Nursing,
University of Prince Edward Island

Mary Martin-Smith, BScN, RN*
Public Health Nursing Consultant, Population Health Branch
Saskatchewan Health, Regina, Saskatchewan

Beth McGinnis, RN, MEd, MN
Project Manager, Public Health
Department of Health and Wellness, Fredericton, New Brunswick

Donna Meagher-Stewart, PhD, RN*
Associate Professor, School of Nursing
Dalhousie University, Halifax, Nova Scotia

Barbara Mildon, RN, MN, CHE*
Chair, Community Health Nursing Standards Committee
President, Community Health Nurses Association of Canada, & VP Nursing Leadership, Saint
    Elizabeth Health Care, Markham, Ontario

Shirley Sterlinger, RN, BScN*
Public Health Nurse
Burnaby, British Columbia

*Member of the Synthesis & Evaluation Subcommittee

Table of contents

Introduction

Evolving from centuries of community care by laywomen and members of religious orders, community health nursing began its journey toward recognition as a nursing specialty in the mid-eighteen hundreds. Community health nursing has been indelibly shaped and influenced by such remarkable nurses as Florence Nightingale and Lillian Wald and organizations such as the Victorian Order of Nurses, the Henry Street Settlement, and the Canadian Red Cross Society. Over the course of the 20th century, public health and home health nursing have emerged from common roots to engender the ideals of community health nursing. Today, community health nurses (CHNs) practice in diverse settings such as homes, schools, shelters, churches, community health centres and on the street. Their position titles may be as varied as their practice settings.

Community health nursing respects its common roots and traditions while embracing advances that promote the ongoing evolution of community health nursing as a dynamic nursing specialty. Community health nursing is concerned with the health of individuals, families, groups, communities and populations, throughout their lifespan in a continuous rather than episodic process (Cradduck, 2000). CHNs collaborate with individuals, families, groups, communities and populations in designing and implementing community development activities, health promotion and disease prevention strategies. CHNs view disease prevention, health protection and health promotion as goals of professional nursing practice (Smith, 1990). Community health nursing is rooted in caring (Canadian

Nurses Association, 1998) and practice is informed by conceptual models and nursing theories and the nursing code of ethics (CNA, 2002a). CHNs embrace the principles of primary health care and these practice standards support the enactment of these principles in their practice. Community health nursing concepts and competencies are essential to community focused nursing practice and are pivotal in guiding the practices of all nurses concerned with promoting and preserving the health of populations. The social conscience expressed in community health nursing has been reflected in public policies such as the Canada Health Act (Government of Canada, 1984), the Ottawa Charter for Health Promotion (World Health Organization, Canadian Public Health Association, Health and Welfare Canada, 1986) and the Jakarta Declaration (World Health Organization, 1997).

Developing community nursing standards

National community health nursing standards have been developed by a representative committee of community health nurses under the auspices of the Community Health Nurses Association of Canada (CHNAC). An interest group of the Canadian Nurses Association, CHNAC was formed in 1987 as a national communication network and forum for community health nurses across Canada. National practice standards for community health nurses have never been developed, although at least one province has developed its own standards (e.g. the 1985 Ontario standards, now out of print). The Canadian Public Health Association's 1990 booklet entitled *Community Health—Public Health Nursing in Canada* remains an excellent reference for community health nursing practice; however it does not explicitly identify practice standards. Input into the development of these standards was invited and gratefully received from community health nurses across Canada.

Purpose of standards

Standards for professional practice are a hallmark of self-regulating professions. Nurses with varied levels of preparation may practice in the community setting. These standards, though, are specifically intended to inform the practice of registered nurses.

Every nurse regardless of practice focus or setting is accountable for the fundamental knowledge and expectations inherent in basic nursing practice. These standards expand upon generic nursing practice expectations and articulate the practice principles and variations specific to community health nursing practice.

Community health nursing practice standards are established to:

- define the scope and depth of community nursing practice and establish criteria, or expectations, for acceptable nursing practice in the provision of safe, ethical care
- support on-going development of community health nursing
- promote community health nursing as a specialty
- serve as a necessary foundation for the development of certification of community health nursing as a specialty by the Canadian Nurses Association
- inspire excellence in and commitment to community nursing practice.

Knowledge of these standards is an expectation of every community health nurse working in any of the domains of practice, education, administration or research. Nurses in clinical practice will use them to guide and evaluate their own practice. Nursing educators will include them in course curricula and nurse administrators will use them to direct policy and guide performance expectations. Nurse researchers can use these standards to guide the development of knowledge specific to community health nursing. It is recognized that nurses may enter community health nursing as novice practitioners and will require experience and additional learning and skill development opportunities to support evolution of their practice. These standards become basic practice expectations after two years of experience. The practice of expert community health nurses will extend beyond these standards.

Community health nursing

Community health nurses are registered nurses whose practice specialty promotes the health of individuals, families, communities, and populations, and an environment that supports health. The practice of community health nurses combines nursing theory and knowledge, social sciences and public health science with primary health care. Whether working with individuals, families, groups, communities or populations, community health nurses identify and promote care decisions that build on the capacity that is inherent in the individual/community. A critical part of community health nursing practice is to marshal resources to support health by co-ordinating care, and planning services, programs and policies with individuals, caregivers, families, other disciplines, organizations, communities and government(s). Community health nurses function within the Canadian Nurses Association's (CNA) *Code of Ethics for Registered Nurses* (2002a).

While community health nursing concepts and competencies are included in the practices of nurses with varied functions and position titles across Canada, this document will have the most direct application in the areas of home health and public health nursing. The differing and distinct client and program emphasis of home health and public health nursing are historically linked through common beliefs and values, traditions, skills, and above all, their unique focus on the promotion and protection of community health.

A home health nurse (HHN) is a community health nurse who synthesizes knowledge from primary health care (including the determinants of health), nursing science, and theory and knowledge of the social sciences to provide clinical care and treatment that is directed towards health restoration, maintenance, or palliation. Home health nursing is a specialized area of nursing practice in which the nurse provides care in the client's home, school or workplace. Clients, their designated caregivers and their families are the focus of home health nursing practice, and HHNs integrate health promotion, teaching and counseling within their clinical care activities. The goal of care is to initiate, manage and evaluate the resources needed to promote the client's optimal level of well-being and function. Nursing activities necessary to achieve this goal may be aimed primarily at prevention, maintenance, restoration, or palliation. The educational preparation for HHNs may be a nursing diploma or a degree; however, a baccalaureate degree is preferred.

A public health nurse (PHN) is a community health nurse who synthesizes knowledge from public health science, primary health care (including the determinants of health), nursing science, and theory and knowledge of the social sciences to promote, protect, and preserve the health of populations. PHNs practice population health promotion in increasingly diverse settings, such as community health centres, schools, street clinics, youth centres and nursing outposts, and with diverse partners, to meet the health needs of specific populations. Although the focus of public health nursing practice is health promotion of populations, public health nurses integrate their personal and clinical understanding and knowledge of the health and illness experiences of individuals, families and communities into their population health promotion practice. That is, public health nurses recognize that a community's health is inextricably linked with the health of its constituent members and is often reflected first in individual and family health experiences. Healthful communities and systems that support health, in turn, contribute to opportunities for health for individuals, families, groups and populations. The educational preparation for entry to practice as a PHN is a baccalaureate degree in nursing.

The relationship between HHN and PHN practice may be thought of in terms of the shifting lens of a camera. The HHN begins with a close-up lens zooming in and focusing on the individual client and family, then shifting to a wide-angle lens to encompass groups and the supports in the community. The move from a wide-angle to close-up lens is useful for PHNs shifting their focus between systems, population health and intersectoral partnership and the health of individual clients and families.

The mission of community health nurses

Community health nurses view health as a resource for functioning on a day-to-day basis. Their practice promotes, protects and preserves the health of individuals, families, groups, communities and populations wherever they live, work, learn, worship and play, in a continuous rather than an episodic process (Cradduck, 2000). Their practice is derived from a unique understanding of the influence of the environmental context on health. Community health nurses work at a high level of autonomy and build partnerships based on a philosophy of primary health care, caring and empowerment. Community health nurses combine specialized nursing, social, and public health science with their experiential knowledge of individuals, families, communities and populations when providing nursing services.

The values and beliefs of community health nurses

The following values and beliefs are based on Canadian Nurses Association's *Code of Ethics for Registered Nurses* (2002a), and are interpreted from the community health nursing perspective. The community health nurse values and believes in:

Caring

Community health nurses recognize that caring is an essential human need but that its expression in practice varies across cultures and domains. The importance of caring in community health nursing is seen as essential and universal. In the Canadian context of community health nursing practice, caring is based on the principle of social justice, in which the nurse brings an awareness of equity and the fundamental right of all humans to accessible, competent health care and essential determinants of health. Caring is expressed through competent practice and the development of a connective relationship that values the individual/community as unique and worthy of a nurse's "presence" and attention. Caring community health nursing practice acknowledges the physical, spiritual, emotional and cognitive nature of individuals, families, groups and communities. Community health nurses enact their belief in caring by preserving, protecting and enhancing human dignity in all of their interactions.

The principles of primary health care

Community health nurses recognize that primary health care is a different way of thinking about health and health care that is fundamental to their practice. Primary health care differs significantly from primary care (first point of access to care) and is an integral part of the Canadian health care system. Community health nurses value the following key principles of primary health care as described by the World Health Organization (1978): 1) universal access to health care services, 2) focus on the determinants of health, 3) active individual and community participation in decisions that affect their health and life, 4) partnership with other disciplines, communities and sectors for health, 5) appropriate use of knowledge, skills, strategies, technology and resources, and 6) focus on health promotion/illness prevention throughout the life experience from birth to death. Community health nurses recognize and incorporate knowledge of the impact of the socio-political-economic environment on the health of individuals and the community, and their own practice.

Multiple ways of knowing

Community health nurses integrate multiple types of knowledge into their practice. Critical examination of this knowledge provides for evidence based community health nursing practice. Four fundamental patterns of knowing in nursing have been identified by Carper (1978): 1) aesthetics, the art of nursing, 2) empirics, the science of nursing, 3) personal knowledge, and 4) ethics, the component of moral knowledge in nursing knowledge. Each pattern is an essential component of the integrated knowledge base of community health nursing practice.

The art of nursing for community health nurses is the adaptation of knowledge and practice to particular rather than universal circumstance. It encourages the exploration of possibilities, promotes individual creativity and style and contributes to the transformative power of community health nursing.

The science of community health nursing includes research, epidemiology, theories and models that include publicly verifiable, factual descriptions, explanations and predictions based on subjective and objective data. Empirical knowledge is generated by and tested by scientific research (Fawcett, Watson, Neuman & Hinton, 2001).

Personal knowledge, the most fundamental way of knowing, evolves from discovery of self, values and morals, and lived experience. It involves continuous learning through reflective practice. Reflective practice in community health nursing involves the critical examination of practice, interpersonal relationships and intuition in order to evaluate, adapt and enhance practice.

Ethical knowledge describes the moral obligations, normative values and goals of community health nursing. It is guided by moral principles and ethical standards set by the Canadian Nurses Association (2002). Ethical inquiry is directed at clarifying values and beliefs and may use dialogue to examine the socio-political impact of community health nursing on the health environment (Fawcett et al, 2001).

White (1995) adds a fifth way of knowing to Carper's typology, socio-political knowing, which goes well beyond personal knowing and nurse-client introspection. It is synonymous with emancipatory knowing in that it situates nursing within the broader social, political, and economic context where nursing and health care happen. It enables the nurse to question the status quo and structures of domination in society that affect the health of persons and communities.

By integrating multiple ways of knowing into the practice of community health nursing, the individual nurse becomes a co-creator of nursing knowledge. Recognition of diverse evidence for practice allows community health nursing to question and move beyond the status quo to evolve and create relevant and effective action for community health.

Individual/community partnership

Community health nurses believe that it is paramount to have the individual/community as an active partner in decisions that affect their health and well-being. Participation is essential throughout all components of the nursing process. In partnership, the community/individual takes an active role in defining their own health needs during assessment, sets their own priorities among health goals, controls the choice and use of various actions to improve their health and lives, and evaluates the efforts made. During assessment and throughout the community health nursing process, community health nurses identify the health values of the individual/community, including what health means to that particular individual or community. Inherent in the nursing process is working with individuals and communities to build capacity to participate in and make decisions concerning their health. For community health nurses, participation is the basis of therapeutic, professional, caring relationships that promote empowerment. Community health nurses also make their expertise available as a resource to those with whom they are working.

Concurrent with capacity building work, community health nurses also have a responsibility as an advocate. Nurses' knowledge and experience equip them to advocate in partnership with clients who are vulnerable or intimidated in a particular situation, to assist them in accessing services (case advocacy). Community health nurses also have an advocacy function in creating policy, system and resource allocation change (class advocacy) to increase opportunities for health within society (Pope, Snyder & Mood, 1995, p. 254).

Empowerment

Community health nurses recognize that empowerment is an active, involved process where people, groups, and communities move towards increased individual and community control, political efficacy, improved quality of community life, and social justice. Empowerment is a community concept because individual empowerment builds from working with others to effect change and includes the desire to increase freedom of choice for others and society. Empowerment is not something that can be done to or for people, but involves people discovering and using their own strengths. Empowering strategies or environments (e.g. healthy workplaces such as those supporting flex time or exercise) build capacity by moving individuals, groups and communities towards the discovery of their strengths and their ability to take action to improve quality of life.

Community health nursing standards

Drawing upon the values and beliefs of community health nursing, nursing knowledge, and the partnerships that are established with people in the community, five interrelated standards of practice form the core expectations for community health nursing practice. These standards are:

1. **Promoting health**
2. **Building individual/community capacity**
3. **Building relationships**
4. **Facilitating access and equity, and**
5. **Demonstrating professional responsibility and accountability.**

The Canadian community health nursing practice model

The prerequisite to community health nursing practice is an understanding of the community health nursing process and its evidence/knowledge base. The Canadian community health nursing practice model (Figure 1) has been developed specifically for this standards document to reflect the knowledge and experience of community health nurses in practice, education, research and administration across Canada. The model depicts the context of community health nursing practice, the foundational values and beliefs held by community health nurses (CHNs), the community health nursing process, and the five standards of practice.

The influence of the legislative, policy and social environment on community health nursing practice is acknowledged. Community health nursing practice is delivered through several agencies and organizations, such as provincial or municipal departments of health, regional health authorities, and non-government organizations. Historically, multiple social, economic, and political forces have impacted upon legislation and public policies that provide the environmental context in which community health nursing and health care happen. CHNs are accountable to a variety of authorities and stakeholders (e.g. public, regulatory body, employer) and the legislative and policy mandates from multiple sources both internal and external to their employment situation. This context influences CHN practice. Most of the legislation and policy sources that are significantly influential are provincial/territorial in nature. The structure and processes of the organization in which community health nurses are employed also influence their practice through the organizational values and principles, policies, goals, objectives, standards and outcomes. It is acknowledged that these forces can serve as enabling factors, or may serve to constrain the scope and manner in which community health nursing is practiced.

The community health nurse works with individuals, families, groups, communities, populations, systems and/or society, but at all times the health of the person or community is the focus and motivation from which nursing actions flow. The standards of practice are applied to practice in all settings where people live, work, learn, worship and play.

The philosophical base and foundational values and beliefs that characterize community health nursing—caring, the principles of primary health care, multiple ways of knowing, individual/community partnerships and empowerment—are embedded in the standards and are reflected in the development and application of the community health nursing process.

The community health nursing process involves the traditional nursing process components of assessment, planning, intervention and evaluation but is enhanced by community health nurses in three dimensions: 1) individual/community participation in each component, 2) multiple ways of knowing, each of which is necessary to understand the complexity and diversity of nursing in the community; knowledge and utilization of all these ways of knowing forms evidence-based practice consistent with these standards, and 3) the inherent influence of the broader environment on the individual/community that is the focus of care (e.g. the community will be affected by provincial/territorial policies, its own economic status and by the actions of its individual citizens).

The standards of practice are founded on the values and beliefs of community health nurses, and utilization of the community health nursing process.

The model (Figure 1) illustrates the dynamic nature of community health nursing practice, embracing the present and projecting into the future. The values and beliefs (or shaded) ground practice in the present yet guide the evolution of community health nursing practice over time. The community health nursing process (unshaded) provides the vehicle through which community health nurses work with people, and supports practice that exemplifies the standards of community health nursing. The standards of practice revolve around both the values and beliefs and the nursing process with the energies of community health nursing always being focussed on improving the health of people in the community and facilitating change in systems or society in support of health. Community health nursing practice does not occur in isolation but rather within an environmental context, such as policies within their workplace and the legislative framework applicable to their work.

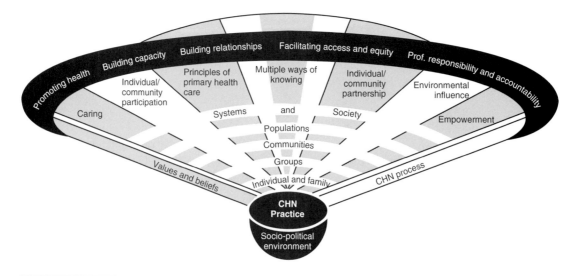

FIGURE 1. The Canadian Community Health Nursing Practice Model.

The Standards of practice

Knowledge of, and adherence to, the following standards is an expectation of every community health nurse working in any of the domains of practice, education, administration or research. These standards serve as a benchmark for novice community health nurses and become basic practice expectations after two years of experience. The practice of expert community health nurses will extend beyond these standards. While each standard is relevant to the practice of both home health nurses and public health nurses, the emphasis in practice on elements of specific standards will vary according to the practice focus.

Standard 1: Promoting health

Community health nurses view health as a dynamic process of physical, mental, spiritual and social well-being. They believe that individuals and/or communities realize aspirations and satisfy needs within their cultural, social, economical and physical environments. Community health nurses consider health as a resource for everyday life that is influenced by circumstances, beliefs and the determinants of health including social, economic and environmental health determinants: a) income and social status, b) social support networks, c) education, d) employment and working conditions, e) social environments, f) physical environments, g) biology and genetic endowment, h) personal health practices and coping skills, i) healthy child development, j) health services, k) gender, and l) culture (Health Canada, 2000). It includes self-determination and a sense of connectedness to the community.

Community health nurses promote health using the following strategies: a) health promotion, b) illness and injury prevention and health protection, and c) health maintenance, restoration, and palliation. It is recognized that it may be relevant to use these strategies in concert with each other when providing care and services. This standard incorporates these strategies by drawing upon the frameworks of primary health care (WHO, 1978), the Ottawa Charter for Health Promotion (WHO, 1986), and the Population Health Promotion Model (Health Canada, 2000).

a) Health promotion

Community health nurses focus on health promotion and the health of populations. Health promotion is a mediating strategy between people and their environments—a positive, dynamic, empowering, and unifying concept that is based in the socio-environmental approach to health. This broad concept is envisioned as bringing together people who recognize that basic resources and prerequisite conditions for health are critical for achieving health. The population's health is closely linked with the health of its constituent members and is often reflected first in individual and family experiences from birth to death. Healthy communities and systems support increased options for well-being in society. Community health nurses consider socio-political issues that may be underlying individual/community problems.

The community health nurse:

1. Collaborates with individual/community and other stakeholders in conducting a holistic assessment of assets and needs of the individual/community.
2. Uses a variety of information sources to access data and research findings related to health at the national, provincial/territorial, regional, and local levels.
3. Identifies and seeks to address root causes of illness and disease.
4. Facilitates planned change with the individual/community/population through the application of the Population Health Promotion Model.
   - Identifies the level of intervention necessary to promote health
   - Identifies which determinants of health require action/change to promote health
   - Utilizes a comprehensive range of strategies to address health-related issues.
5. Demonstrates knowledge of and effectively implements health promotion strategies based on the Ottawa Charter for Health Promotion.
   - Incorporates multiple strategies addressing: a) healthy public policy; b) strengthening community action; c) creating supportive environments; d) developing personal skills, and e) re-orienting the health system
   - Identifies strategies for change that will make it easier for people to make a healthier choice.
6. Collaborates with the individual/community to assist them in taking responsibility for maintaining or improving their health by increasing their knowledge, influence and control over the determinants of health.
7. Understands and uses social marketing and media advocacy strategies to raise consciousness of health issues, place issues on the public agenda, shift social norms, and change behaviours if other enabling factors are present.
8. Assists the individual/community to identify their strengths and available resources and take action to address their needs.
9. Recognizes the broad impact of specific issues such as political climate and will, values and culture, individual/community readiness, and social and systemic structure on health promotion.
10. Evaluates and modifies population health promotion programs in partnership with the individual/community and other stakeholders.

b) Prevention and health protection

The community health nurse adopts the principles of prevention and protection and applies a repertoire of activities to minimize the occurrence of diseases or injuries and their consequences to individuals/communities. Health protection strategies often become mandated programs and laws by governments for the larger geo-political entity.

The community health nurse:

1. Recognizes the differences between the levels of prevention (primary, secondary, tertiary).
2. Selects the appropriate level of preventative intervention.
3. Helps individuals/communities make informed choices about protective and preventative health measures such as immunization, birth control, breastfeeding, and palliative care.

4. Assists individuals, groups, families, and communities to identify potential risks to health.

5. Utilizes harm reduction principles to identify, reduce or remove risk factors in a variety of contexts including home, neighbourhood, workplace, school and street.

6. Applies epidemiological principles in using strategies such as screening, surveillance, immunization, communicable disease response and outbreak management and education.

7. Engages collaborative, interdisciplinary and intersectoral partnerships to address risks to the individual, family, community, or population health and to address prevention and protection issues such as communicable disease, injury and chronic disease.

8. Collaborates in developing and using follow-up systems within the practice setting to ensure that the individual/community receives appropriate and effective service.

9. Practices in accordance with legislation relevant to community health practice (e.g. public health legislation, child protection).

10. Evaluates collaborative practice (personal, team, and/or intersectoral) in achieving individual/community outcomes such as reductions in communicable disease, injury and chronic disease or reducing the impacts of a disease process.

c) Health maintenance, restoration and palliation

Community health nurses provide clinical nursing care, health teaching and counselling in health centres, homes, schools and other community based settings to individuals, families, groups, and populations whether they are seeking to maintain their health or dealing with acute, chronic or terminal illness. The community health nurse links people to community resources and co-ordinates/facilitates other care needs and supports. The activities of the community health nurse may range from health screening and care planning at an individual level to the forming of intersectoral collaborations and resource development at the community and population level.

The community health nurse:

1. Assesses the individual/family/population's health status and functional competence within the context of their environmental and social supports.

2. Develops a mutually agreed upon plan and priorities for care with the individual/family.

3. Identifies a range of interventions including health promotion, disease prevention and direct clinical care strategies (including those related to palliation), along with short and long term goals and outcomes.

4. Maximizes the ability of an individual/family/community to take responsibility for and manage their health needs according to resources and personal skills available.

5. Supports informed choice and respects the individual/family/community's specific requests while acknowledging diversity, unique characteristics and abilities.

6. Adapts community health nursing techniques, approaches and procedures as appropriate to the challenges inherent to the particular community situation/setting.

7. Uses knowledge of the community to link with, refer to or develop appropriate community resources.

8. Recognizes patterns and trends in epidemiological data and service delivery and initiates improvement strategies.
9. Facilitates maintenance of health and the healing process for individuals/families/communities in response to significant health emergencies or other diverse community situations that negatively impact upon health.
10. Evaluates individual/family/community outcomes systematically and continuously in collaboration with the individuals/families, significant others, other health practitioners and community partners.

Standard 2: Building individual/community capacity

Building capacity is the process of actively involving individuals, groups, organizations and communities in all phases of planned change for the purpose of increasing their skills, knowledge and willingness to take action on their own in the future. The community health nurse works collaboratively both with the individual/community affected by health compromising situations and the people and organizations who control resources. Community health nurses start where the individual/community is at to identify relevant issues and assess resources and strengths. They determine the individual's or community's stage of readiness for change and priorities for action. They take collaborative action by building on identified strengths and facilitate the involvement of key stakeholders: individuals, organizations, community leaders and opinion leaders. They work with people to improve the determinants of health and "make it easier to make the healthier choice." Community health nurses use supportive and empowering strategies to move individuals and communities toward maximum autonomy.

The community health nurse:

1. Works collaboratively with the individual/community, other professionals, agencies and sectors to identify needs, strengths and available resources.
2. Facilitates action in support of the five priorities of the Jakarta Declaration to:
   - Promote social responsibility for health
   - Increase investments for health development
   - Expand partnerships for health promotion
   - Increase individual and community capacity
   - Secure an infrastructure for health promotion.
3. Uses community development principles:
   - Engages the individual/community in a consultative process
   - Recognizes and builds on the group/community readiness for participation
   - Uses empowering strategies such as mutual goal setting, visioning and facilitation
   - Understands group dynamics and effectively uses facilitation skills to support group development
   - Enables the individual/community to participate in the resolution of their issues
   - Assists the group/community to marshal available resources to support taking action on their health issues.
4. Utilizes a comprehensive mix of community/population based strategies such as coalition building, intersectoral partnerships and networking to address issues of concern to groups or populations.

5. Supports the individual/family/community/population in developing skills for self-advocacy.
6. Applies principles of social justice and engages in advocacy in support of those who are as yet unable to take action for themselves.
7. Uses a comprehensive mix of interventions and strategies to customize actions to address unique needs and build individual/community capacity.
8. Supports community action to influence policy change in support of health.
9. Actively works to build capacity for health promotion with health professionals and community partners.
10. Evaluates the impact of change on individual/community control and health outcomes.

Standard 3: Building relationships

Building relationships within community health nursing is based upon the principles of connecting and caring. Connecting is the establishment and nurturing of a caring relationship and a supportive environment that promotes the maximum participation of the individual/community, and their own self-determination. Caring involves the development of empowering relationships, which preserve, protect, and enhance human dignity. Community health nurses build caring relationships based on mutual respect and on an understanding of the power inherent in their position and its potential impact on relationships and practice.

The community health nurse's most unique challenge is building a network of relationships and partnerships with a variety of relevant groups, communities, and organizations. These relationships occur within a complex, changing, undefined and often ambiguous environment that may present conflicting and unpredictable circumstances.

The community health nurse:
1. Recognizes her/his personal attitudes, beliefs, assumptions, feelings and values about health and their potential effect on interventions with individuals/communities.
2. Identifies the individual/community beliefs, attitudes, feelings and values about health and their potential effect on the relationship and intervention.
3. Is aware of and utilizes culturally relevant communication in building relationships. Communication may be verbal or non-verbal, written or pictorial. It may involve face-to-face, telephone, group facilitation, print or electronic means.
4. Respects and trusts the family's/community's ability to know the issue they are addressing and solve their own problems.
5. Involves the individual/community as an active partner in identifying relevant needs, perspectives and expectations.
6. Establishes connections and collaborative relationships with health professionals, community organizations, businesses, faith communities, volunteer service organizations, and other sectors to address health related issues.
7. Maintains awareness of community resources, values and characteristics.
8. Promotes and facilitates linkages with appropriate community resources when the individual/community is ready to receive them (e.g. hospice/palliative care, parenting groups).

9. Maintains professional boundaries within an often long-term relationship in the home or other community setting where professional and social relationships may become blurred.

10. Negotiates an end to the relationship when appropriate, e.g. when the client assumes self-care, or when the goals for the relationship have been achieved.

Standard 4: Facilitating access and equity

Community health nurses embrace the philosophy of primary health care and collaboratively identify and facilitate universal and equitable access to available services. Community health nurses engage in advocacy by analyzing the full range of possibilities for action, acting on affected determinants of health, and influencing other sectors to ensure their policies and programs have a positive impact on health. Community health nurses collaborate with colleagues and with other members of the health care team to promote effective working relationships that contribute to comprehensive client care and the achievement of optimal client care outcomes. Community health nurses use advocacy as a key strategy to meet identified needs and enhance individual and/or community capacity for self-advocacy. They are keenly aware of the impact of the determinants of health on individuals, families, groups, communities and populations. The practice of community health nursing occurs with consideration for the financial resources, geography and culture of the individual/ community.

The community health nurse:

1. Assesses and understands individual and community capacities including norms, values, beliefs, knowledge, resources and power structure.
2. Provides culturally sensitive care in diverse communities and settings.
3. Supports individuals/communities in their choice to access alternate health care options.
4. Advocates for appropriate resource allocation for individuals, groups and populations to facilitate access to conditions for health and health services.
5. Refers, co-ordinates or facilitates access to service within health and other sectors.
6. Adapts practice in response to the changing health needs of the individual/ community.
7. Collaborates with individuals and communities to identify and provide programs and delivery methods that are acceptable to them and responsive to their needs across the life span and in different circumstances.
8. Uses strategies such as home visits, outreach and case finding to ensure access to services and health-supporting conditions for potentially vulnerable populations (e.g. persons who are ill, elderly, young, poor, immigrants, isolated, or have communication barriers).
9. Assesses the impact of the determinants of health on the opportunity for health for individuals/families/communities/populations.
10. Advocates for healthy public policy by participating in legislative and policymaking activities that influence health determinants and access to services.
11. Takes action with and for individuals/communities at the organizational, municipal, provincial/territorial and federal levels to address service gaps and accessibility issues.

12. Monitors and evaluates changes/progress in access to the determinants of health and appropriate community services.

Standard 5: Demonstrating professional responsibility and accountability

Community health nurses work with a high degree of autonomy in providing programs and services. They are accountable to strive for excellence, to ensure that their knowledge is evidence-based, current and maintains competence, and for the overall quality of their own practice. Community health nurses are accountable to initiate strategies that will help address the determinants of health and generate a positive impact on people and systems.

Within a complex environment, community health nurses are accountable to a variety of authorities and stakeholders as well as to the individual/community they serve. This places them in a variety of situations with unique ethical dilemmas. These include whether responsibility for an issue lies with the individual/family/community/population, or with the nurse or the nurse's employer, the priority of one individual's rights over another's, individual or societal good, allocation of scarce resources and dealing with issues related to quality versus quantity of life.

The community health nurse:
1. Takes preventive and/or corrective action individually or in partnership with others to protect individuals/communities from unsafe or unethical circumstances.
2. Advocates for societal change in support of health for all.
3. Utilizes nursing informatics (information and communication technology) to generate, manage and process relevant data to support nursing practice.
4. Identifies and takes action on factors which impinge on autonomy of practice and quality of care.
5. Participates in the advancement of community health nursing by mentoring students and novice practitioners.
6. Participates in research and professional activities.
7. Makes decisions using ethical standards/principles, taking into consideration the tension between individual versus societal good and the responsibility to uphold the greater good of all people or the population as a whole.
8. Seeks assistance with problem solving as needed to determine the best course of action in response to ethical dilemmas and risks to human rights and freedoms, new situations, and new knowledge.
9. Identifies and works proactively to address nursing issues that will affect the population through personal advocacy and participation in relevant professional associations.
10. Contributes proactively to the quality of the work environment by identifying needs/issues and solutions, mobilizing colleagues, and actively participating in team and organizational structures and mechanisms.
11. Provides constructive feedback to peers as appropriate to enhance community health nursing practice.
12. Documents community health nursing activities in a timely and thorough manner, including telephone advice and work with communities and groups.
13. Advocates for effective and efficient use of community health nurse resources.

14. Utilizes reflective practice as a means of continually assessing and seeking to improve personal community health nursing practice.
15. Seeks professional development experiences that are consistent with current community health nursing practice, new and emerging issues, the changing needs of the population, the evolving impact of the determinants of health and emerging research.
16. Acts upon legal obligations to report to appropriate authorities situations of unsafe or unethical care provided by family, friends or other individuals to children or vulnerable adults.
17. Uses available resources to systematically evaluate the availability, acceptability, quality, efficiency and effectiveness of community health nursing practice.

Definitions

Access: Accessibility of health care refers to the extent to which community health nursing services reach people who need them most and how equitably those services are distributed throughout the population. (Stanhope & Lancaster, 2001)

Advocacy: A combination of individual and social actions designed to gain political commitment, policy support, social acceptance and systems support for a particular health goal or programme. (WHO, 1998, p. 5)

Collaboration: An approach to community care built on the principles of partnership and maximizing participation in decision-making. Collaboration includes shared identification of issues, capacities and strategies.

Intersectoral collaboration:
A recognized relationship between part or parts of different sectors of society which has been formed to take action on an issue to achieve health outcomes or intermediate health outcomes in a way which is more effective, efficient or sustainable than might be achieved by the health sector acting alone. (WHO, 1998, p. 14)

Community: A specific group of people, often living in a defined geographical area, who share a common culture, values and norms, are arranged in a social structure according to relationships which the community has developed over a period of time. Members of a community gain their personal and social identity by sharing common beliefs, values and norms which have been developed by the community in the past and may be modified in the future. They exhibit some awareness of their identity as a group, and share common needs and a commitment to meeting them. (WHO, 1998, p. 5)

Community Development: The process is based on the philosophical belief that people and communities are entitled to have control over factors that affect their lives. It is grounded in valuing absolute worth of the individual and starting where they are. It is a process that is used frequently (although not exclusively) with the most disenfranchised groups in society. It is a process of involving a community in the identification and reinforcement of those aspects of everyday life, culture and political activity that are conducive to health. This might include support for political action to modify the total environment and strengthen resources for healthy living, as well as reinforcing social networks and social support within a community and developing the material resources and economic base available to the community. (CPHA, 1990)

Connecting: The establishment of a perception of connection, engagement, attachment, or bonding between the nurse and the family member(s). There are three components: making the connection, sustaining the connection, and breaking the connection. (Davis and Oberle, 1990)

Determinants of health: The Federal, Provincial, Territorial Advisory Committee on Population Health (1999) identifies the following determinants or prerequisites to health: a) socio-economic determinants including income, education and literacy, employment, and working conditions; and b) social determinants including social support, safety in the home and community, participation in civic activities; healthy child development; c) physical environmental determinants including the state of the natural environment, the presence of environmental tobacco smoke, availability of transportation, affordable and adequate housing; personal health practices; health services; and biology and genetic endowment. (Health Canada, 1999)

Epidemiology: The study of the distribution and determinants of health-states or events in specified populations, and the application of this study to the control of health problems. (Last, 2000)

Equity: Accessible services to promote the health of populations most at risk of health problems. (Stanhope & Lancaster, 2001)

> *Equity* means fairness. Equity in health means that people's needs guide the distribution of opportunities for well-being; all people have an equal opportunity to develop and maintain their health, through fair and just access to resources for health. (WHO, 1998, p. 7)

Evidence based practice: Nursing practice is based on various types of evidence, including experimental and non-experimental research, expert opinion, and historical and experiential knowledge, shaped by theories, values, client choice, clinical judgement, ethics, legislation, and work environments. Evidence-based decision-making is a continuous interactive process involving the explicit, conscientious and judicious consideration of the best available evidence to provide care. (Canadian Nurses Association, 2002b)

Group: People who interact and share a common purpose or purposes. Note: There is no clear distinction between a group and a community except that groups tend to have fewer members than a community. The means used to plan and provide programs or activities for both are similar except for scale.

Health promotion: Health promotion is the process of enabling people to increase control over, and to improve their health. (WHO, CPHA, Health and Welfare Canada, 1986)

Health outcomes: A change in the health status of an individual, group or population which is attributable to a planned intervention or series of interventions, regardless of whether such an intervention was intended to change health status. Outcomes may be for individuals, groups or whole populations. (WHO, 1998, p. 20)

> *Intermediate health outcomes:*
> Intermediate health outcomes are changes in the determinants of health, notably changes in lifestyles, and living conditions which are attributable to a planned

intervention or interventions, including health promotion, disease prevention and primary health care. (WHO, 1998, p. 14)

Maintenance: Designed or adequate to maintain a patient in a stable condition: serving to maintain a gradual process of healing or to prevent a relapse. (Merriam-Webster, 2003)

Nursing informatics: Integrates nursing science, computer science, and information science to manage and communicate data, information, and knowledge in nursing practice. Nursing informatics facilitates the integration of data, information, and knowledge to support clients, nurses, and other providers in their decision-making in all roles and settings. (Staggers & Bagley-Thompson, 2002)

Palliation: The combination of active and compassionate therapies intended to comfort and support individuals and families who are living with, or dying from, a progressive life-threatening illness, or are bereaved. This includes attending to physical, psychological, psychosocial, and spiritual needs. (adapted from: Canadian Palliative Care Association, 1995)

Partnerships: Relationships between individuals, groups or organizations wherein the different participants in the relationship work together to achieve shared goals. Involves active and flexible collaboration between health care providers and clients/individuals and communities, which includes choice, accountability, dignity and respect, and is focused on increasing clients' capacities for self-reliance using empowering strategies. (Hitchcock, Schubert & Thomas, 1999)

Population: A collection of individuals who have one or more personal or environmental characteristics in common. (Stanhope & Lancaster, 2002, p. 24)

Population health: The health of a population as measured by health status indicators and as influenced by the determinants of health. As an approach, population health focuses on the interrelated conditions and factors that influence the health of a population over the life course, identifies systematic variations in their patterns of occurrence, and applies the resulting knowledge to develop and implement policies and actions to improve the health and well being of these populations. (Health Canada, 2000)

Prevention: Disease prevention covers measures not only to prevent the occurrence of disease, such as risk factor reduction, but also to arrest its progress and reduce its consequences once established. Primary prevention is directed towards preventing the initial occurrence of a disorder. Secondary prevention seeks to arrest or retard existing disease and its effects through early detection and appropriate treatment; tertiary prevention reduces the occurrence of relapses and the establishment of chronic conditions through, for example, effective rehabilitation.

Disease prevention is sometimes used as a complementary term alongside health promotion. Although there is frequent overlap between the content and strategies, disease prevention is defined separately. Disease prevention in this context is considered to be action which usually emanates from the health sector, dealing with individuals and populations identified as exhibiting identifiable risk factors, often associated with different risk behaviours. (WHO, 1998, p. 4)

Primary Care: First contact care, continuous, comprehensive and co-coordinated care provided to populations undifferentiated by gender, disease, or organ system. (Starfield, 1994)

Primary Health Care: "Essential health care based on practical, scientifically sound and socially acceptable methods and technology made universally accessible to individuals and families in the community through their full participation and at a cost that the community and country can afford to maintain at every stage of their development in the spirit of self-reliance and self-determination. It forms an integral part both of the country's health system, of which it is the central function and main focus, and of the overall social and economic development of the community. It is the first level of contact of individuals, the family and community with the national health system bringing health care as close as possible to where the people live and work, and constitutes the first element of a continuing health care system." This definition of Primary Health Care was approved at the 1978 WHO conference at Alma Ata. (WHO, 1978, p. 21)

Public health science: Areas of knowledge deemed essential for preparation of community health nurses which include epidemiology, biostatistics, nursing theory, change theory, economics, politics, public health administration, community assessment, management theory, program planning and evaluation, population health and community development theory, history of public health and issues in public health. (Stanhope & Lancaster, 2001)

Restoration: Returning to a normal or healthy condition. (Merriam-Webster, 2003)

REFERENCES

Canadian Nurses Association. (1998). *A national framework for the development of standards for the practice of nursing: A discussion paper.* Ottawa: Author.

Canadian Nurses Association. (2002a). *Code of ethics for registered nurses.* Ottawa: Author.

Canadian Nurses Association. (2002b). *Position statement: Evidence-based decision-making and nursing practice.* Ottawa: Author. Retrieved April 7, 2003, from http://www.cna-nurses.ca/_frames/policies/policiesmainframe.htm.

Canadian Palliative Care Association. (1995). *Palliative care: Towards a consensus in standardized principles of practice.* Ottawa, ON: Author.

Canadian Public Health Association. (1990). *Community health—Public health nursing in Canada: Preparation & practice.* Ottawa: Author.

Carper, B. A. (1978). Fundamental patterns of knowing in nursing. *Advances in Nursing Science, 1*(1), 13–23.

Cradduck, G. R. (2000) Primary health care practice. In M. Stewart (Ed), *Community nursing: promoting Canadian's health* (2nd ed., pp. 352–369). Toronto: W.B. Saunders.

Davies, B. & Oberle, K. (1990). Dimensions of the supportive role of the nurse in palliative care. *Oncology Nursing Forum, 17*(1), 87–94.

Fawcett, J., Watson, J., Neuman, B., & Hinton, P. (2001) On nursing theories and evidence. *Journal of Nursing Scholarship, 33*(2), 115–120.

Health Canada. (1999). *Toward a healthy future: Second report on the health of Canadians.* Federal, Provincial and Territorial Committee on Population Health. Ottawa: Author.

Health Canada. (2000). *Population health approach.* Ottawa: Author. Retrieved April 7, 2003, from http://www.hc-sc.gc.ca/hppb/phdd/approach/index.html.

Hitchcock, J. E., Schubert, P. E., & Thomas, S.A. (1999). *Community health nursing: Caring in action.* Albany: Delmar Publishers.

Government of Canada. (1984). *Canada Health Act.* R.S.C. 1984, c. C-6. Ottawa: Department of National Health and Welfare.

Last, J. M. (Ed.). (2000). *A dictionary of epidemiology* (4th ed.). New York: Oxford University Press, Inc.

Merriam-Webster Medical Dictionary. (2003). Springfield, MA: Merriam-Webster Inc. [Electronic version]. Retrieved April 7, 2003, from http://www.intelihealth.com/IH/ihtIH/WSIHW000/9276/9276.html.

Pope, A., Snyder, M. & Mood, L. (Eds.). (1995). *Nursing, health and the environment: Strengthening the relationship to improve the public's health.* Washington, DC: National Academy Press. Retrieved April 7, 2003, from http://books.nap.edu/books/030905298X/html/index.htm.

Smith, M. C. (1990). Nursing's unique focus on health promotion. *Nursing Science Quarterly, 3*(3), 105–106.

Staggers, N., & Bagley-Thompson, C. (2002). The evolution of definitions for nursing informatics: A critical analysis and revised definition. *Journal of the American Medical Informatics Association, 9*(3), 255–262.

Stanhope, M. & Lancaster, J. (2001). *Community and public health nursing* (5th ed.). St. Louis: Mosby.

Starfield, B. (1994). Is primary care essential? *Lancet, 344*(8930), 1129–1133.

White, J. (1995). Patterns of knowing: Review, critique, and update. *Advances in Nursing Science, 17*(4), 73–86.

World Health Organization. (1978). *Alma-Ata 1978: Report of the international conference on primary health care.* Geneva: Author.

World Health Organization, Canadian Public Health Association, Health and Welfare Canada. (1986). *The Ottawa charter for health promotion.* Ottawa: Canadian Public Health Association.

World Health Organization. (1997). *The Jakarta declaration on leading health promotion into the 21st century.* Geneva: Author.

World Health Organization. (1998). *Health promotion glossary.* Geneva: Author.

BIBLIOGRAPHY

Alexander, J., & Kroposki, M. (1999). Outcomes for community health nursing practice. *Journal of Nursing Administration, 29*(5), 49–56.

Allender, J. A., & Spradley, B. W. (2001). *Community health nursing: Concepts and practice.* Philadelphia: Lippincott.

Anderson, E. T., & McFarlane, J. (2000). *Community as partner: Theory and practice in nursing* (3rd ed.). Philadelphia: Lippincott.

Baum, F. (1999). *The new public health: An Australian perspective.* Melbourne: Oxford University Press.

Benefield, L. E. (1998). Competencies of effective and efficient home care nurses. *Homecare Manager, 2*(3), 25–28.

Benner, P., & Wrubel, J. (1989). *The primacy of caring.* Menlo Park, CA: Addison Wesley.

Bramadat, I. J., Chalmers, K., & Andrusyszyn, M. (1996). Knowledge, skills and experiences for community health nursing practice: The perceptions of community nurses, administrators and educators. *Journal of Advanced Nursing, 24,* 1224–1233.

Burbach, C. A., & Brown, B. E. (1988). Community health and home health nursing: Keeping the concepts clear. *Nursing and Health Care, 9*(2), 97–100.

Chinn, P., & Kramer, M. K. (1999). *Theory and nursing: Integrated knowledge development* (5th ed.). St. Louis: Mosby

Clarke, P. M. & Cody, W. K. (1994). Nursing theory-based practice in the home and community: The crux of professional nursing education. *Advances in Nursing Science, 17*(2), 41–53.

Coffman, S. (1997). Home care nurses as strangers in the family. *Western Journal of Nursing Research, 19*(1), 82–96

Clark, M. J. (1998). *Nursing in the community: Dimensions of community health nursing.* Stamford, CT: Appleton & Lange.

Community Health Nurses' Interest Group. (1998). *Position statement on public health nursing.* Retrieved April 7, 2003, from www.chnig.org (http://action.web.ca/home/chnig/readingroom. shtml?sh_itm=b7eaaac7469d96d29623e0fc41c21414).

Courtney, R., Ballard, E., Fauver, S., Gariota, M., & Holland, L. (1996). The partnership model: Working with individuals, families, and communities toward a new vision of health. *Public Health Nursing, 13*(3), 177–186.

Ehrlich, A., & Galloway, T. (2000). *Community health nursing standards in the U.S., the U.K. and Canada: A review of literature.* Unpublished manuscript. Prepared for the Ontario Community Health Nursing Standards Task Force.

Falk Rafael, A. (2000). Watson's philosophy, science, and theory of human caring as a framework for guiding community health nursing practice. *Advanced Nursing Science, 23*(2), 34–49.

Forker, J. E. (1996). Perspectives on assessment: Assessing competency for community-focused nursing practice. *Nurse Educator, 21*(3), 6–7.

Hamilton, N., & Bhatti, T. (1996). *Population health promotion: An integrated model of population health and health promotion.* Ottawa: Health Canada. Retrieved April 7, 2003, from http:// www.hc-sc.gc.ca/hppb/phdd/php/php.htm.

Helvie, C. O. (1998). Advanced practice nursing in the community. California: Sage Publications.

Kaiser, K. L., & Rudolph, E. J. (1996). In search of meaning: Identifying competencies relevant to evaluation of the community health nurse generalist. *Journal of Nursing Education, 35*(4), 157–162.

Klug, R. M. (1994). Setting home care standards. *Pediatric Nursing, 20*(4), 404–406.

Koch, M. (1997). Going home: Is home health care for you? *Nursing97,* October, 49.

Labonte, R. (1993). Health promotion and empowerment: Practice frameworks. *Issues in health promotion series, 3.* (HP-10–0102). Toronto: Centre for Health Promotion, University of Toronto & ParticipACTION.

McKenzie, J., McKenzie, C., & Smeltzer, J. *Planning, implementing and evaluating health promotion programs: A primer* (3rd ed.). Needham Heights, MA: Allyn and Bacon.

McMurray, A. (1999). *Community health and wellness: A socioecological approach.* Sydney: Mosby.

Meyer, K. A. (1997). An educational program to prepare acute care nurses for a transition to home health nursing. *The Journal of Continuing Education in Nursing, 28*(3), 124–129.

Moch, S. D. (1990). Personal knowing: Evolving research and practice. *Scholarly Inquiry for Nursing Practice: An International Journal, 4*(2), 155–163.

Naidoo, J., & Wills, J. (2000). *Health promotion: Foundations for practice.* London: Bailliere Tindall.

Palmer, A., Burns, S., & Bulman, C. (Eds). (1994). *Reflective practice in nursing: The growth of the professional practitioner.* London, U.K.: Blackwell Scientific Publications.

Pender, N. J., Murdaugh, C., & Parsons, M. A. (2001). *Health promotion in nursing practice.* (4th ed.). New Jersey: Prentice Hall.

Reid-Haughian, C., Diem, E. & Ontario Community Health Nursing Standards Team. (2000). *Draft core standards #4 for community health nursing.* Unpublished manuscript prepared for the Community Health Nurses Initiatives Group, affiliated with the Registered Nurses Association of Ontario.

Rice, R. (1998). Implementing undergraduate student learning in home care. *Geriatric Nursing, 19*(2), 106–108.

Saskatchewan Health. (1999). *A population health promotion framework for Saskatchewan health districts.* Regina: Author.

Shields, L., & Lindsey, A. E. (1998). Community health promotion nursing practice. *Advances in Nursing Science, 20*(4), 23–36.

Stewart, M. J. (Ed.). (2000). *Community nursing: Promoting Canadian's health* (2nd ed.). Toronto: W.B. Saunders, Canada.

Thompson, R. (2001). *Draft mission statement and values for community health nurses* (prepared for provincial consultation). British Columbia Community Health Nurses Association.

University of Kansas. (2002). *Community tool box*. Retrieved April 7, 2003, from http://ctb.lsi.ukans.edu/.

Valanis, B. (1999). *Epidemiology in health care* (3rd ed.). Stamford, CT: Appleton & Lange.

Vandall-Walker, V. (2002). Nursing support with family members of the critically ill: A framework to guide practice. In L. Young & V. Hayes (Eds.), *Transforming health promotion practice: Concepts, issues, and applications.* Philadelphia, PA: F.A. Davis.

Wass, A. (1999). Assessing the community. In J. E. Hitchcock, P. E. Schubert, & S. A. Thomas (Eds.), *Community health nursing: Caring in action* (pp. 245–265). New York: Delmar Publishers.

Watson, J. (1985). *Nursing: The philosophy and science of caring.* Boulder, CO: Associated University Press.

World Health Organization. (1998). *Health for all in the twenty-first century.* Geneva: Author.

World Health Organization. (2002). Various publications on primary health care and health promotion. Geneva: Author. Available: http://www.who.int/hpr/archive/docs/index.html.

Index

A

Ability objectives, 166
Access, 424
Accessibility to health care services, 12–13
Accomplishment objectives, 166–167
Achievement, sense of, 20–21
Action statements, 125–143
Action steps, 146
  step 1) plan, 147–177
  step 2) take action, 178–207
  step 3) determine results/impact, 208–233
  step 4) evaluate teamwork, 169–171, 203–204,
    228–230
  see also Collaborative action and evaluation;
    Determine results/impact; Take action;
    Workplan steps in assessment
Action timeline form, 404
Action workplan form, 405
Adult learners, assumptions about, 288
Advocacy, 424
Advocates for change, 325, 327
AIDS, 90
Alma-Ata Declaration, World Health Organization
  (WHO), 12
American Association of Colleges of Nursing, 8
Analysis of evaluation data, 211
Appreciation, showing, 217
Appreciation objectives, 166
Appropriate use of resources, 13–14
Assessment
  definition of, 58
  see also Collaborative community assessment
Assessment methods, 86–89
Assessment steps, 61, 62
  step 1) establish relationships within project
    and community, 61–65
    community contacts, 63
    contact list, 65
    project organizers, 62–63
    rationale/issue/population group of the project,
      63–64

  step 2) secondary data, 66–79, 117–119
    census data, 69
    health status and the determinants,
      72–73
    key determinants of health, 75–77
    local surveys and program statistics, 78
    policy documents, 67–68
    population-based or issue-based, 69
    regional and local data, 69–70
    review of literature, 73–74
    sociodemographic data, 69
    sources and types list, 66
    systematic process for managing the
      information and references,
      79, 80
  step 3) community assessment, 86, 89–96, 97
    community mapping, 89–92
    key informant interviews, 94–96
  step 4) specific assessment, 86, 96–114
    community (group) meetings, 102–105,
      123
    focused discussions, 105–107, 119–121
    progressive inquiry, 99–101
    questionnaires, 107–111
  step 5) action statements, 125–143
    analyze data, 125–128
    assessment report, 136–139, 142–143
    draft action statements, 132–136
    validation and presentation, 128–132
  workplans, 85–86
    beginning, 71
    completed step 3, 97
    form for, 405
    see also Action steps
Assessment timeline form, 400–401
Assessment tools, 112
Assessment workplan form, 402
Associated theories, 158–159
Assumptions about adult learners, 288
Audience, 214–215
Awareness objectives, 165–166

NOTES

NOTES

NOTES

NOTES

NOTES

NOTES

NOTES

NOTES

NOTES

NOTES

NOTES

NOTES

examples of pgms

7 demographics   dads⊂ c. kids
    eg young   ⊂ kids
                      fathers +
         vs.   sons
      older men

project goal

which DOH addressing? p 75-6